1

Nutrition for Sport and Exercise

Second Edition

Jacqueline R. Berning, PhD, RD

Assistant Professor
University of Colorado—Colorado Springs
Colorado Springs, Colorado

Suzanne Nelson Steen, DSc, RD

Sports Nutritionist
Department of Intercollegiate Athletics
Husky Sports Nutrition Services
University of Washington
Seattle, Washington

AN ASPEN PUBLICATION®
Aspen Publishers, Inc.
Gaithersburg, Maryland
1998

First edition published as *Sports Nutrition for the 90s*

The authors have made every effort to ensure the accuracy of the information herein. However, appropriate information sources should be consulted, especially for new or unfamiliar procedures. It is the responsibility of every practitioner to evaluate the appropriateness of a particular opinion in the context of actual clinical situations and with due considerations to new developments. Authors, editors, and the publisher cannot be held responsible for any typographical or other errors found in this book.
Aspen Publishers, Inc., is not affiliated with the American Society of Parenteral and Enteral Nutrition.

Library of Congress Cataloging-in-Publication Data
Berning, Jacqueline R.
Nutrition for sport and exercise/
Jacqueline R. Berning, Suzanne Nelson Steen.
p. cm.
Includes bibliographical references and index.
ISBN 0-8342-0882-2
1. Athletes—Nutrition.
2. Physical fitness—Nutritional aspects.
3. Exercise—Physiological aspects.
I. Steen, Suzanne Nelson. II. Title.
TX361.A8B47 1998
613.2'024' 796—dc21
98-11758
CIP

Orders: (800) 638-8437
Customer Service: (800) 234-1660

About Aspen Publishers • For more than 35 years, Aspen has been a leading professional publisher in a variety of disciplines. Aspen's vast information resources are available in both print and electronic formats. We are committed to providing the highest quality information available in the most appropriate format for our customers. Visit Aspen's Internet site for more information resources, directories, articles, and a searchable version of Aspen's full catalog, including the most recent publications: **http://www.aspenpublishers.com**
Aspen Publishers, Inc. • The hallmark of quality in publishing
Member of the worldwide Wolters Kluwer group.

Editorial Services: Ruth Bloom

Library of Congress Catalog Card Number: 98-11758
ISBN: 0-8342-0882-2

Printed in the United States of America

2   3   4   5

Table of Contents

Contributors

Jacqueline R. Berning, PhD, RD
Assistant Professor
University of Colorado—Colorado Springs
Colorado Springs, Colorado

Edmund R. Burke, PhD
Professor
Exercise Science Program
Biology Department
University of Colorado—Colorado Springs
Colorado Springs, Colorado

Priscilla M. Clarkson, PhD
Professor
Department of Exercise Science
University of Massachusetts
Amherst, Massachusetts

Ellen J. Coleman, MA, MPH, RD
Sports Nutrition Consultant
The Sport Clinic
Riverside, California

Emily M. Haymes, PhD
Professor
Department of Nutrition,
    Food and Movement Sciences
Tallahassee, Florida

Linda B. Houtkooper, PhD, RD
Nutrition Specialist
Department of Nutritional Sciences

Special Assistant to Directors
Cooperative Extension and Arizona Prevention
    Center
University of Arizona
Tucson, Arizona

Asker E. Jeukendrup, PhD
Nutrition Research Center
Department of Human Biology
Maastricht University
Maastricht, The Netherlands

Mitchell Kanter, PhD
Principal Scientist
Quaker Oats Clinical Nutrition Research
The Quaker Oats Company
Barrington, Illinois

Zebulon V. Kendrick, PhD
Professor, Department of Physical Education
Director, Biokinetics Research Laboratory
Temple University
Philadelphia, Pennsylvania

Melinda Manore, PhD, RD
Professor
Department of Family Resources and Human
    Development
Arizona State University
Tempe, Arizona

Robert Murray, PhD
Director
Gatorade Exercise Physiology Laboratory
Barrington, Illinois

Jay Naik, MS
Research Specialist
Department of Human Kinetics
University of Wisconsin—Milwaukee
Milwaukee, Wisconsin

David L. Nichols, PhD
Center for Research on Women's Health
Texas Woman's University
Denton, Texas

Charlotte F. Sanborn, PhD
Director
Center for Research on Women's Health
Texas Woman's University
Denton, Texas

Wim H. M. Saris, PhD, MD
Nutrition Research Center
Department of Human Biology
Maastricht University
Maastricht, The Netherlands

Ann C. Snyder, PhD
Professor and Chair
Department of Human Kinetics
University of Wisconsin—Milwaukee
Milwaukee, Wisconsin

Suzanne Nelson Steen, DSc, RD
Chair
Department of Nutrition Education
Graduate Division
Immaculata College
Immaculata, Pennsylvania

Jorunn Sundgot-Borgen, PhD
Associate Professor
Department of Biology and Sports Medicine
The Norwegian University of Sport and
    Physical Education
Oslo, Norway

Janice L. Thompson, PhD
Assistant Professor
Department of Health Promotion and
    Kinesiology
The University of North Carolina
Charlotte, North Carolina

Foreword

The President's Council on Physical Activity, Healthy People 2010, and the National Institutes of Health have all encouraged Americans to increase their physical activity to improve their overall health. However, the effects of this increased activity on the need for nutrients has fostered a whole new industry of sports foods and drinks, many of which arc not always based on fact. Whether for a weekend "warrior" or an elite athlete, interest in sports nutrition and how it might be used to optimize performance is at an all-time high. Unfortunately, accurate and up-to-date information concerning optimal nutrition for the active person is not readily available for the athlete or for the health professional practicing in the sports and fitness arena. On the other hand, mythology about what will improve performance is rampant in every magazine or newspaper one picks up. Because optimal nutrition varies among athletes of different genders, among those participating in different sports, and across the lifespan of the individual, there is a need for health professionals who can answer questions truthfully and assist the athlete in making healthful decisions. Designing an optimal dict for an athlete requires knowledge of the basic fundamentals of sports nutrition, as well as information based on practical and personal experience and an understanding of the individual athlete. *Nutrition for Sport and Exercise* provides an accurate and effective resource for health professionals involved in the care of athletes. The editors are scientists conducting research in the field, and as a consequence they know not only where the gaps in the knowledge are, but who best to ask to tell as much as they know. They have pulled together an outstanding group of authors, well respected for their scholarly activity, as well as for their ability to apply their knowledge in a practical manner. The combination of efforts has resulted in an outstanding blend of science and practice that will give the health practitioner a very useful resource.

Outstanding in this regard are the case studies, which set this book apart from any other. These case studies will be very useful not only to the nutritionist working with athletes, but to other allied health professionals who give basic nutrition advice to their clients.

I congratulate the editors and the authors for their perseverance in the fields of nutrition and exercise science. The authors should be commended for practically applying the science through integration with their experience and producing a book that will be a daily resource for health professionals involved in the care of athletes. Their wisdom will assist us all in improving the performance and health of all physically active people.

Gail Butterfield, PhD, RD, FACSM
Director, Nutrition Studies
Palo Alto Veterans Affairs Health
Care System
Director of Sports Nutrition
Program in Sports Medicine
Stanford University Medical School

Preface

While athletes today embrace high-tech equipment and materials for improved results, many need only look to their diet to enhance performance quickly, easily, and dramatically. Indeed, no amount of motivation, training, or natural ability will ensure victory without proper "fuel" for the engine. Yet despite the wealth of knowledge regarding nutrition and the specific needs of the human body in training, few athletes, coaches, or even allied health professionals have bridged the gap between laboratory and clinical research and the practical application of these findings.

As a result, athletes and coaches will often blindly attempt any dietary regimen or nutritional supplement to gain a competitive edge. For example, fad products featured in glossy advertisements, though they are not regulated for efficacy or safety, remain attractive to athletes with little or no nutrition education. Thus, any health professional dedicated to working with athletes—be they elite or recreational—must keep abreast of valid *and* invalid nutrition claims and practices. Nothing would discredit a member of the sports medicine team faster than pronouncing an unfamiliar supplement as useless when the coach has already looked into the scientific basis for the product. Concerned health professionals must be prepared to offer education rather than mysterious training mandates.

Many professionals, especially dietitions, working with athletes would like to become more involved with sports nutrition, yet they may not have received the necessary training to assess the special needs of athletes or to counsel them effectively regarding their dietary intake. *Nutrition for Sport and Exercise* was developed to provide health care professionals with a comprehensive resource on sports nutrition and exercise science. Each chapter provides the inclusion of both current research and the translation of research findings into practical advice that is sensitive to the needs and concerns of coaches and athletes. In addition, all chapters have been prepared by professionals who conduct research in nutrition and exercise, work closely with elite athletes or teams, or are elite athletes themselves educated in the science of sports nutrition and exercise physiology. Thus, the entire book offers unique insights on how to effectively design and implement the optimal diet for individual athletes, and how nutrition can be used to achieve peak performance.

We hope that the authors will answer your questions on sports nutrition and exercise science and will offer you new ideas for educating athletes, coaches, and parents about the importance of making wise food choices for health and performance—and we wish you success as you meet the challenges and enjoy the rewards of working with athletes!

Jacqueline R. Berning, PhD, RD
Suzanne Nelson Steen, DSc, RD

CHAPTER 1

Exercise Physiology: Implications for Sports Nutrition

Zebulon V. Kendrick

Almost half of the adolescents and young adults of the United States do not participate in vigorous physical activity. The percent of those who are inactive increases with increasing age.[1] This large percent of the population that is inactive is of particular concern, because lack of regular physical activity or exercise is recognized as a risk factor for heart disease.[1-3] Participation in physical activities has been associated with a reduction in risk for all-cause mortality,[2-5] cardiovascular disease,[6-8] diabetes,[9,10] colon cancer,[11-13] and depression and anxiety,[14,15] as well as improved mental health[14,15] (Exhibit 1–1). Regular physical activity may also reduce other risk factors such as hypertension,[16,17] hyperlipidemia,[18,19] glucose intolerance,[20] and obesity.[21-24]

Prescriptive exercise programs are often used in conjunction with weight-management programs for athletes, special populations, and the general public. To gain overall improvements in functional capacity and reduce risk factors associated with the disease state, both aerobic (that is, endurance exercise) and resistive (that is, strength exercises) modes of exercise may be prescribed. The sports nutritionist needs to be aware of regular activity patterns of adolescents and adults, the bioenergetics of exercise for optimal physiologic and performance gains, skeletal muscle responses to regular exercise, the exercise prescription, special considerations of exercise and nutrient balance and metabolism interactions, and pertinent, special concerns of pediatric and aging populations.

PHYSICAL ACTIVITY PATTERNS IN THE UNITED STATES

Nearly 50% of those persons between 12 and 21 years of age are not vigorously active, with sharp decreases in activity occurring during adolescence[1,25,26] (Exhibit 1–2). Sixty percent of adults do not participate in regular physical activity, with 25% being not active at all[1,27] (Exhibit 1–3). In adolescent, young adult, and adult populations, inactivity is more prevalent in women than men, in blacks than other ethnic groups, and in less affluent than more affluent persons.[25,27] Equally troublesome to the high incidence of inactivity are the increasing number of states that no longer require mandatory daily physical education classes and the decreasing number of students enrolled in such classes.[1]

The National Health Promotion Interview Survey of 1985 found that only 7.5% of Americans 65 years of age or older participated in aerobic activity. In surveys with rigorous definitions that classify physical activity by intensity, the type of activity, and the physical fitness level of the exerciser, it was estimated that only up to 22% of older Americans were "active." When less rigorous definitions were used, 30% to 47% of the population were considered active.[28]

Because almost 85% of adults who are older suffer from at least one chronic degenerative disease,[29] both health care resources and the personal independence and vitality of the person who is older are challenged. Exercise and proper

Exhibit 1–1 Effect of Regular Exercise on Risk for Disease

All-Cause Mortality

Lower mortality rates for both older and younger adults

Cardiovascular Disease

Decreases the risk of cardiovascular disease

May prevent or delay development of high blood pressure

May reduce blood pressure in persons with hypertension

Diabetes Mellitus

May lower the risk of noninsulin-dependent diabetes

May be useful in management of insulin-dependent diabetes

Body Fat

May favorably affect the distribution of body fat

Cancer

May decrease the risk of colon cancer

Mental Health and Health-Related Quality of Life

May relieve symptoms of depression and anxiety

May improve mood state

May enhance psychological well-being

May improve physical functioning in persons with compromised health

Source: Reprinted from *Physical Activity and Health: A Report of the Surgeon General*, 1996, U.S. Department of Health and Human Services, Centers for Disease Control and Prevention, National Center for Chronic Disease Prevention and Health Promotion.

nutrition may delay the clinical manifestations of many of these diseases. Clearly, inactivity and disuse account for a significant portion of many age-associated changes in physiologic function.[30] Increasing physical activity has been shown to improve physiologic function and to reduce all-cause mortality.[2–6]

Lower all-cause mortality rates are seen more often in persons who participate regularly in moderate to vigorous exercise than in those persons who are sedentary or with low cardiovascular function.[2–6] Paffenbarger et al,[2] in their epidemiologic study of physical activity and mortality among men, found that the relative risk of all-cause mortality was reduced from 1.00 for persons who expended fewer than 500 kcal · week^{-1} to 0.63 for persons who expended between 1500 and 1999 kcal · week^{-1}. To achieve the weekly

Exhibit 1–2 Physical Activity Patterns of Adolescents and Young Adults

Activity Patterns

50% engage in vigorous activity during leisure time

25% engage in regular activity during leisure time

25% report no activity during leisure time

Physical Inactivity Is More Prevalent:

In females than males

Among black females than white females

With increasing grade level

Physical Activity in Schools

Daily attendance in physical education classes has declined from 42% to 25% in the 1990s

Only 19% of high school students are active more than 20 minutes in daily physical education classes

Source: Reprinted from *Physical Activity and Health: A Report of the Surgeon General*, 1996, U.S. Department of Health and Human Services, Centers for Disease Control and Prevention, National Center for Chronic Disease Prevention and Health Promotion.

Exhibit 1–3 Physical Activity Patterns of Adults

Activity Patterns

15% engage in vigorous activity during leisure time

22% engage in regular activity during leisure time

25% report no activity during leisure time

Physical Inactivity Is More Prevalent:

In women than men

Among blacks and Hispanics than whites
In older than younger adults
In less affluent than more affluent persons

Most Popular Physical Activities

Walking
Gardening or yard work

Source: Reprinted from *Physical Activity and Health: A Report of the Surgeon General*, 1996, U.S. Department of Health and Human Services, Centers for Disease Control and Prevention, National Center for Chronic Disease Prevention and Health Promotion.

1500 kcal expenditure, a person would need to expend a little more than 200 kcal daily for activity or exercise. Some activities expressed in metabolic equivalents (METs) that may be used to expend 1500 kcal a week are listed in Table 1–1.[1,31,32]

Because resting energy expenditure (REE) is approximately 0.0175 kcal · min^{-1} · kg body weight, the energy cost of an activity may be expressed in multiples of REE or METs.[31,32] The following equation may be used to estimate the energy cost of an activity in kcal given a person's body weight:

Assigned MET value × body weight$_{kg}$ × (duration of activity/60 min)

For example, for a person weighing 70 kg exercising at an activity level of 5 METs for 40 minutes, the kcal cost of the activity is the following:

[5 METs × 70 kg × (40 min/60 min)] = 233 kcal or 5.8 kcal · min^{-1}

Caloric equivalents for MET cost of activithÁs for different body masses are listed in Table 1–2.

BIOENERGETICS OF EXERCISE

Because muscle cells store limited amounts of adenosine triphosphate (ATP) and depend upon metabolic pathways to provide sufficient ATP for muscle function during activity, activities of muscular work may be classified according to the predominant energy system used. Physical activities may be classified as power, speed, or endurance depending upon the duration of the event, the rate of energy production, and the enzyme system used[33] (Table 1–3). Both power and speed events are considered nonoxidative, whereas endurance events are considered oxidative. Power events use the hydrolysis of high-energy phosphogens [that is, intracellular ATP and adenosine diphosphate (ADP) and creatine phosphate]; speed events use nonoxidative glycogenolysis and glycolysis; and endurance events oxidatively metabolize carbohydrates, lipids, and amino acids (for long-duration activities).[33]

Few athletic events are considered solely power events. Power events are of a very short duration of several seconds and include heavy weight lifting, field events in track and field sports, and vaulting in gymnastics, which use the ATP-creatine phosphate energy system.[34,35] These events require the rapid hydrolysis of ATP to ADP. The one-step reaction of hydrolyzing creatine phosphate to release energy and a phosphate and to allow reconstitution of ATP from ADP is critical for supplying the energy requirement of the cell.[35,36] For short-term, high-intensity exercise such as a 40- or a 100-m sprint, the ATP-creatine phosphate system can produce energy at high rates. However, the ATP-creatine phosphate system is significantly

Table 1–1 Activities in METs That May Be Used To Expend 1500 kcal a Week

Activity	Rate of Effort	MET Equivalent
Bicycling	< 10 mph	4.0
	10–11.9 mph	6.0
	12–13.9 mph	8.0
	14–15.9 mph	10.0
Walking	3 mph	3.5
	3.5–4 mph	4.0
	3.5 mph uphill	6.0
Running	5 mph	8.0
	6 mph	10.0
	7 mph	11.5
	8 mph	13.5
Lap Swimming	Slow freestyle	8.0
	Fast freestyle	10.0
Sport	Tennis, singles	8.0
	Tennis, doubles	6.0
	Volleyball, noncompetitive	3.0
	Volleyball, competitive	4.0
	Soccer	10.0
	Basketball	8.0
	Shooting baskets	4.5
	Football, competitive	9.0
	Football, flag	8.0
	Softball/baseball	5.0
	Golf/Pulling clubs	5.0
	Golf/Carrying clubs	5.5
	Golf/Using vehicle	3.5
	Ice hockey	8.0
	Field hockey	8.0
	Roller skating	7.0
Lawn and gardening	Raking lawn	4.0
	Planting trees	
	Walking power mower	4.5
	Clearing land	
	Hauling branches	5.5
	Shoveling < 10 lb	6.0
	Shoveling > 10 lb	7.0
	Using heavy power tools	6.0

Note: METs = metabolic equivalents

Source: Adapted with permission from B.E. Ainsworth et al., Compendium of Physical Activities: Classification of Energy Costs of Human Physical Activities, *Medicine and Science in Sports and Exercise*, Vol. 25, pp. 71–80, © 1993, Williams & Wilkins.

depleted within 10 to 20 seconds of high-intensity activity,[34,35] which limits the extent that creatine phosphate can be used to adequately supply energy to the working muscle under these conditions.

Although the ATP-creatine phosphate system is used at the initiation of speed events, cytosolic glucose and glycogen are metabolized to provide suitable intracellular ATP to maintain the activity. As a person exercises at high intensities be-

Table 1–2 Caloric Equivalents Based on Body Mass for MET Cost of Activities

Caloric Expenditure (kcal · min⁻¹)

MET Cost	50 kg	60 kg	70 kg	80 kg	90 kg	100 kg
2	1.8	2.1	2.5	2.8	3.2	3.5
3	2.6	3.2	3.7	4.2	4.7	5.3
4	3.5	4.2	4.9	5.6	6.3	7.0
5	4.4	5.3	6.1	7.0	7.9	8.8
6	5.3	6.3	7.4	8.4	9.5	10.5
7	6.1	7.4	8.0	9.8	11.0	12.3
8	7.0	8.4	9.8	11.2	12.6	14.0
9	7.9	9.5	11.0	12.6	14.2	15.8
≥10	≥8.7	≥10.5	≥12.3	≥14.0	≥15.8	≥17.5

Note: Calculation of kcal · min⁻¹ by body mass is based on the following equation:

$$kcal \cdot min^{-1} = MET \times [(body\ mass_{kg} \times 3.5)/200]$$

This equation is found in American College of Sport Medicine. *ACSM's Guidelines for Exercise Testing and Prescription.* 5th ed. Baltimore, MD: Williams & Wilkins; 1995.

MET = metabolic weight

Table 1–3 Energy Sources for Muscular Work

Metabolic Activity	Exercise Duration	Enzyme System/Location	Energy Storage Form	Sport Activities
Power	0–4 sec	Single enzyme/ Cytosol	ATP, Creatine phosphate	Field events, weight lifting
Speed	5–60 sec	One complex pathway/Cytosol	Muscle glycogen and glucose	Track sprints < 400 m Swim sprints < 100 m
Endurance	> 2 min	Several complex pathways/Cytosol and mitochondria	Muscle and liver glucose and glycogen; muscle, blood, and adipose lipids; muscle, blood and liver amino acids	> 1500-m run

Note: ATP = adenosine triphosphate

Source: Modified from *Exercise Physiology: Human Bioenergetics and Its Application, Second Edition* by George A. Brooks, Thomas D. Fahey, and Timothy P. White. Copyright © 1996 by Mayfield Publishing Company. Reprinted by permission of the publisher.

yond several seconds, a greater proportion of the energy used for the activity comes from the glycolytic energy system. The glycolytic pathway catabolizes glucose (or glycogen through glycogenolysis) to form two molecules of either pyruvic acid or lactic acid. The glycolytic pathway extracts energy stored in glucose to be used to rejoin inorganic phosphate to ADP to form ATP.

When glycolysis becomes the major producer of ATP, hydrogens are transferred from NADH to pyruvic acid to form lactic acid through lactate dehydrogenase, allowing for the "recycling" of the intermediate energy carrier, NAD+, so that glycolysis can continue. The accumulation of lactic acid reduces the intracellular pH, which may influence the ability of the working muscle to continue to produce ATP from glycolysis. The rate-limiting enzyme of glycolysis, phosphofructokinase,[37] as well as other glycolytic enzymes, are sensitive to reductions in pH. Cessation of energy production through inhibition of glycolytic enzymes has been demonstrated to occur when muscle pH decreases below 6.4 to 6.6.[38]

Speed events that depend upon glycolysis for ATP production include activities that require rapid energy production lasting from several seconds to about 2 minutes. Such activities include sprint events between 200 to 800m in track and between 50 and 100m in swimming.

Endurance exercise includes activities with durations greater than several minutes that use both cytosolic and mitochondrial processes for energy production. The requirement for both cytosolic and mitochondrial energy production is due to the limited rate of mitochondrial processes that do not operate at a sufficient rate to sustain energy production for high-intensity events such as sprint events. However, these sites of energy production may be sufficient for lower intensities of activity. Mitochondrial ATP production involves the interaction of two cooperating metabolic pathways—the Krebs cycle (that is, citric acid cycle) and the electron transport chain.

The primary function of the Krebs cycle is to complete the oxidation of carbohydrate, lipid, or amino acid precursors using the intermediate energy carriers, NAD and flavin adenine dinucleotide (FAD), which carry hydrogen and its electrons. These intermediate energy carriers, in turn, donate pairs of electrons to the electron transport chain. The energy from each pair of electrons taken by NADH and FADH to the electron transport chain can be used to generate three and two molecules of ATP, respectively.

MUSCLE FIBER TYPE AND BIOENERGETICS

Muscle fiber motor units predispose the ability of a person to do specific physical activities at competitive levels. Muscle fiber motor units

are classified based upon their contractile machinery (that is, myofibrillar isoforms and ATPases), rate of contraction (that is, fast-twitch or slow-twitch muscle fibers),[39-41] and by their metabolic characteristics (that is, fast glycolytic, white muscle; fast glycolytic-oxidative, fast red muscle; and slow oxidative, slow red muscle)[39-42] (Table 1–4).

Fast-twitch white muscle fibers have a high glycolytic capacity, a rapid increase to peak tension, and a quick relaxation time. Types IIb and IIa are two subtypes of fast-twitch muscles in humans.[41] Type IIb fibers are also referred to as fast-glycolytic fibers because their myosin ATPase activity and speed of contraction are the greatest of all fiber types, and these fibers also have a high concentration of glycolytic enzymes.[39,40] Type IIa fibers are also referred to as fast-oxidative-glycolytic, fast-twitch red, or intermediate fibers. Because these fibers contain significant oxidative and glycolytic properties, type IIa fibers are biochemically between type IIb and type I fibers and are adaptable to exercise stress.[39-41] Slow-twitch muscle fibers experience a slow increase to peak tension, relax slower, have a high oxidative capacity (that is, contain large amounts of oxidative enzymes and have a high mitochondrial volume), have a large concentration of myoglobin, and have a high capillary density.[39-42]

Fast-twitch muscle fibers are predominately used for power and speed events, whereas slow-twitch fibers are predominately used for endurance events. Because muscle fiber type is genetically determined, athletes with predominately slow-twitch muscle fibers will not become elite sprinters nor will sprinters with predominately fast-twitch muscle fibers become elite marathon runners. Sprinters possess a large percent of fast-twitch fibers, whereas endurance athletes generally have a large percent of slow-twitch fibers.[39,43]

THE EXERCISE PRESCRIPTION

The following factors need to be considered when designing an exercise prescription: (1) the mode (type) of exercise to be done; (2) the frequency of the training session; (3) the duration of each training session; (4) the intensity of the

Table 1–4 Contractile and Histochemical Comparisons of Slow-Twitch and Fast-Twitch Muscle Motor Units

	Slow-Twitch	Fast-Twitch	
Variable	*I*	*IIa*	*IIb*
Other classification schemes	Slow	Fast oxidative-glycolytic	Fast glycolytic
Visual appearance	Pink to red	Red	White (pale)
Speed of contraction	Slowest	Intermediate	Highest
Myofibrillar-ATPase activity	Low	High	Highest
Specific tension developed	Moderate	High	High
Number of mitochondria	High	Moderate to high	Low
Predominant energy system	Oxidative	Oxidative/nonoxidative	Nonoxidative
Resistance to fatigue	High	Moderate to high	Low

Source: Data from F. Booth and D. Thompson, *Physiology Review*, Vol. 71, pp. 541–585, © 1991; D. Pette and R.S. Staron, *Reviews of Physiology, Biochemistry and Pharmacology*, Vol. 116, pp. 1–76, © 1990; D. Pette and C. Spamer, *Federation Proceedings*, Vol. 45, pp. 2910–2914, © 1986; K.M. Baldwin et al., *American Journal of Physiology*, Vol. 222, pp. 373–378, © 1972; and D. Costill et al., *Medicine and Science in Sports and Exercise*, Vol. 8, pp. 96–100, © 1976.

work effort of the training session[44]; and (5) appropriate nutrition and hydration (fluid intake) for optimal performance. (Appropriate nutrition and fluid replacement for optimal performance are addressed elsewhere in this book.) Further, when designing an exercise prescription, one must be aware of the health status (risk factors and symptomatology), current state of functional capacity and conditioning, and interests and skills required for activities the participant may do. For those persons with significant risk factors or men 45 years old or older or women 55 years old or older (who have not experienced early menopause), medical clearance should be obtained before beginning an exercise program.[44] To best evaluate a person who wants to begin to exercise, especially a person whose health status is of concern, the results of a comprehensive physical examination, laboratory studies, and both a resting and an exercise stress electrocardiogram (EKG) may be required to design a safe and suitable exercise prescription. A summary of the components of physical fitness, principles of training, and general conditioning guidelines is found in Exhibit 1–4.

General Guidelines

The position papers by the American College of Sports Medicine[45] and the *Report of the Sur-geon General*[1] recommend that, for a person to develop and maintain cardiorespiratory fitness, muscular strength and endurance, and optimal body composition, he or she should have an exercise frequency of 3 to 5 days per week at a duration that may be for several minutes for special populations or between 20 and 60 minutes for healthy persons, depending upon the modality of the exercise, the functional capacity of the participant, and the desired threshold intensity to improve performance. Both warm-up and cooldown periods are important components of an exercise prescription.[44] The warm-up period should last at least 5 minutes (longer for persons who are older and persons with low functional capacity) and should consist of activities that will elicit a gradual increase in metabolism and heart rate toward the desired exercise range. The cooldown period should be at least 5 minutes and represents a period for the metabolism and heart rate to gradually return to their resting levels.

Exercise Intensity

During the exercise session, neither the peak intensity of effort nor the average intensity of effort as outlined by the exercise prescription should be exceeded.[44] The peak intensity of exercise should not exceed 90% of the functional capacity of the participant and should average

Exhibit 1–4 General Guidelines of a Physical Fitness Program

Duration and Frequency of Exercise

Normal, healthy persons—15 to 60 minutes, three to five sessions/week

Persons with low exercise tolerance—5 to 10 minutes daily or twice daily

Persons with weight-control problems—low intensity, 45 to 60 minutes, five to six times a week

Exercise Intensity

Peak should never exceed 90% of functional capacity with an exception for highly trained athletes

Exercise intensity should average about 60% to 70% of the functional capacity

70% of functional capacity *is not* the same as 70% of VO_{2max}

Prescription by Heart Rate

Peak = heart rate at 90% functional capacity

Average = heart rate at 60% to 70% functional capacity

Heart rate average at 70% of functional capacity is about 60% of functional capacity in METs

Exercise training session format should consist of:

Warm-up of approximately 5 minutes

Training for 20 to 60 minutes

Modes of exercise training (jogging, walking, cycling, etc.)

Suitable duration and intensity of exercise for each mode

Cool-down of approximately 5 minutes

METs = metabolic equivalents

Source: Data from American College of Sports Medicine, *ACSM's Guidelines for Exercise Testing and Prescription.* 5th ed., © 1995, Williams & Wilkins.

---

between 60% and 70% of her or his functional capacity. Well-conditioned participants and athletes may be exceptions to the peak intensity guideline and may exercise at higher intensities.

A desired exercise intensity may be between 60% and 85% of the maximal oxygen consumption (VO_{2max}) for the general population and 85% to 100% VO_{2max} for well-conditioned athletes. Determination of the VO_{2max} is usually done in a laboratory and may not be a feasible method to estimate the exercise intensity of activity. Therefore, other methods of estimating exercise intensity are used. Exercise intensity may be prescribed as a percent of functional capacity by calculating 60% and 90% (higher for athletes) of the maximal heart rate, maximal heart rate reserve, or MET cost of activity (that is, multiples of sitting REE, approximately equal to 3.5 ml O_2 · kg body wt^{-1} · min^{-1}). Methods to calculate exercise intensity by percent of maximal heart rate and percent of maximal heart rate reserve are as follows:

$$\text{percent of maximal heart rate} = \text{maximal heart rate}$$
$$\times$$
$$\text{desired percent of exercise intensity}$$

$$\text{maximal heart rate reserve} =$$
$$[\text{maximal heart rate} - \text{resting heart rate}$$
$$\times$$
$$\text{desired percent exercise intensity}]$$
$$+$$
$$\text{resting heart rate}$$

The exercise intensity is prescribed differently for resistive training because resistive training usually uses smaller muscle groups. The use of a percent of the VO_{2max}, a percent of the maximal heart rate, or a percent of the heart rate reserve may not adequately reflect true resistive exercise intensity. The exercise intensity for resistive training is often prescribed as a percent of the 1-repetition maximum (1-RM) for a predetermined number of repetitions and sets (see Exhibit 1–5 for terms of resistive training).

Exhibit 1–5 Definitions and Terms of Resistive Exercise

Concentric (myometric) muscular exercise—The application of muscular tension while the muscle shortens.

Eccentric muscular exercise—The application of muscular tension while the muscle lengthens (is stretched).

Isokinetic muscular exercise—The application of muscular tension at a constant speed of muscle movement.

Isometric muscular exercise—The application of muscular tension without muscular movement.

Isotonic exercise—The application of muscular tension with muscular movement. Isotonic exercise may be classified as concentric or eccentric.

Load or resistance—The mass (weight) to be moved.

Overload—The effort beyond what a body system or tissue is accustomed to achieve a training effect.

Overtraining—Declines in exercise performance and prolonged sensation of fatigue due to training sessions that are too long, intense, and/or frequent, which minimize the ability of the body to adequately recover from the exercise.

Plyometric exercise—The rapid application of tension as a muscle is being stretched before the muscle can contract to elicit movement.

Repetition—The number of work efforts within one set.

1-Repetition Maximum (1-RM)—The maximal amount of weight that can be moved through a full range of motion one time.

Reversibility—The loss of improvements acquired from overload when the overload is removed.

Set—Specified number of work efforts done as a unit.

Specificity—The training effect is specific to the muscle group used.

Expected Responses to Exercise

When following an exercise prescription, the participant should expect to experience an increase in heart rate and strength in heart-pumping action[33,38,44] (Exhibit 1–6 and see also Case Study 1). Although not usually monitored except in clinical settings, one would expect the systolic blood pressure and the frequency and depth of breathing to increase as the intensity of the effort increases. After the exercise session, a person may experience some muscle and general body tiredness. This tiredness should quickly subside in persons who have been regularly exercising. If the tiredness is prolonged or becomes chronic, the person is likely overtraining. With overtraining, the exercise bouts are usually too long or too strenuous and may ultimately result in injury. Overtraining is also associated with decreased exercise performance, loss of body weight, depressed immune function, and increased heart rate and systolic blood pressure during the exercise session as compared to the normal exercise response and response at rest, and psychological staleness.[46,47] Clearly, it is paramount that modifications in the exercise prescription occur if overtraining persists.

RESISTIVE TRAINING EXERCISES TO IMPROVE MUSCULAR STRENGTH

Methods of resistive training to improve muscular strength may be classified as isomet-

Exhibit 1–6 Expected Responses to Acute Exercise

Increased heart rate
Increased strength of heart action
Increase in systolic blood pressure
Increased depth and rate of breathing
Some muscle tiredness during recovery from exercise
Some general body tiredness during recovery from exercise

Case Study 1

17-year old male honor student; height—71 inches; weight—138 pounds.

Clinical Status: Complains of fatigue and has recurring respiratory infections.

Exercise Referral: Prolonged fatigue following training regimen for a marathon. Athlete has noticed that his heart rate is higher than he is accustomed during training. He runs 90+ miles weekly.

It is likely that this person is overtraining. Indicators that he is overtraining are the recurring respiratory infections, prolonged fatigue following training sessions, and elevated heart rate during exercise. By interview, it was found that he was consuming about 45 to 50% of his calories from carbohydrates. It is also likely that he may also be experiencing glycogen depletion due to the high weekly training mileage.

Recommendations: Decrease weekly mileage by at least 15 miles. Increase carbohydrate intake to about 60% of the caloric intake. Consume carbohydrates (fluid drinks) during exercise on days running long distances.

---

ric, isotonic (constant-load exercise using a barbell, dumbbell, or variable-resistance exercise using specially designed machines), or isokinetic.[33,38,48,49] These classifications are based on the relationship between the application of muscular tension and muscular movement in response to the load (resistance) placed upon the muscle. With isometric exercise, the application of muscular tension occurs without muscular movement.[50] Isotonic exercise occurs when the muscle either shortens (myometric or concentric) or lengthens (plyometric or eccentric) with either constant-load or variable-resistance exercise.[48,51-53] Plyometric loading involves a sudden eccentric stress and muscle stretch, which is immediately followed by a rapid concentric contraction.[33,52] Isokinetic exercise occurs when the muscle exerts tension at a constant speed.

Because isometric training does not involve muscular movement through its range of motion and does not improve the ability of the muscle to exert force at any other muscle position, increases in muscular strength are limited only to the static joint angle of the muscle. Therefore, isometric training is used more for rehabilitative purposes than for training.

The most common mode of resistive training is isotonic. Eccentric training has been demonstrated to increase recruitment of type IIb fibers and may improve muscular strength more than concentric training.[49] However, eccentric training results in greater tension-induced damage to muscle than concentric training. A more recent modification of resistive training is plyometric training, which has been shown to improve jumping ability of athletes. Plyometric training uses the elastic properties of muscle by applying a quick stretch to the muscle as the tension for contraction is being generated, immediately followed by a rapid concentric contraction.[52,53]

General guidelines for resistive exercise for the development of muscular strength and endurance are presented in Exhibit 1–7. To achieve improvements in both general body muscular strength and endurance, a person should exercise multiple muscle groups of the upper and lower body at 65% to 70% and 75% to 80% of the 1-RM, respectively, for two or three sets of 8 to 12 repetitions for each muscle group. To develop greater muscular strength, usually four to eight repetitions using greater percents of the 1-RM are done for four to six sets.

Many athletes participating in strength and power sports prefer constant-resistance exercise using free weights over the use of variable-resistance machines.[33] However, there is little definitive evidence that one method of training is superior to the other, although free weights may produce greater strength gains during the short

Exhibit 1–7 Development of Muscular Strength and Muscular Endurance

---

Generally, small muscle groups are exercised:
  Lower body about 75% to 80% of 1-RM
  Upper body about 65 to 70% of 1-RM
  10 to 12 or more repetitions per muscle
  group
Use up to 8 to 12 weight training stations:
  First 3 weeks—complete one set
  4th to 6th week—complete two sets
  Thereafter, three sets if needed

1-RM = 1-repetition maximum

---

term and may allow a greater specificity of training.[54] (See Case Study 2 for an example.)

For special populations and the elderly, a person may use a 3-RM instead of a 1-RM to reduce the stress of determining the exercise intensity and minimizing the chance of injury. Resistive exercise can be done using free weights, machines, or by water exercises in a pool.

Water exercise has been used as an exercise modality to improve musculoskeletal and cardiorespiratory functions in special populations.[55,56] (See Case Study 3 for an example.) Recently, water-exercise programs have been used as a resistive modality to improve muscular endurance[57] and peak torque of knee extensors[58] of elderly men and women (Figure 1–1). In a group of elderly black women, both the biceps curl and leg press performances were shown to significantly increase after participation in a water-exercise program (unpublished data) (Figure 1–1). Because water is approximately 1000 times denser than air, the movement of segments of the body or the entire body through water creates sufficient drag (resistance) to the development of muscular strength and endurance.[59] This modality for resistive training may be excellent for persons with musculoskeletal limitations or contraindications for doing land exercise.

Whenever performing resistive exercise, one must be aware of the potential of a pressor effect of an increased heart rate and blood pressure (Exhibit 1–8). As a result of the pressor effect, the exercise heart rate during resistive training may not accurately reflect the true intensity of training. In addition, the pressor effect may be more profound for unsupported arm exercise than for supported arm exercise.

Outcomes of resistive training are listed in Exhibit 1–9. Heavy resistive training may increase lean body mass through increases in muscle protein content resulting in greater strength and muscle hypertrophy.[60,61] Resistive training also interacts with the nervous system to optimize motor unit involvement for recruitment of muscles that enable an activity to be done.[62,63] Improving muscular strength not only helps a person to reach his or her performance goals, but may also lessen the incidence and severity of injury from falls,[64–67] improve ambulation and

---

Case Study 2

35-year old female; height—65 inches; weight—157 pounds.

Clinical Status: Normal

Exercise Referral: To begin to exercise. Wants to improve general fitness and reduce health risks.

Recommendations: Determine sport and individual exercise activities the person enjoys (Table 1–1 has the MET cost of a variety of activities that may be chosen). Refer to Table 1–2 to determine the kcal/min from the MET cost of activity by body weight. Target a caloric expenditure of at least 1500 kcal/week from all exercise activities. To design a general fitness program, refer to Exhibits 1–4 and 1–7. Aerobic training may be performed 3 days/week and resistive training 2 days/week.

Case Study 3

66-year old female; height—64 inches; weight—175 pounds.

Clinical Status: Blood pressure 134/86 with medication; arthritic hip.

Exercise Referral: Complaints of leg fatigue when walking and problems climbing stairs.

This woman was an excellent candidate for a water exercise program because of her arthritic hip, which limited her weight-bearing activities on land. Following medical clearance, this woman participated in a 12-week water exercise program including exercises of walking in water at a mid-chest depth, repetitive horizontal and vertical jumping activities, and exercises for the upper body. A brief description of the water exercise program is found in Ruoti et al.[57]

Outcomes: Improved strength of knee extensors and hip muscles, improved ambulation, and ability to walk up a flight of stairs without undue pain; improved aerobic capacity; and reduction in blood pressure medication.

---

gait,[65,67,68] improve ease of changing body positions,[68] and lessen the dependence of persons who are elderly upon others during activities of daily living.[68–97]

TRAINING TO IMPROVE AEROBIC POWER

Generally, training to improve aerobic power involves rhythmic activities of 20 to 60 minutes duration using large muscle groups (Exhibit 1–10). Common methods for aerobic training and for aerobic athletic competitions include interval training and long, slow, distance training (over-distance training).[33] High-intensity continuous training when the athlete trains at an intensity between 80% to 90% of his or her VO_{2max} has been found to provide an excellent training stimulus for improvements in VO_{2max} and the respiratory capacity of muscle.[72–74] Nonathletes most likely will not be able to sustain activity at

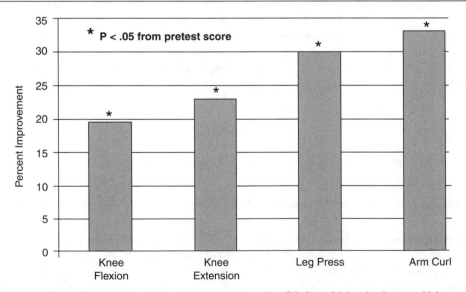

Figure 1–1 Effect of Water Exercise on Muscular Strength of Selected Muscle Groups. Values are percent improvement above that for control subjects. Knee flexor and extensor peak torque was determined using a Cybex dynamometer. Leg press and arm curl were determined from a 1-repetition maximum (1-RM) using universal machines.

Exhibit 1–8 Pressor Response and Resistive Training

> At about 20% of a maximal skeletal muscle contraction, a pressor response may occur.
> The pressor response will result in an increased heart rate and blood pressure.
> Unsupported arm exercise usually elicits greater physiologic responses than supported arm exercise.

Exhibit 1–10 Exercise for Aerobic Fitness

> Use large muscle groups
> Use rhythmic exercises for 15 to 60 minutes
> Activities include the following:
>   Walking
>   Cycling
>   Dancing
>   Skiing or home use of ski machines
>   Water exercise

80% to 90% of their VO_{2max} for a suitable duration to receive the positive training benefits from high-intensity continuous training. Regardless of the training method chosen, the intensity of training generally has a greater effect on improving VO_{2max} compared to the duration of training.

Interval training includes repeated exercise bouts interspersed with short recovery periods of light exercise for a specific number of sets (work intervals done).[75] For aerobic power, the distance or length of the work interval usually lasts more than 60 seconds with a target exercise heart rate between 85% and 100% for athletes, which is lower for nonathletes. The rest interval is usually done for the same duration as the work interval or in a ratio with the work interval. For persons who are not highly trained, the rest interval may be two or three times the duration of the work interval. One major advantage to interval training is that the participant learns the pace of the event to be done.[33]

Long, slow training or over-distance training is a method of aerobic training for endurance

Exhibit 1–9 Outcomes of Regular Resistive Exercise

> Increased lean body mass
> Improved muscular strength
> Improved motor unit recruitment of muscle to do activity
> Improved muscular endurance
> Reduced ambulatory time to complete a walking task
> More ease in changing body positions
> Greater functional capacity for instrumental activities of daily living

events such as long-distance running, cycling, and swimming because of increases in VO_{2max} and tissue respiratory capacity.[33,76] During this type of training, athletes exercise below their competitive pace or about 70% of their maximal heart rate for durations longer than their specific competition. Although this method of training increases the respiratory capacity of muscle,[76] the limitation of over-distance training is that the lower-than-competition intensity (pace) of the exercise lacks the specificity of the athlete's learning pace and skill at the intensity the event will be done.

The expected outcomes of aerobic training are found in Exhibit 1–11. Aerobic training improves myocardial efficiency with submaximal stroke volume increasing and a concomitant decrease in exercise heart rate.[33] There is also an improved blood-pressure response to exercise, particularly in those persons with hypertension. In fact, the improved blood pressure may last for several hours after the exercise session in persons with hypertension. Aerobic training will also improve capillary density within the working muscles, improve work capacity, reduce serum lipids if they are high, and reduce body fat. For adults who are older and for adults who are deconditioned, regular aerobic activity has been shown to improve functional capacity.

ANAEROBIC TRAINING TO IMPROVE ANAEROBIC POWER

Athletic events of short durations (less than 60 seconds) depend upon anaerobic energy production through the immediate ATP-creatine phos-

Exhibit 1–11 Outcomes of Regular Aerobic Training

Reduction in resting heart rate

Reduction in submaximal heart rate for a given exercise test

Increased myocardial efficiency at given submaximal workloads

Improved blood-pressure response to exercise

Increase in functional capillaries (capillary density) in muscles

Increased physical work capacity

Improved serum lipid levels

---

phate system and nonoxidative or anaerobic glycolysis.[33] To train the ATP-creatine phosphate system, athletes need to perform high-intensity exercise that lasts less than 10 seconds with rest intervals of two to three times the work (exercise) interval.[33] For example, football players may train using repeated 30- or 40-yard dashes with rest intervals of about 30 seconds; hockey players may train by repeated all-out sprints with changing direction between the lines across the ice rink with 30-second rests between sprints; and basketball players may complete similar sprints using the end lines and the center court line. Athletes need to train at high intensities for intervals less than 60 seconds to improve nonoxidative glycolysis.[33]

DAILY ENERGY REQUIREMENTS

Three distinct components that constitute the daily energy requirements[77–83] are the REE, the thermic effect of food, and the thermic effect of activity. The REE composes about 65% to 70% of the total daily energy expenditure.[78,80] The thermic effects of activity and thermic effect of food compose about 20% to 35% and 10% to 15% of the daily energy expenditure, respectively.[78,79] REE is well-correlated to body weight and to lean body mass, which represent metabolically active tissues.[78,80–83]

One important factor that influences REE is the level of physical activity. The thermic effect of physical activity and the REE are usually con-

sidered independent components of daily energy expenditure. Regular aerobic exercise-training regimens performed by both young and old adults[84] and middle-distance female runners,[85] as well as acute strenuous exercise,[86] have been shown to increase the REE (Table 1–5). It has been demonstrated, in both calorie-restricted[83] and noncalorie-restricted[85,87] young male and female populations, that strenuous exercise training may increase REE. In unpublished work, it was demonstrated that resistive exercise training reversed a 6-week low-calorie, protein-supplemented diet-induced decrease in REE. In this study, female subjects were randomly divided into the following four groups: no diet, no resistive exercise training; diet alone; resistive exercise training alone; and diet and resistive exercise training. Subjects in the diet alone and diet and resistive exercise-training groups lost about 4 and 5 kg of body weight, respectively. On the basis of the regression equation of Owen[79] using body mass, the diet-induced reduction of REE should be 29 and 36 kcal $\cdot$ day^{-1} for the diet alone and the diet and resistive exercise-training groups of subjects, respectively. The actual reductions in REE for diet alone and the diet and resistive exercise-training subjects were 166 and 16 kcal $\cdot$ day^{-1} greater than predicted, respectively. These findings suggest that resistive exercise training attenuated the diet-induced reduction in REE. Acute heavy resistance training has also been shown to increase REE by about 3% (Figure 1–2) for at least 48 hours after the exercise (unpublished data).

Resistive training may help to preserve or increase metabolically active lean body mass, which has been shown to decrease with increasing age.[60,61,84,88,89] It has been demonstrated that adults who are older and who have participated in weight-training regimens increased their muscular strength and muscle size.[90–92] Improvements in muscular strength have also been strongly correlated to improvements in ambulation.[66,68,69,92,93] Resistive exercise-induced increases in REE and the further increases of caloric expenditure due to the thermic effect of physical activity in active adults should also

Table 1–5 Effect of Exercise Training on Resting Energy Expenditure (REE)

Condition/Gender	Age (yrs)	Activity	Change in REE	Reference
Diet and Exercise				
Male and female	22–52	Jogging, cycling, swimming, and/or weight circuit	Reversed diet-induced decrease	82
Female	25–45	Dieting, sedentary	–193 kcal/day	Unpublished
Female	19–39	Dieting, weight training	–52 kcal/day	Unpublished
Exercise				
Male	20–23	3-hour treadmill at 50% VO_{2max}	4.7% increase	85
Male	Not given	Football—game and hard practice	25% increase	86
Female	25.9 ± 2.4	Middle-distance runners	8% increase	84

contribute to the reduction of body fat and increase in lean body mass that is often seen after resistive training.

The third component of daily energy expenditure is the thermic effect of food, which is the energy expended for the digestion, absorption, transportation, and storage of nutrients. Although the thermic effect of food represents a smaller percentage of the daily energy expenditure relative to REE than the thermic effect of physical activity, it is thought to be of importance in the long-term regulation of body weight.[78,94] Regular strenuous physical activity may influence the thermic effect of food, as sug-

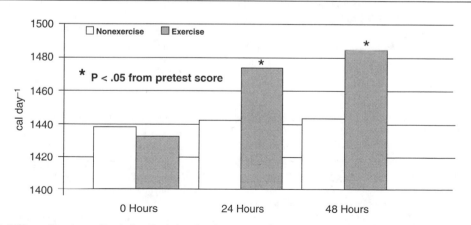

Figure 1–2 Effect of an Acute Resistive Training Session on Resting Metabolic Rate of Women Who Are Untrained. The 11 women did two sets of 10 to 12 repetitions of a 12-station resistive training circuit immediately after the determination of the resting metabolic rate at 0 hours.

gested by a study[95] in which the effects of a 1600-kcal meal on the thermic effect of food in eight trained and eight untrained male subjects were examined. Postprandial thermic effect of food was lower in the trained than in the untrained male subjects of this study. This finding has been confirmed in men who were trained[96,97] but not in women who were trained.[79,98] It is doubtful that the exercise-induced change in the thermic effect of food is as pronounced as its effects on REE and increased caloric requirement from physical activity.

REFERENCES

1. U.S. Department of Health and Human Services. *Physical Activity and Health: A Report of the Surgeon General*. Atlanta, GA: Department of Health and Human Services, Centers for Disease Control and Prevention, National Center for Chronic Disease Prevention and Health Promotion; 1996.

2. Paffenbarger RS Jr, Hyde RT, Wing AL, Lee IM, Jung DL, Kampert JB. The association of changes in physical activity level and other lifestyle characteristics with mortality among men. *N Engl J Med*. 1993;328:538–545.

3. Blair SN, Kohl HW III, Barlow CE, Paffenbarger RS Jr, Gibbons LW, Macera CA. Changes in physical fitness and all-cause mortality: a prospective study of healthy and unhealthy men. *JAMA*. 1995;273:1093–1098.

4. Paffenbarger RS Jr, Hyde RT, Wing AL, Hsieh C-C. Physical activity, all-cause mortality, and longevity of college alumni. *N Engl J Med*. 1986;314:605–613.

5. Slattery ML, Jacobs DR. Physical fitness and cardiovascular disease mortality: the U.S. Railroad Study. *Am J Epidemiol*. 1988;127:571–580.

6. Blair SN, Kohl HW III, Paffenbarger RS Jr, Clark DG, Cooper KH, Gibbons LW. Physical fitness and all-cause mortality: a prospective study of healthy men and women. *JAMA*. 1989;262:2392–2401.

7. Kannel WB, Belanger A, D'Agostino R, Israel I. Physical activity and physical demand on the job and risk of cardiovascular disease and death. The Framingham Study. *Am Heart J*. 1986;112:820–825.

8. LaCroix AZ, Leveille SG, Hecht JA, Grothaus LC, Wanger EH. Does walking decrease the risk of cardiovascular disease hospitalizations and death in older adults? *J Am Geriatr Soc*. 1996;44:113–120.

9. Kriska AM, Blair SN, Pereira MA. The potential role of physical activity in the prevention of non-insulin-dependent diabetes mellitus: the epidemiological evidence. *Exerc Sport Sci Rev*. 1994;22:121–143.

10. Zimmet PZ. Kelly West Lecture: 1991 challenges in diabetes epidemiology—from West to the rest. *Diabetes Care*. 1992;15:232–252.

11. Wu AH, Paganini-Hill A, Ross RK, Henderson BE. Alcohol, physical activity, and other risk factors for colorectal cancer: a prospective study. *Br J Cancer*. 1987;55:687–694.

12. Chow W-H, Dosemeci M, Zheng W, et al. Physical activity and occupational risks of colon cancer in Shanghai, China. *Int J Epidemiol*. 1993;22:23–29.

13. Fraser G, Pearce N. Occupational physical activity and risk of cancer of the colon and rectum in New Zealand males. *Cancer Causes Control*. 1993;4:45–50.

14. McAuly E. Physical activity and psychosocial outcomes. In: Bouchard C, Shepard RJ, Stephens T, eds. *Physical Activity, Fitness, and Health: International Proceedings and Consensus Statement*. Champaign, IL: Human Kinetics Publishers; 1994:551–568.

15. Morgan WP. Physical activity, fitness, and depression. In: Bouchard C, Shepard RJ, Stephens T, eds. *Physical Activity, Fitness, and Health: International Proceedings and Consensus Statement*. Champaign, IL: Human Kinetics Publishers; 1994:851–867.

16. Stamler R, Stamler J, Gosch FC, et al. Primary prevention of hypertension by nutritional-hygienic means: final report of randomized, controlled trial. *JAMA*. 1989;262:1801–1807.

17. Kelly G, McClellan P. Antihypertensive effects of aerobic exercise: a brief meta-analytic review of randomized controlled trials. *Am J Hypertens*. 1994;7:115–119.

18. Durstine JL, Haskell WL. Effects of exercise training on plasma lipids and lipoproteins. *Exerc Sport Sci Rev*. 1994;22:477–521.

19. Leon AS. Effects of exercise conditioning on physiologic precursors of coronary heart disease. *J Cardiopulm Rehabil*. 1991;11:46–57.

20. Eriksson KF, Lindgarde F. Prevention of type 2 (non-insulin-dependent) diabetes mellitus by diet and physical exercise. *Diabetologia*. 1991;34:891–898.

21. DiPietro L. Physical activity, body weight, and adiposity: an epidemiologic perspective. *Exerc Sport Sci Rev*. 1995;23:275–303.

22. Ching PL, Willett WC, Rimm EB, Colditz GA, Gortmaker SL, Stampfer MJ. Activity level and risk of overweight in male health professionals. *Am J Public Health*. 1996;86:25–30.

23. Tremblay A, Despres J-P, Leblanc C, et al. Effect of intensity of physical activity on body fatness and fat distribution. *Am J Clin Nutr.* 1990;51:153–157.

24. Kaye SA, Folsom AR, Prineas RJ, Potter JD, Gapstur SM. The association of body fat distribution with lifestyle and reproductive factors in a population study of postmenopausal women. *Int J Obes.* 1990;14:583–591.

25. Centers for Disease Control and Prevention. *Youth Risk Behavior Survey*, 1993 data tape. Atlanta, GA: U.S. Department of Health and Human Services, Public Health Service, Centers for Disease Control and Prevention, National Center for Chronic Disease Prevention and Health Promotion; 1993.

26. Kolbe LJ, Kann L, Collins JL. Overview of the youth behavior surveillance system. *Public Health Rep.* 1993;108(suppl 1):2–10.

27. National Center for Health Statistics. Plan and operation of the Third National Health and Nutritional Examination Survey, 1988–94. *Vital and Health Statistics, Series 1, No. 32.* Hyattsville, MD: U.S. Department of Health and Human Services, Public Health Service, Centers for Disease Control and Prevention, National Center for Health Statistics; 1994: DHHS Publication No. (PHS)94-1308.

28. National Center for Health Statistics, Schoenborn CA. Health promotion and disease prevention: United States, 1985. *Vital and Health Statistics, Series 10, No. 163.* Hyattsville, MD: U.S. Department of Health and Human Services, Public Health Service, Centers for Disease Control and Prevention, National Center for Health Statistics; 1988: DHHS Publication No. (PHS)88-1591.

29. Jette AM, Branch LG. The Framingham disability study: II. Physical disability among the aging. *Am J Public Health.* 1981;71:1211–1216.

30. Rodgers MA, Evans WJ. Changes in skeletal muscle with aging: effects of exercise training. *Exerc Sport Sci Rev.* 1993;21:65–102.

31. Ainsworth BE, Haskell WL, Leon AS, et al. Compendium of physical activities: classification of energy costs of human physical activities. *Med Sci Sports Exerc.* 1993;25:71–80.

32. Fox SM 3rd, Naughton JP, Gorman PA. Physical activity and cardiovascular health. III. The exercise prescription, frequency, and type of activity. *Mod Concepts Cardiovas Dis.* 1972;41:25–30.

33. Brooks GA, Fahey TD, White TP. *Exercise Physiology: Human Bioenergetics and Its Applications.* 2nd ed. Mountain View, CA: Mayfield Publishing Company; 1996.

34. Bessman S, Carpenter CL. The creatine phosphate shuttle. *Annu Rev Biochem.* 1985;54:831–862.

35. Conley K. Cellular energetics during exercise. *Adv Vet Sci Comp Med.* 1994;38A:1–39.

36. di Prampero P, Boutellier U, Pietsch P. Oxygen deficit and stores at onset of muscular exercise in humans. *J Appl Physiol: Respir, Enviro Exercise Physiol.* 1983; 55:146–153.

37. Spriet L. Phosphofructokinase activity and acidosis during short-term tetanic contractions. *Can J Physiol Pharmacol.* 1991;69:298–304.

38. Wilmore JH, Costill DL. *Physiology of Sport and Exercise.* Champaign, IL: Human Kinetics; 1994.

39. Booth F, Thompson D. Molecular and cellular adaptation of muscle in response to exercise: perspectives of various models. *Physiol Rev.* 1991;71:541–585.

40. Pette D, Staron RS. Cellular and molecular diversities of mammalian skeletal muscle fibers. *Rev Physiol Biochem Pharmacol.* 1990;116:1–76.

41. Pette D, Spamer C. Metabolic properties of muscle fibers. *Fed Proc.* 1986;45:2910–2914.

42. Baldwin KM, Klinkerfuss GH, Terjung RL, Mole PA, Holloszy JO. Respiratory capacity of white, red, and intermediate muscle, adaptive response to exercise. *Am J Physiol.* 1972;222:373–378.

43. Costill D, Fink WJ, Pollock ML. Muscle fiber composition and enzyme activities of elite distance runners. *Med Sci Sports.* 1976;8:96–100.

44. American College of Sport Medicine. *ACSM's Guidelines for Exercise Testing and Prescription.* 5th ed. Baltimore, MD: Williams and Wilkins; 1995.

45. American College of Sports Medicine. Position stand, physical activity, physical fitness, and hypertension. *Med Sci Sports Exerc.* 1993;25(10):i–x.

46. Hooper SL, Mackinnon LT, Howard A, Gordon RD, Baachmann AW. Markers for monitoring overtraining and recovery. *Med Sci Sports Exerc.* 1995;27:106–112.

47. Fry RW, Morton AR, Keast D. Overtraining in athletes: an update. *Sports Med.* 1991;12:32–65.

48. Komi PV. Physiological and biomechanical correlates of muscle function: effects of muscle structure and stretch-shortening cycle on force and speed. *Exerc Sport Sci Rev.* 1981;12:81–121.

49. Gonyea WJ, Sale D. Physiology of weight lifting. *Arch Phys Med Rehabil.* 1982;63:235–237.

50. Hettinger TL, Muller EA. Muskelleistung und muskeltraining. *Arbeits Physiologie.* 1953;15:111–126.

51. Manning RJ, Graves JE, Carpenter DM, Leggett SH, Pollock ML. Constant vs. variable resistance knee extension training. *Med Sci Sports Exerc.* 1990;22:397–401.

52. Bobbert MF, Huijing PA, van Ingen Schenau GJ. Drop jumping. I. The influence of jumping technique on the biomechanics of jumping. *Med Sci Sports Exerc.* 1987;19:332–338.

53. Kramer JF, Morrow A, Leger A. Changes in rowing ergometer, weight lifting, vertical jump and isokinetic per-

formance in response to standard and standard plus plyometric training programs. *Int J Sports Med.* 1993;14:449–454.

54. Stone M, O'Bryant H. *Weight Training: A Scientific Approach.* Minneapolis, MN: Burgess; 1986.

55. Danneskiold-Samsoe B, Lyngberg K, Risum T, Telling M. The effect of water exercise therapy given to patients with rheumatoid arthritis. *Scand J Appl Physiol.* 1987;19:31–35.

56. Gehlsen GM, Grigsby SA, Winant DM. Effects of an aquatic fitness program on the muscular strength and endurance of patients with multiple sclerosis. *Phys Ther.* 1984;64:653–657.

57. Ruoti RG, Troup JT, Berger RA. The effects of nonswimming exercise on older adults. *J Orthop Sports Phys Ther.* 1994;19(3):140–145.

58. Kendrick ZV, McGettigan JC, Paolone AM, Ruoti RG. Effect of water exercise on knee flexor and extensor peak torque, resting metabolic rate, and body composition in elderly adults. *Age.* 1996;19:173.

59. Costill DL, Maglischo EW, Richardson AB. *Swimming.* Oxford, England: Blackwell Scientific; 1992.

60. Alway S, Strat-Gundersen J, Grumbt WH, Gonyea WJ. Muscle cross sectional area and torque in resistance-trained subjects. *Eur J Appl Physiol.* 1990;60:86–90.

61. Costill DL, Coyle EF, Fink WF, Lesmes GR, Witzmann FA. Adaptations in skeletal muscle following strength training. *J Appl Physiol.* 1979;46:96–99.

62. Moritani T, deVries HA. Neural factors versus hypertrophy in the time course of muscle strength gain. *Am J Phys Med.* 1979;58:115–119.

63. Rube N, Secher NH. Effect of training on central factors in fatigue following two- and one-leg on static exercise in man. *Acta Physiol Scand.* 1991;141:87–95.

64. Tinetti ME, Baker DI, McAvay G, et al. A multifactoral intervention to reduce the risk of falling among elderly people living in the community. *N Engl J Med.* 1994;331:821–827.

65. Tinetti ME, Powell L. Fear of falling and low self-efficacy: a cause of dependence in elderly persons. *J Gerontol.* 1993;48:35–38.

66. Gryfe CI, Amies A, Ashley MJ. A longitudinal study of falls in an elderly population. I. *Age Ageing.* 1977;6:201–210.

67. Isskrant I. The etiology of fractured hips in females. *Am J Public Health.* 1968;58:485–490.

68. Fiatarone MA, Evans WJ. The etiology and reversibility of muscle dysfunction in the aged. *J Gerontol.* 1993;48:77–83.

69. Minor MA. Physical activity and management of arthritis. *Ann Behav Med.* 1991;13:117–121.

70. Stauffer RN, Chao EY, Gyory A. Biomechanical gait analysis of the diseased knee joint. *Clin Orthop.* 1977;126:246–255.

71. Greenleaf JE, Kuzlowski S. Physiological consequences of reduced physical activity during bed rest. *Exerc Sport Sci Rev.* 1982;10:84–119.

72. Hickson RC, Bomze HA, Holloszy JO. Linear increase in aerobic power induced by a strenuous program of endurance exercise. *J Appl Physiol: Respir, Envir, Exercise Physiol.* 1977;42:372–376.

73. Dudley G, Abraham W, Terjung R. Influence of exercise intensity and duration on biochemical adaptations in skeletal muscle. *J Appl Physiol: Respir, Envir, Exercise Physiol.* 1982;53:844–850.

74. Farrell PA, Wilmore JH, Coyle EF, Biling JE, Costill DL. Plasma lactate accumulation and distance running performance. *Med Sci Sports.* 1979;11:338–344.

75. Fox EL, Mathews D. *Interval Training: Conditioning for Sports and General Fitness.* Philadelphia, PA: WB Saunders; 1974.

76. Poehlman ET, Horton ES. Regulation of energy expenditure in aging humans. *Annu Rev Nutr.* 1990;10:255–275.

77. Poehlman ET. A review: exercise and its influence on resting energy metabolism in man. *Med Sci Sports Exerc.* 1989;21:515–525.

78. D'Alessio DA, Kavle EC, Mozzoli MA, et al. Thermic effect of food in lean and obese men. *J Clin Invest.* 1988;81:1781–1789.

79. Owen OE, Kavle E, Owen RS, et al. A reappraisal of caloric requirements in healthy women. *Am J Clin Nutr.* 1986;44:1–19.

80. Owen OE, Holup JL, D'Alessio DA, et al. A reappraisal of the caloric requirements of men. *Am J Clin Nutr.* 1987;46:875–885.

81. Kendrick ZV, Bezilla TA, Paolone VJ. Resting energy expenditure of undergraduate and graduate college women. *Ann Sports Med.* 1990;5:166–170.

82. Kendrick ZV, McPeek CK, Young KF. Prediction of the resting energy expenditure of women following 12 to 18 weeks of very-low-calorie-dieting. *Ann Sports Med.* 1990;5:118–123.

83. Mole PA, Stern JS, Schultz CL, Bernauer EM, Holcomb BJ. Exercise reverses depressed metabolic rate produced by severe caloric restriction. *Med Sci Sports Exerc.* 1989;21:29–33.

84. Bielinski R, Schutz Y, Jequier E. Energy metabolism during the postexercise recovery in man. *Am J Clin Nutr.* 1985;42:69–82.

85. Edwards HT, Thorndike AA, Dill DR. The energy requirement in strenuous muscular exercise. *New Engl J Med.* 1935;213:532–536.

86. Herring JL, Mole PA, Meredith CN, Stern JS. Effect of suspending exercise training on resting metabolic rate in women. *Med Sci Sports Exerc.* 1992;24:59–65.

87. Poehlman ET, McAuliffe TL, Van Houten DR, Danforth E Jr. Influence of age and endurance training on metabolic rate and hormones in healthy men. *Am J Physiol: Endocrin Metab.* 1990;259:E66–E72.

88. Forbes GB, Holloran E. The adult decline in lean body mass. *Hum Biol.* 1976;48:162–173.

89. Forbes GB, Reina JC. Adult lean body mass declines with age: some longitudinal observations. *Metabolism.* 1970;19:653–663.

90. Moritani T, deVries HA. Potential for gross muscle hypertrophy in older men. *J Gerontol.* 1980;35:672–682.

91. Frontera WR, Meredith CN, O'Reilly KP, Knuttgen HG, Evans WJ. Strength conditioning in older men: skeletal muscle hypertrophy and improved function. *J Appl Physiol: Respir, Envir, Exercise Physiol.* 1988;64:1038–1044.

92. Fiatarone MA, Marks EC, Ryan ND, Meredith CN, Lipsitz LA, Evans WJ. High-intensity strength training in nonagenarians. Effects on skeletal muscle. *JAMA.* 1990;263:3029–3034.

93. Evans WJ: Exercise, nutrition, and aging. *J Nutr.* 1992;122(suppl):796–801.

94. Tremblay A, Fontaine E, Poehlman ET, Mitchell D, Perron L, Bouchard C. The effect of exercise training on resting metabolic rate in lean and moderately obese individuals. *Int J Obes.* 1986;10:511–517.

95. Tremblay A, Cote J, LeBlanc J. Diminished dietary thermogenesis in exercise-trained human subjects. *Eur J Appl Physiol.* 1983;52:1–4.

96. LeBlanc J, Diamond P, Cote J, Labrie A. Hormonal factors in reduced postprandial heat production of exercise trained subjects. *J Appl Physiol.* 1984;56:772–776.

97. Poehlman ET, Melby CL, Badylak SF. Resting metabolic rate and postprandial thermogenesis in highly trained and untrained males. *Am J Clin Nutr.* 1988;47:793–798.

98. LeBlanc J, Mercier P, Samsom P. Diet-induced thermogenesis with relation to training state in female subjects. *Canad J Physiol Pharmacol.* 1984;62:334–337.

CHAPTER 2

Carbohydrate—The Master Fuel

Ellen J. Coleman

The availability of bodily carbohydrate stores (muscle and liver glycogen and blood glucose) plays a critical role in athletic performance. Consuming carbohydrate before endurance exercise can help performance by "topping off" muscle and liver glycogen stores. Consuming carbohydrate during endurance exercise can improve performance by maintaining blood glucose levels and carbohydrate oxidation. Also, consuming adequate carbohydrate after exercise is necessary to replenish muscle and liver glycogen between daily exercise sessions or competitive events.

DETERMINANTS OF EXERCISE FUEL USAGE

A variety of factors determine which type of fuel the muscles will use during exercise. These include the intensity of the exercise, the duration of the exercise, the person's training state, and the composition of the diet.[1] Of these factors, the exercise intensity and duration of the athletic event are particularly important.

Intensity

The energy demands of exercise dictate that carbohydrates are the preferred fuel for high-intensity work. High-intensity, short-duration exercise (such as sprinting 400 m) relies on the glycolytic (lactic acid) pathway for the production of adenosine triphosphate (ATP). Only glucose, derived primarily from the breakdown of muscle glycogen, can be used as fuel.

When glucose is broken down through glycolysis, muscle glycogen is used 18 times faster than when glucose is fully oxidized. A more rapid rate of muscle glycogen breakdown will also occur during high-intensity exercise (for example, over 70% of VO_{2max}) when the glycolytic pathway is pulled in to assist the aerobic energy system to provide adequate ATP. Extended mixed anaerobic–aerobic intermittent exercise like soccer, basketball, football drills, and running or swimming also result in a greater breakdown of muscle glycogen. The use of muscle glycogen is most rapid during the early stages of exercise and is exponentially related to exercise intensity.

During endurance exercise, muscle glycogen supplies half of the energy for a moderate workout (60% VO_{2max}) and nearly all of the energy during an intense workout ($\geq$ 80% VO_{2max}).

Exercise of low to moderate intensity (up to 60% of VO_{2max}) can be fueled almost entirely aerobically. During exercise, the sympathetic nervous system is stimulated and the adrenal medulla releases the catecholamines epinephrine and norepinephrine into the bloodstream. Exercise also causes the anterior pituitary to secrete growth hormone. These hormones block the release of insulin from the pancreas.

The hormonal changes that occur during exercise—increased epinephrine, norepinephrine, and growth hormone, and decreased insulin—promote greater fat oxidation and prompt the adipose tissue to release fatty acids into the bloodstream. These, combined with intramuscular triglycerides, supply about half of the energy during low- to moderate-intensity exercise (40–60% of VO_{2max}). Muscle glycogen and blood glucose supply the rest.

Muscle glycogen breakdown is required for high-intensity exercise (>70% of VO_{2max}) because fat utilization is limited above 60% of VO_{2max}. The breakdown of fat to ATP is a slow process and doesn't supply ATP fast enough to provide energy for high-intensity exercise. Also, the oxidation of glucose provides more calories per liter of oxygen than does fat. Glucose delivers 5.10 kcal per liter of oxygen and fat delivers 4.62 kcal per liter of oxygen.[1]

There would be a greater total yield of ATP from fat than from carbohydrate if the muscle could oxidize fat at a sufficiently high rate during intense exercise. A six-carbon glucose molecule produces 36 ATP, whereas an 18-carbon fatty acid (stearic acid) produces 147 ATP—a 1.3 greater yield of ATP per carbon molecule. However, 6 molecules of oxygen are required to oxidize a glucose molecule, whereas 26 oxygen molecules are required to oxidize stearic acid. Thus, the oxygen requirement for glucose is 77% less than the oxygen requirement for stearic acid.[2]

When less oxygen becomes available, as during high-intensity exercise, it is a distinct advantage for the muscles to use glucose because less oxygen is required to produce energy. During endurance exercise, the lower oxygen requirement for the oxidation of carbohydrate produces a lower cardiovascular stress than does the oxidation of fat.

The shift in fuel from fat to glycogen as the exercise intensity increases is also partly due to the accumulation of lactic acid, which occurs during high-intensity exercise. Lactic acid hinders the mobilization of fat from the adipose tissue. Thus, the muscles must rely more on glycogen for ATP production.

Duration

The duration of exercise also defines whether the fuel used will be mostly carbohydrate or fat. The longer the time spent exercising, the greater the contribution of fat as fuel. Fat can supply as much as 60% to 70% of the energy needs for moderate-intensity exercise (60% of VO_{2max}) lasting 4 to 6 hours.

As the duration of the exercise increases, the intensity must decrease, because there is a limited supply of stored glycogen. When muscle glycogen stores are low, fat breakdown supplies most of the energy needed for exercise. However, fat oxidation is limited above 60% of VO_{2max}. Also, a certain level of carbohydrate breakdown is necessary for fats to be used continually for energy. To this extent, "fat burns in a carbohydrate flame."

It must be noted that muscle glycogen is the predominant fuel for most types of exercise. It takes at least 20 minutes for fat to be available to the muscles as fuel in the form of free fatty acids. Most athletes don't work out long enough to burn significant amounts of fat as fuel during exercise. Also, most athletes train at an exercise intensity of 70% of VO_{2max} or above, limiting the use of fat as fuel.

This does not mean that a person needs to work out for a long time at a low intensity to lose body fat. When the workout creates a caloric deficit, the body will pull from its fat stores at a later time to make up that caloric deficit.

Training State

Endurance training causes several major adaptations that facilitate fat utilization.[1] When more fat is burned, less muscle glycogen is used. This "glycogen sparing" effect aids endurance because muscle glycogen stores are limited and fat stores are abundant.

First, endurance training increases VO_{2max} by increasing the maximum cardiac output and improving the extraction of oxygen from the blood by the muscles. This translates into greater fat utilization because the athlete can perform more aerobically at the same absolute level of exercise.

Second, endurance training raises the threshold at which lactic acid accumulates in the blood. Persons who are untrained accumulate lactic acid at about 50% of VO_{2max}, whereas endurance athletes accumulate lactic acid at about 70% of VO_{2max}. Lactic acid speeds up the rate of muscle glycogen breakdown by interfering with fat mobilization. A higher blood lactate threshold enables athletes to use more fat as fuel.

Third, endurance training increases the muscle's capillary density and mitochondrial density, which increases fat oxidation.

Endurance training also increases the capacity of the muscles to store glycogen. Persons who are untrained have muscle glycogen stores that are roughly 80 to 90 mmol/kg. Endurance athletes have muscle glycogen stores of 130 to 135 mmol/kg. Thus, endurance training confers a dual performance advantage—the muscle glycogen stores are higher at the onset of exercise and the athlete depletes them at a slower rate.[1]

Diet

The percentages of carbohydrate and fat in the diet also determine the amount of glycogen and fat used as fuel. A high-carbohydrate diet increases the use of glycogen as fuel. A high-fat diet increases the use of fat as fuel. However, a high-fat diet reduces the athlete's ability to sustain high-intensity exercise and decreases endurance due to low muscle glycogen stores. Although there is no performance advantage to a high-fat diet, there is a performance advantage when fat utilization is increased through endurance training. The ability to use fat will spare muscle glycogen and improve endurance.

CARBOHYDRATE RECOMMENDATIONS FOR TRAINING

Building up and maintaining glycogen stores during training require a carbohydrate-rich diet.

Glycogen depletion can occur gradually over repeated days of heavy training when muscle glycogen breakdown exceeds its replacement. When adequate carbohydrate is not consumed on a daily basis between training sessions, the muscle glycogen content before exercise gradually declines, and training or competitive performance may be impaired. The feeling of sluggishness associated with muscle glycogen depletion is often referred to as "staleness" and blamed on overtraining.

Costill and colleagues evaluated glycogen synthesis of persons following a 45% carbohydrate diet during 3 successive days of running 16.1 kilometers at 80% of VO_{2max}.[3] Muscle glycogen levels before exercise started at 110 mmol/kg and decreased to 88 mmol/kg on day 2 and 66 mmol/kg on day 3. Another study of Costill and colleagues found that a diet providing 525 to 648 g of carbohydrate promoted glycogen synthesis of 70 to 80 mmol/kg and provided near maximal repletion of muscle glycogen within 24 hours.[4] This corresponds to a carbohydrate intake of about 8 to 10 g/kg daily.

Fallowfield and Williams also evaluated the importance of a high-carbohydrate intake on recovery from prolonged exercise.[5] Their subjects ran at 70% of VO_{2max} for 90 minutes, or until volitional fatigue, whichever came first. During the next 22.5 hours, the runners consumed isocaloric diets containing either 5.8 or 8.8 g of carbohydrate per kilogram. After the rest period, the runners ran at the same intensity so that endurance capacity could be assessed. Those that consumed 8.8 g/kg of carbohydrate were able to match their running time of the first race. Even though the two diets were isocaloric, the running time of those who consumed only 5.8 g/kg of carbohydrate decreased by more than 15 minutes.

Some athletes do not voluntarily increase caloric intake to meet the energy demands of increased training. Costill and colleagues studied the effects of 10 days of increased training volume at a high intensity on muscle glycogen and swimming performance.[6] Six swimmers selected a diet containing 4700 calories/day and 8.2 g of carbohydrate/kg/day, whereas four swimmers selected a diet containing only 3700 calories/day and 5.3 g of carbohydrate/kg/day. These four swimmers couldn't tolerate the heavier training demands and swam at significantly slower speeds, presumably due to a 20% decline in muscle glycogen.

Athletes who train exhaustively on successive days must consume adequate carbohydrate and energy to minimize the threat of chronic fatigue associated with the cumulative depletion of muscle glycogen.

Glycogen depletion can occur during training in sports that require repeated, near maximal bursts of effort (such as football, basketball, and soccer) as well as during endurance exercise. A telltale sign of glycogen depletion associated with training is when the athlete has difficulty maintaining a normal exercise intensity. A sudden weight loss of several pounds (due to glycogen and water loss) may accompany glycogen depletion associated with training. Athletes who don't consume enough carbohydrate or calories and/or who don't rest for full days are prime candidates.

A review of the literature by Sherman and Wimer questions the belief that low dietary carbohydrate intake during training causes reduced muscle glycogen with subsequent fatigue.[7] However, they note that it is well-established that low blood glucose, muscle, and/or liver glycogen concentrations can contribute to fatigue during certain types of exercise.

Because dietary carbohydrate contributes directly to maintenance of body carbohydrate reserves, Sherman and Wimer recommend continuing to advise athletes to eat a high-carbohydrate diet. They also recommend watching for signs of staleness during training and taking note of those athletes whose dietary habits make them more prone to glycogen depletion associated with training.

Glycogen depletion associated with training can be prevented by a carbohydrate-rich diet (6–10 g/kg/day) and periodic rest days to give the muscles time to rebuild their stores. The typical American diet (46% carbohydrate—about 4 g/kg) doesn't supply enough carbohydrate. Carbohydrate is essential for glycogen synthesis and should provide at least 6 g/kg of body weight daily (about 60% of total calories.) A diet containing 8 to 10 g of carbohydrate/kg is recommended when the athlete partakes in intense exercise (70% of VO_{2max}) for several hours or more daily. If the athlete exercises for an hour or less, a diet providing 6 g of carbohydrate/kg should be sufficient to replenish muscle glycogen stores. Endurance athletes undergoing heavy training will need to reduce fat intake to about 20% to 25% of total calories to obtain 8 to 10 g of carbohydrate/kg/day.

These guidelines for carbohydrate intake assume that the athlete is consuming adequate calories. Consumption of a reduced energy diet will impair endurance performance because of muscle and liver glycogen depletion. Walberg-Rankin notes that adequate carbohydrate intake is also important for athletes participating in high-power activities (for example, wrestling, gymnastics, and dance) who have lost weight because of negative energy balances.[8] Desire for weight loss and consumption of low-energy diets are prevalent among athletes participating in high-power activities. Negative energy balance can harm high-power performance because of impaired acid–base balance, reduced glycolytic enzyme levels, selective atrophy of type II muscle fibers, and abnormal sarcoplasmic reticulum function. Adequate dietary carbohydrate may ameliorate some of the damaging effects of energy restriction on the muscle.[8]

Athletes participating in ultra-endurance events (those lasting more than 4 hours) have the greatest dietary carbohydrate requirements. Saris and colleagues studied food intake and energy expenditure during the Tour de France.[9] During this demanding 22-day, 2400-mile race, the cyclists consumed an average of 850 g of carbohydrate per day or 12.3 g/kg/day. About 30% of the total energy consumed was provided by high-carbohydrate beverages.

Brouns and associates evaluated the effect of a simulated Tour de France study on food and fluid intake, energy balance, and substrate oxidation.[10,11] Although the cyclists consumed 630 g of carbohydrate (8.6 g/kg/day), they oxidized 850 g of carbohydrate per day (11.6 g/kg/day). In spite of ad libitum intake of conventional foods, the cyclists were unable to ingest sufficient carbohydrate and calories to compensate for their increased energy expenditure. When the diet was supplemented with a 20% carbohydrate beverage, carbohydrate intake increased to 16 g/kg/day and carbohydrate oxidation increased to 13 g/kg/day.

Ultra-endurance athletes who require more than 600 g of carbohydrate/day may need to supplement their dietary intake with high-carbohydrate beverages because it is unlikely that they can eat enough conventional foods to meet their carbohydrate and energy requirements.[11] Saris and colleagues recommend that ultra-endurance athletes participating in training or competition consume 12 to 13 g of carbohydrate/kg/day. They also suggest that this range represents the maximum contribution of carbohydrate to energy metabolism during extreme ultra-endurance exercise.[9]

In addition to providing proper muscle glycogen stores, the athlete's diet should help to prevent chronic diseases such as cardiovascular disease and cancer. Both of these objectives can be met by following the 1995 *Dietary Guidelines for Americans*[12] and the *Food Guide Pyramid*.[13]

TYPE OF CARBOHYDRATE

The primary advantage of complex carbohydrates over simple carbohydrates is that they are more nutrient-dense. They provide more B vitamins necessary for energy metabolism as well as more fiber and iron, thereby contributing to a nutritionally balanced diet. However, many sugary baked goods and candies are also high in fat. Sugar intake may be increased to meet increased carbohydrate requirements, but the majority of the carbohydrate should come from complex carbohydrates (Table 2–1).

FORM OF CARBOHYDRATE

Each carbohydrate form (liquid versus solid) offers certain advantages for the athlete.[14] Sports drinks and other liquids encourage the consumption of water needed to maintain hydration during exercise. Also, carbohydrate must be in a liquid or semiliquid state before leaving the stomach. However, compared to liquids, high-carbohydrate foods can be easily carried by the athlete during exercise and provide both variety and satiety.

GLYCEMIC INDEX

The glycemic index indicates how much a food increases the blood glucose level relative to glucose, which has a glycemic index value of 100. In practical terms, the glycemic index is influenced by the form (liquid or solid) in which the food is eaten, its fiber content, the presence of protein and fat, and food-processing and food-preparation methods.

The glycemic index is not simply a function of whether the carbohydrate is in a liquid or solid form. An orange has a glycemic index that is almost identical to the value for orange juice. The glycemic index is also not a function of whether the food is a starch (for example, pasta) or simple carbohydrate (for example, table sugar). For instance, a baked potato has a glycemic index that is close to the value for glucose.

The glycemic index concept has limitations. The numbers that are available are largely based on tests using single foods. High glycemic foods often don't affect the glycemic response when combined with other foods. Also, the glycemic index is based on equal grams of carbohydrate, not average serving sizes.

FOOD-EXCHANGE SYSTEM

In practical terms, a high-carbohydrate diet can be created by using the food-exchange sys-

Table 2–1 High Carbohydrate Foods with Gram Weights

Food Group	Calories	Carbohydrate (g)
Milk		
Low-fat (2%) milk (1 cup)	121	12
Skim milk (1 cup)	86	12
Chocolate milk (1 cup)	208	26
Pudding, any flavor (1/2 cup)	161	30
Frozen yogurt, low-fat (1 cup)	220	34
Fruit-flavored low-fat yogurt (1 cup)	225	42
Meat		
Blackeye peas (1/2 cup)	134	22
Pinto beans (1 cup)	235	42
Navy beans (1 cup)	259	48
Refried beans (1/2 cup)	142	26
Meat loaf (3 oz)	230	13
Fruits and vegetables		
Fruits		
Apple (1 medium)	81	21
Apple juice (1 cup)	111	28
Applesauce (1 cup)	232	60
Banana (1)	105	27
Cantaloupe (1 cup)	57	14
Cherries, raw (10)	49	11
Cranberry juice cocktail (1 cup)	147	37
Dates, dried (10)	228	61
Fruit cocktail, packed in own juice (1/2 cup)	56	15
Fruit Roll-Ups (1 roll)	50	12
Grapes (1 cup)	114	28
Grape juice (1 cup)	96	23
Orange (1)	65	16
Orange juice (1 cup)	112	26
Pear (1)	98	25
Pineapple (1 cup)	77	19
Prunes, dried (10)	201	53
Raisins (2/3 cup)	302	79
Raspberries (1 cup)	61	14
Strawberries (1 cup)	45	11
Watermelon (1 cup)	50	12
Vegetables		
Three-bean salad (1/2 cup)	90	20
Carrots (1 medium)	31	8
Corn (1/2 cup)	89	21
Garbanzo beans (chickpeas) (1 cup)	269	45
Lima beans (1 cup)	217	39
Peas, green (1/2 cup)	63	12
Potato (1 large)	220	50

continues

Table 2–1 continued

Food Group	Calories	Carbohydrate (g)
Vegetables (continued)		
Sweet potato (1 large)	118	28
Water chestnuts (1/2 cup)	66	15
White beans (1 cup)	249	45
Grain		
Bagel (1)	165	31
Biscuit (1)	103	13
White bread (1 slice)	61	12
Whole wheat bread (1 slice)	55	11
Breadsticks (2 sticks)	77	15
Cornbread (1 square)	178	28
Cereal, ready-to-eat (1 cup)	110	24
Oatmeal (1/2 cup)	66	12
Cream of Rice (3/4 cup)	95	21
Cream of Wheat (3/4 cup)	96	20
Malto-Meal (3/4 cup)	92	19
Flavored oatmeal, Quaker instant (1 packet)	110	25
Graham crackers (2 squares)	60	11
Saltines (5 crackers)	60	10
Triscuit crackers (3 crackers)	60	10
Pancake (4″ diameter)	61	9
Waffles (2, 3.5″ × 5.5″)	130	17
Rice (1 cup)	223	50
Rice, brown (1 cup)	232	50
Hamburger bun (1)	119	21
Hot dog bun (1)	119	21
Noodles, spaghetti (1 cup)	159	34
Flour tortilla (1)	85	15

tem. The 1986 exchange lists are the basis of a meal-planning system designed by a committee of the American Diabetes Association and the American Dietetic Association (Exhibit 2–1).[15]

The following are the six exchange lists: meat, vegetables, fruit, starch/bread, milk, and fat. Each lists foods that have about the same amount of carbohydrate, protein, fat, and calories. Any food on a list can be exchanged or traded for any other food on the same list.

Exchange plans are provided for different calorie levels (from 1500 to 4000). These exchange plans are designed to supply about 60% carbohydrate, 15% to 20% protein, and less than 25% fat (Exhibit 2–2).

Because the milk, bread, and fruit exchanges have the most carbohydrate per serving, they are emphasized. These exchange plans will meet the carbohydrate needs of most athletes. Exchange plans supplying 496 g and 605 g of carbohydrate are also provided for periods of heavy training and carbohydrate loading (Exhibit 2–3).

HIGH-CARBOHYDRATE SUPPLEMENTS

Some athletes train so heavily that they have difficulty eating enough food to obtain the amount of carbohydrate needed for optimum

Exhibit 2–1 Food-Group–Exchange System

MILK   *90–150 calories*
Nonfat
   12 g carbohydrate
   8 g protein
   0 g fat
   • 1 cup skim milk, nonfat yogurt
Low-Fat
   12 g carbohydrate
   8 g protein
   5 g fat
   • 1 cup 2% milk, plain low-fat yogurt
High-Fat
   2 g carbohydrate
   8 g protein
   8 g fat
   • 1 cup whole milk

MEAT AND SUBSTITUTES
Lean Meat   *55 calories*
   0 g carbohydrate
   7 g protein
   3 g fat
   • 1 oz lean beef (eg, sirloin)
   • 1 oz lean pork (eg, tenderloin)
   • 1 oz poultry without skin
   • 1 oz fish
Medium-Fat Meat   *75 calories*
   0 g carbohydrate
   7 g protein
   5 g fat
   • 1 oz ground beef
   • 1 oz skim/part mozzarella, ricotta
   • 4 oz tofu
   • 1 egg
High-Fat Meat   *100 calories*
   0 g carbohydrate
   7 g protein
   8 g fat
   • 1 oz corned beef
   • 1 oz spare ribs
   • 1 oz cheese (eg, cheddar, swiss)
   • 1 oz cold cuts
   • 1 hot dog
   • 1 tbsp peanut butter

BREAD/GRAINS   *80 calories*
   15 g carbohydrate
   3 g protein
   0 g fat
   • 1 slice whole wheat bread
   • 1/2 bagel, English muffin
   • 1 6-inch tortilla
   • 1/2 cup pasta
   • 3 cups popcorn, popped, no added fat
   • 1/2 cup bran flakes
   • 1/2 cup corn
   • 1 small potato
   • 2 pancakes (add 1 fat)
   • 1 waffle (add 1 fat)

FRUITS   *60 calories*
   15 g carbohydrate
   0 g protein
   0 g fat
   • 1 small apple
   • 1/2 banana
   • 1/3 cantaloupe
   • 1/2 cup grapefruit juice
   • 1 small orange
   • 1 cup watermelon

VEGETABLES   *25 calories*
   5 g carbohydrate
   2 g protein
   0 g fat
   • 1/2 cup cooked vegetables
   • 1 cup raw vegetables
   • 1/2 cup vegetable juice

FAT   *45 calories*
   0 g carbohydrate
   0 g protein
   5 g fat
   • 20 small peanuts
   • 1 tsp oil
   • 1 slice bacon
   • 2 tsp mayonnaise
   • 1 tsp butter, margarine
   • 1 tbsp cream cheese
   • 2 tbsp sour cream

Source: Copyright © 1995 by the American Diabetes Association and the American Dietetic Association. Reproduction of the Exchange Lists in whole or in part, without permission of the American Dietetic Association or the American Diabetes Association, is a violation of federal law. This material has been modified from *Exchange Lists for Meal Planning*, which is the basis of a meal planning system designed by a committee of the American Diabetes Association and the American Dietetic Association. While designed primarily for people with diabetes and others who must follow special diets, the Exchange Lists are based on principles of good nutrition that apply to everyone.

Exhibit 2–2 Calculations for Training Diets

| | *Number of Exchanges* | | | | | |
| | | | *Calorie Level* | | | |
Food Group	*1500*	*2000*	*2500*	*3000*	*3500*	*4000*
Milk	3	3	4	4	4	4
Meat	5	5	5	5	6	6
Fruit	5	6	7	9	10	12
Vegetable	3	3	3	5	6	7
Grain	7	11	16	18	20	24
Fat	2	3	5	6	8	10

Example: 3000 calorie training diet—source of carbohydrate:

Milk	4	exchanges × 12 g carbohydrates =	48 g
Fruit	9	exchanges × 15 g carbohydrates =	135 g
Vegetables	5	exchanges × 5 g carbohydrates =	25 g
Grains	18	exchanges × 15 g carbohydrates =	270 g

478 g carbohydrate × 4 cal/g = 1912 calories from carbohydrates

$$\frac{1912}{3000} = .637 \times 100 = 63.7\% \text{ carbohydrates}$$

performance. Athletes, such as those participating in ultra-endurance events, may have difficulty consuming adequate amounts of carbohydrate for several reasons.

To get 4000 calories per day, the athlete would have to eat 24 servings of grains, 12 of fruits and 7 of vegetables. It is difficult to eat that much food regularly for several reasons.[11] Often, the stress of intense training can decrease appetite, resulting in reduced consumption of calories and carbohydrate. Consuming a large volume of food can cause gastrointestinal (GI) distress and interfere with training. And, the athlete may be spending so much time training there aren't many rest hours available for replenishment.

Athletes who have difficulty consuming enough carbohydrate can use a commercial high-carbohydrate supplement.[11] Most products are 18% to 24% carbohydrate and contain glucose polymers (maltodextrins) to reduce the solution's osmolality and potential for GI distress. High-carbohydrate supplements do not replace regular food, but are designed to supply supplemental calories and carbohydrate when needed (Tables 2–2 and 2–3). If the athlete has no difficulty eating enough food, these products are unnecessary.

High-carbohydrate supplements can be consumed before or after exercise (for example, with meals or between meals). Though ultra-endurance athletes may also use them during exercise, they are too concentrated in carbohydrate to double for use as a fluid-replacement beverage.

CARBOHYDRATE LOADING

During endurance exercise that exceeds 90 to 120 minutes, such as marathon running, muscle glycogen stores become progressively lower. When they decrease to critically low levels (the

Exhibit 2–3 Carbohydrate-Loading Meal Plans

60%	Exchanges	Carbohydrate (g)	Calories
Milk (nonfat)	6	72	540
Meat (lean)	6	0	330
Fruit	10	150	600
Vegetables	4	20	100
Bread	17	255	1360
Fat	6	—	270
TOTALS:		497	3200

Distribution of Calories: **Protein: 19%**   **Carbohydrate: 62%**   **Fat: 19%**

70%	Exchanges	Carbohydrate (g)	Calories
Milk (nonfat)	5	60	450
Meat (lean)	5	0	275
Fruit	15	225	900
Vegetables	4	20	100
Bread	20	300	1600
Fat	4	0	180
TOTALS:		605	3505

Distribution of Calories: **Protein: 16%**   **Carbohydrate: 70%**   **Fat: 14%**

Source: Reprinted with permission from Nutrition Dimension, © 1996.

point of glycogen depletion), high-intensity exercise cannot be maintained. In practical terms, the athlete is exhausted and must either stop exercising or drastically reduce the pace.

Muscle glycogen depletion is a well-recognized limitation to endurance exercise. Athletes using glycogen supercompensation techniques (carbohydrate loading) can nearly double their muscle glycogen stores. The greater the glycogen content before exercise, the greater the endurance potential.

The classic study on carbohydrate loading by Bergstrom and associates compared the exercise time to exhaustion at 75% of VO_{2max} after 3 days of three diets varying in carbohydrate content—a low-carbohydrate diet (less than 5% carbohydrate calories), a normal diet (50% carbohydrate calories), and a high-carbohydrate diet (at or above 82% carbohydrate calories).[16]

The low-carbohydrate diet provided muscle glycogen stores of 38 mmol/kg, which sustained only an hour of exercise. The mixed diet provided muscle glycogen stores of 106 mmol/kg, which sustained 115 minutes of exercise. The high-carbohydrate diet provided 204 mmol/kg of muscle glycogen, which sustained 170 minutes of the high-intensity exercise.

After additional research, the carbohydrate loading sequence developed into a week-long regimen starting with an exhaustive training session 1 week before competition. For the next 3 days, the athlete consumed a low-carbohydrate

Table 2–2 High-Carbohydrate Beverage Comparison Chart

Beverage	Flavors	Carbohydrate Ingredient	Carbohydrate (g)	Sodium (mg)	Calories
GatorLode® High-carbohydrate— loading and recovery drink The Gatorade Company	Citrus	Maltodextrin, dextrose	71	90	280
Carbo Power® Nature's Best	Fruit Punch, Tea, Grape	Glucose polymers from maltodextrin, fructose	100	0	400
Ultra Fuel® Twin Labs	Fruit Punch, Lemon-Lime, Grape, Orange	Maltodextrin, high fructose corn syrup	100	30	400

Courtesy of Gatorade Sports Science Institute, Chicago, Illinois.

Table 2–3 Nutrition Beverage Comparison Chart

Beverage	Flavors	Calories (per 8-oz serving)	Carbohydrates (g)	Protein (g)	Fat
GatorPro® Sports nutrition supplement The Gatorade Company	Chocolate, Vanilla	360	59	17	6
Sport Shake® Mid-America Farms	Chocolate, Vanilla, Strawberry, Cafe Mocha, Pina Colada	430	63	13	13
Metabolol II® Champion Nutrition	Plain, Orange Smoothie, Chocolate	260	36	20	4

Courtesy of Gatorade Sports Science Institute, Chicago, Illinois.

diet, yet continued exercising, to decrease muscle glycogen stores even further.

Then, for 3 days before competition, the athlete rested and ate a high-carbohydrate diet to promote glycogen supercompensation. For years, this week-long sequence was considered the best way to achieve maximum glycogen storage.

This regimen has many drawbacks. Three days of reduced carbohydrate intake can cause hypoglycemia (low blood sugar) and ketosis (increased blood acids) with associated nausea, fatigue, dizziness, and irritability. The dietary manipulations prove to be too cumbersome for many athletes, and an exhaustive training session the week before competition may predispose the athlete to injury. A revised method of carbohydrate loading that eliminates many of the problems associated with the old regimen has been proposed by Sherman and colleagues.[17]

Six days before competition, the athlete participates in intense exercise (70% to 75% of aerobic capacity) for 90 minutes. On that day and the next 2 days, the athlete consumes a normal diet providing 4 g/kg of body weight. On the 2nd and 3rd days, training is decreased to 40 minutes at 70% to 75% of aerobic capacity. On the next 2 days, the athlete eats a high-carbohydrate diet providing 10 g/kg of body weight and reduces training to 20 minutes at 70% to 75% of aerobic capacity. On the last day, the athlete rests, but maintains the high-carbohydrate diet. This modified regimen results in muscle glycogen stores equal to those provided by the classic carbohydrate-loading regimen.[17]

Carbohydrate loading enables the athlete to maintain high-intensity exercise longer, but will not affect pace for the first hour of the event. In a field study conducted by Karlsson and Saltin, runners participated in a 30 K race after eating a normal diet or high-carbohydrate diet.[18] The high-carbohydrate diet provided muscle glycogen levels of 193 mmol/kg, compared to 94 mmol/kg for the normal diet. All runners covered the 30 K distance faster (by approximately 8 minutes) when they began the race with high muscle glycogen stores.

The increased muscle glycogen stores did not help the runners go faster for the first hour of the race, but kept them from slowing down toward the end. Thus, carbohydrate loading will not enable athletes to go out faster, but the athletes will be able to maintain the same pace longer.

Loading Considerations

The classic carbohydrate-loading technique used a low-carbohydrate diet because it was believed that this was necessary to achieve the maximum levels of muscle glycogen storage. It is now known that endurance training is the primary stimulus for increased muscle glycogen synthesis. Endurance training increases the activity of glycogen synthase, the enzyme responsible for glycogen storage.[1]

This means that the athlete must be endurance-trained or carbohydrate loading will not work. Also, the exercise to deplete the stores must be the same as the athlete's competitive event because glycogen stores are specific to the muscle groups used. For example, a runner needs to deplete his or her stores by running rather than cycling.

It is essential that training is reduced during the 3 days before competition. Too much exercise during this period will use too much of the stored glycogen and defeat the purpose of the whole process. The final 3 days, when the athlete tapers and eats a high-carbohydrate diet, is the real "loading" phase of the regimen.

If the athlete has difficulty consuming enough carbohydrate through food, a commercial high-carbohydrate supplement can be added. Athletes who have diabetes or high triglycerides may have medical complications if they carbohydrate load. They should check with their physician before attempting the regimen.

For each gram of glycogen stored, additional water is stored. Some athletes note a feeling of stiffness and heaviness associated with the increased glycogen storage. These sensations will dissipate with exercise.

Carbohydrate loading will only help athletes engaged in continuous endurance exercise lasting longer than 90 minutes. Glycogen stores greater than usual won't enable the athlete to exercise more intensely during shorter duration exercise. In fact, the stiffness and heaviness associated with the increased glycogen stores may hurt performance during shorter events.

CARBOHYDRATE IN THE HOUR BEFORE EXERCISE

Athletes have been warned not to eat large amounts of carbohydrate before exercise. This admonition was based on the results of a study conducted during the late 1970s by Foster and colleagues that indicated that consuming 75 g of glucose (300 kcal) 30 minutes before exercise reduced endurance by causing hypoglycemia (low blood sugar).[19] This chain of events was thought to occur because of the high blood insulin levels induced by the carbohydrate feeding before exercise.

The pancreas secretes insulin in response to an increase in blood sugar. Insulin lowers blood sugar and promotes the uptake of glucose into the cells. When the blood sugar decreases, some persons suffer from symptoms indicative of hypoglycemia (dizziness, nausea, confusion, and partial blackout) or become exhausted sooner. Fortunately, these insulin and glucose responses are transient and probably won't harm performance, unless the athlete is sensitive to a decrease in blood glucose.

A 1987 study by Hargreaves and colleagues contradicts the findings of Foster.[20] Cyclists consumed 75 g of glucose or water 45 minutes before bicycling until exhausted. Although the carbohydrate feeding caused high blood insulin and low blood glucose levels, there were no differences in the exercise time to exhaustion between the rides when glucose and water were consumed.

Consuming carbohydrate an hour before exercise may actually help performance. Sherman and colleagues compared the ingestion of 1.1 g/kg and 2.2 g/kg of a carbohydrate beverage 1 hour before exercise.[21] The subjects cycled at 70% of VO_{2max} for 90 minutes and then underwent a performance trial. Serum insulin was initially increased at the start of and during exercise, and blood glucose initially decreased. Time trial performance was significantly increased 12.5% by the carbohydrate feedings, presumably through increased carbohydrate oxidation.

Does the glycemic index of the carbohydrate before exercise influence performance? Thomas and colleagues compared the consumption of 1 g of carbohydrate per kilogram of lentils (low glycemic), potato (high glycemic), and glucose 1 hour before cycling until exhausted at 65% to 70% of VO_{2max}.[22] Compared to the potato and glucose, the lentil feeding caused a more gradual increase and decrease in blood glucose. Endurance time was 20 minutes longer for the lentils trial than for all other trials, which were not significantly different from each other. The lentils caused a more gradual increase and decrease in blood glucose, thereby maintaining blood glucose levels at higher levels during critical periods of exercise.

The Thomas study results suggest that a low-glycemic solid carbohydrate is the preferred meal before exercise. However, the Sherman study results indicate that performance is also improved after consumption of a high-glycemic liquid carbohydrate. There is also the obvious consideration of whether certain foods (liquid or solid) cause GI distress. Some athletes cannot eat solid food an hour before exercise without risking needing a bathroom break later and/or gut distress in the form of nausea, cramps, or diarrhea.

Because the research is not clear on this issue, athletes should experiment (during training) with different liquid and solid carbohydrates with high and low glycemic indexes to find out what works the best. The research by Sherman and Thomas suggests a carbohydrate feeding of 1 g per kilogram of body weight an hour before exercise to improve performance.

Athletes who are sensitive to having blood glucose decreased have several options in addition to consuming a low-glycemic carbohydrate.

They can consume carbohydrate 5 minutes before exercise or wait until they are exercising.[23] The exercise-induced increase in epinephrine, norepinephrine, and growth hormone inhibits the release of insulin and so counters insulin's effect in decreasing blood sugar.

Consuming sugar immediately before anaerobic exercise such as sprinting or weight lifting will not improve performance because there is already enough ATP, creatine phosphate (CP), and muscle glycogen stored for these tasks. It will not provide athletes with a quick burst of energy, allowing them to exercise more intensely. Eating too much sugar before exercise can increase the risk of GI distress in the form of cramps, nausea, diarrhea, and bloating.

THE MEAL BEFORE EXERCISE

Athletes are often advised to eat 2 to 3 hours before exercise to allow adequate time for gastric emptying. The rationale is that if any food remains in the stomach at the start of exercise, the athlete may become nauseated or uncomfortable when blood is diverted from the GI tract to the exercising muscles. Rather than getting up at the crack of dawn to eat, many athletes who train or compete in the morning simply forgo eating. This overnight fast decreases their liver glycogen stores (the body's main source of blood glucose) by about 80% and can impair performance, especially if the athlete attempts to train or compete in a prolonged endurance event (over an hour) that relies heavily on blood glucose.

During exercise, athletes rely primarily on their pre-existing glycogen and fat stores. Although the meal before exercise doesn't contribute immediate energy for exercise, it can provide energy when the athlete exercises longer than an hour. It can also prevent athletes from feeling hungry, which in itself may impair performance. The carbohydrate from the meal can increase blood glucose to provide energy for the exercising muscles.

Eating a high-carbohydrate meal 2 to 3 hours before morning exercise helps to restore suboptimal liver glycogen stores, which will aid performance during prolonged exercise. If muscle glycogen levels are also low, the meal consumed 2 to 3 hours beforehand can increase these levels as well. The performance benefits of a carbohydrate feeding before exercise appear to be additive to those of consuming carbohydrate during exercise. This implies that these two nutritional strategies operate by different mechanisms.[24]

Does the form of the meal before exercise influence performance? Probably not. Sherman and colleagues evaluated the effect of a 312-g, 156-g, and 45-g liquid carbohydrate feeding 4 hours before exercise.[25] The liquid carbohydrate feedings provided 4.5 g/kg, 2 g/kg, and 0.6 g/kg, respectively. Interval cycling was undertaken for 95 minutes, followed by a performance trial after a 5-minute rest. The 312-g carbohydrate feeding improved performance by 15%, despite increased insulin levels at the start of exercise. Neufer and colleagues found that performance was also improved when a mixed meal (cereal, bread, milk, and fruit juice) was consumed 4 hours before exercise.[23]

How much carbohydrate should the meal before exercise contain? The research by Sherman and colleagues suggests 1 to 4.5 g of carbohydrate per kilogram of body weight, consumed 1 to 4 hours before exercise.[21,25] To avoid potential GI distress, the carbohydrate and calorie content of the meal should be reduced the closer the meal is consumed to exercise. For example, a carbohydrate feeding of 1 g/kg is appropriate an hour before exercise, whereas 4.5 g/kg can be consumed 4 hours before exercise. If gastric emptying is a concern, liquid meals should be considered.

Good examples of solid high-carbohydrate foods for meals before exercise include fruit, bread products (adding jam or jelly increases the carbohydrate content) and low-fat or nonfat yogurt. Fruit juices and nonfat milk are good high-carbohydrate beverages. The athlete may also incorporate commercial high-carbohydrate supplements.

LIQUID MEALS

A number of commercially formulated liquid meals are available to the athlete. Some of these were initially designed for patients who are hospitalized (for example, Sustacal and Ensure), whereas others have been specifically created for and marketed to the athlete (for example, Nutrament, Exceed Nutritional Beverage, and GatorPro). Twelve ounces of Nutrament supplies 360 calories, 16 g of protein, 52 g of carbohydrate, and 10 g of fat. Eight ounces of Exceed Nutritional Beverage supplies 360 calories, 14 g of protein, 54 g of carbohydrate, and 9.5 g of fat. GatorPro and other products are listed in Table 2–3.

These products satisfy the requirements for food before exercise—they are high in carbohydrate and palatable, and they contribute to both caloric intake and hydration. They have several advantages over conventional meals. Liquid meals can be consumed closer to competition than regular meals because of their shorter gastric emptying time. This may help to avoid nausea before competition for those athletes who are tense and have an associated delay in gastric emptying.

Liquid meals also produce a low stool residue, therefore, and help to keep immediate weight gain after the meal to a minimum. This is especially advantageous for wrestlers who need to "make weight." Liquid meals can provide a convenient alternative to solid meals for athletes competing in day-long competitions, tournaments, and multiple events.

Liquid meals can be used for nutritional supplementation during heavy training when caloric requirements are extremely increased. They supply a significant amount of calories and contribute to satiety.

Homemade liquid meals can be concocted by mixing milk, nonfat milk powder, and fruit in a blender (athletes with lactose intolerance can use Lact-Aid milk and skip the milk powder). For added variety, cereal, yogurt, and flavoring (for example, vanilla or chocolate) can be added. Sugar or honey may be added for additional sweetness and carbohydrate.

Both conventional and liquid meals aid in hydration, increase suboptimal muscle and liver glycogen stores, and maintain blood glucose levels during prolonged exercise. If the athlete has no difficulty consuming conventional meals before exercise and/or obtaining adequate calories, liquid meals confer no advantages other than convenience. The ideal meal before exercise, whether liquid or solid, commercial or homemade, is high in carbohydrate and palatable, and does not cause GI distress.

CARBOHYDRATE DURING EXERCISE

Carbohydrate feedings during endurance exercise lasting an hour or longer may enhance performance by providing glucose for the muscles to use when their glycogen stores have decreased to low levels. Coyle and colleagues have shown that consuming carbohydrate during cycling exercise at 70% of VO_{2max} can delay fatigue by 30 to 60 minutes.[26,27]

As the muscles run out of glycogen, they take up more blood glucose, placing a drain on the liver glycogen stores. The longer the run, the more the muscles use blood glucose for energy. When the liver glycogen is depleted, the blood glucose level decreases. Though a few people experience central nervous system (CNS) symptoms indicative of hypoglycemia, most athletes note local muscular fatigue and have to reduce their exercise intensity.

The improved performance associated with carbohydrate feedings probably occurs because of the maintenance of blood glucose levels. Dietary carbohydrate supplies glucose for the muscles at a time when their glycogen stores are diminished. Thus, carbohydrate utilization (and, therefore, ATP production) can continue at a high rate and endurance is enhanced.

Coyle and associates compared the effects of carbohydrate feedings on the onset of fatigue and decrease in work capacity of cyclists.[26] The carbohydrate feedings enabled the cyclists to exercise an average of 33 minutes longer (159 minutes compared to 126 minutes) before reaching the point of fatigue. The carbohydrate feedings maintained blood glucose at higher levels, thereby increasing the utilization of blood glucose for energy.

Coyle and colleagues also measured performance during strenuous prolonged bicycling with and without carbohydrate feedings.[27] During the ride without carbohydrate feedings, fatigue occurred after 3 hours and was preceded by a decrease in blood glucose. During the ride when the cyclists were fed carbohydrate, blood glucose levels were maintained and the cyclists were able to ride an additional hour before reaching the point of fatigue. Both groups used muscle glycogen at the same rate, indicating that endurance was improved by maintaining blood glucose levels, rather than by glycogen sparing.

Running performances with and without carbohydrate feedings have also recently been evaluated. Millard-Stafford and colleagues found that a carbohydrate feeding (55 g per hour) increased blood glucose levels and enabled runners, during a 40-km run in the heat, to finish the last 5 km significantly faster compared to the run without carbohydrate.[28] Wilber and Moffatt found that the run time when runners were fed carbohydrate (35 g per hour) during a treadmill run at 80% of VO_{2max} was 23 minutes longer (115 minutes) compared to the run without carbohydrate (92 minutes).[29]

Carbohydrate's primary role in fluid-replacement drinks is to maintain blood glucose concentration and enhance carbohydrate oxidation. Carbohydrate feedings enhance performance during exercise lasting an hour or longer, especially when muscle glycogen stores are low.[30] In fact, carbohydrate ingestion and fluid replacement independently improve performance and their beneficial effects are additive.

Below and Coyle evaluated the effects of fluid and carbohydrate ingestion, alone or in combination, during 1 hour of intense cycling exercise.[31] In the four trials, the subjects ingested either (1) 1330 mL of water, which replaced 79% of sweat loss, (2) 1330 mL of fluid with 79 g of carbohydrate, (3) 200 mL of water, which replaced 13% of sweat loss, or (4) 200 mL of fluid with 79 g of carbohydrate. When a large volume of fluid or 79 g of carbohydrate was ingested individually, each improved performance by about 6% compared to the placebo trial. When both the large volumes of fluid and carbohydrate were combined, performance was improved by 12%.

How much carbohydrate should the athlete consume during exercise to improve endurance? Coyle and Montain suggest that athletes consume 30 to 60 g (120 to 240 kcal) of carbohydrate every hour.[32] This amount can be obtained through either carbohydrate-rich foods or fluids. Lugo and colleagues found that liquid and solid carbohydrate feedings were equally effective in increasing blood glucose levels and improving cycling performance.[33]

Sports drinks are a practical source of carbohydrate because they replace fluid losses as well. Drinking 5 to 10 oz (150 to 300 mL) of a sports drink containing 4% to 8% carbohydrate (for example, Gatorade, Allsport, and Powerade) every 15 to 20 minutes can provide the proper amount of carbohydrate. For example, drinking 20 oz each hour of a sports drink that contains 6% carbohydrate provides 36 g of carbohydrate. Drinking the same quantity each hour of a sports drink containing 8% carbohydrate provides 48 g of carbohydrate.

High-carbohydrate foods provide a feeling of satiety that athletes will not get from drinking fluids. Eating one banana (30 g), one Power Bar (47 g), or three large graham crackers (66 g) every hour also supplies the necessary amount of carbohydrate.

Sports bars, fig bars, and cookies have a very low water content and, therefore, are more compact and easily carried. By comparison, high-carbohydrate foods that have a high water content, such as fruit, take up more room. For example, to get the amount of carbohydrate supplied by one Power Bar (47 g), one and one-half bananas (45 g) would have to be eaten.

However, the low water content of some solid high-carbohydrate foods also has a disadvantage. Athletes should drink plenty of water when they eat solid food, especially a sports bar. Otherwise, the product will settle poorly and athletes may feel there is a rock in their gut. In addition to aiding digestion, drinking water while eating solid foods encourages the athlete to hydrate adequately.

The athlete should eat or drink carbohydrate before feeling hungry or tired, usually within 30 to 60 minutes of exercise. Consuming small amounts at frequent intervals (every 30 to 60 minutes) helps to prevent GI upset. The athlete's foods and fluids should be easily digested, familiar (tested during training), and enjoyable (to encourage eating and drinking).

The performance benefit of a carbohydrate feeding before exercise appears to be additive to those of consuming carbohydrate during exercise. In a study by Wright and colleagues, cyclists that received carbohydrate both 3 hours before and during exercise were able to exercise longer (289 minutes) than when receiving carbohydrate either before exercise (236 minutes) or during exercise (266 minutes).[34]

This study demonstrates that combining carbohydrate feedings improves performance more than either feeding alone. It is important to note, however, that the improvement in performance with carbohydrate feedings before exercise is less than when smaller quantities of carbohydrate are consumed during exercise. So, if the goal is to provide a continuous supply of glucose during exercise, the athlete should consume carbohydrate during exercise.[24,34]

The American College of Sports Medicine suggests that both fluid and carbohydrate requirements can be met by consuming 600 to 1200 mL per hour (20 to 40 oz) of beverages containing 4% to 8% carbohydrate.[29]

FRUCTOSE

Some athletes consume fructose during exercise. Fructose causes a lower blood glucose and insulin response than glucose, which has led some athletes to think that it is a superior energy source to glucose. It isn't.

Murray and colleagues compared the physiologic, sensory, and exercise performance responses to the ingestion of 6% glucose, 6% sucrose, and 6% fructose solutions during cycling exercise.[35] Blood insulin levels were lower with fructose, as expected. However, fructose was associated with greater GI distress, higher perceived exertion ratings, and higher serum cortisol levels (indicating greater physiologic stress) than glucose or sucrose. Cycling performance times were also significantly better with sucrose and glucose than fructose.

Thus, fructose ingestion not only fails to improve performance, it may actually harm performance. The greater incidence of GI distress with fructose consumption may be due to slower intestinal absorption rate, compared to glucose. This may account for the bloating, cramping, and diarrhea often reported with high fructose intakes.

The lower blood glucose levels associated with fructose feeding may also explain why fructose does not improve performance. Fructose metabolism occurs primarily in the liver, where it is converted to liver glycogen. It is possible that fructose cannot be converted to glucose and released fast enough by the liver to provide adequate amounts for the exercising muscles.

In contrast, blood glucose is maintained or increased by feedings of glucose, sucrose, or glucose polymers. These feedings have been shown to enhance performance and, therefore, are the predominant carbohydrates in sports drinks.

CARBOHYDRATE FEEDINGS AFTER EXERCISE

The restoration of glycogen stores after strenuous training is important to minimize fatigue associated with repeated days of heavy training. Athletes consuming 8 to 10 g of carbohydrate per day will almost replace their muscle glycogen stores during successive days of intense workouts.

The period during which carbohydrate is consumed relative to exercise is also important. Ivy and colleagues evaluated glycogen repletion after exercise.[36] When 2 g of carbohydrate per kilogram was consumed immediately after exercise, muscle glycogen synthesis was 15 mmol/

kg. When the carbohydrate feeding was delayed for 2 hours, muscle glycogen synthesis was decreased by 66% to 5 mmol/kg. By 4 hours after exercise, total muscle glycogen synthesis for the delayed feeding was still 45% slower than that for the feeding given immediately after exercise.

This means that delaying carbohydrate intake for too long after exercise will reduce muscle glycogen storage and impair recovery. However, most athletes aren't hungry after exercising. If this is the case, they can consume a high-carbohydrate drink, such as a sports drink, fruit juice, or a commercial high-carbohydrate beverage. This will also aid in rehydration.

Replenishing muscle glycogen stores after exercise is particularly beneficial for athletes who train intensely several times a day. This will enable them to get the most out of their second workout.

How much carbohydrate should the athlete consume after heavy exercise? Ivy and colleagues suggest taking in 1.5 g of carbohydrate per kilogram immediately (within 30 minutes of exercise), followed by additional 1.5 g/kg feedings every 2 hours thereafter.[37] The first carbohydrate feeding can be a high-carbohydrate beverage and the following feedings can be high-carbohydrate meals.

Why does glycogen repletion occur faster immediately after exercise? There are several possibilities. The blood flow to the muscles immediately after exercise is much greater and the muscle cell is more likely to take up glucose. Also, during the period immediately after exercise, the muscle cells are more sensitive to the effects of insulin, which promotes glycogen synthesis.

Glucose and sucrose are twice as effective as fructose in restoring muscle glycogen after exercise.[38] The difference may be attributed to how the body metabolizes these sugars. Most fructose is converted to liver glycogen, whereas glucose appears to bypass the liver and is stored as muscle glycogen.

Does the type of carbohydrate (simple or complex) have an effect on muscle glycogen storage? Costill and associates compared the effects of simple and complex carbohydrates during a 48-hour period after glycogen-depleting exercise.[4] During the first 24 hours, no differences were found in muscle glycogen synthesis between the two types of carbohydrate (75 mmol/kg for starch, 70 mmol/kg for glucose). However, at 48 hours, the starch diet resulted in significantly greater muscle glycogen synthesis than did the glucose diet (22 mmol/kg for starch, 8 mmol/kg for glucose).

However, in a similar comparison of simple and complex carbohydrate intake during both glycogen depleted and nondepleted states, Roberts and colleagues found that significant increases in muscle glycogen could be achieved with a diet high in simple or complex carbohydrates.[39]

Does the form of carbohydrate influence glycogen repletion? Probably not. Reed and associates provided 3 g of carbohydrate per kilogram in liquid or solid form to subjects after these subjects participated in 2 hours of cycling at 60% to 75% of VO_{2max}. The subjects received half of the carbohydrate immediately after exercise and half 2 hours after exercise. There was no difference in muscle-glycogen-storage rates between the liquid or solid carbohydrate feedings at 2 hours after exercise and at 4 hours after exercise. This indicates that providing liquid or solid carbohydrate with equal carbohydrate contents after exercise produces similar glycogen repletion rates.[40]

Does the glycemic index of the carbohydrate influence glycogen repletion? Burke and colleagues investigated the effect of the glycemic index of carbohydrate intake after exercise on muscle glycogen storage.[41] The subjects cycled for 2 hours at 75% of VO_{2max} to deplete muscle glycogen, then consumed foods with either a high glycemic index or low glycemic index. The total carbohydrate feeding over 24 hours was 10 g/kg, evenly distributed between meals eaten at 0, 4, 8, and 21 hours after exercise. The increase in muscle glycogen content after 24 hours of recovery was greater with the high glycemic diet (106 mmol/kg) than with the low glycemic diet (71.5 mmol/kg). This suggests that the most rapid increase in muscle glycogen content during the first 24 hours of recovery is achieved by consuming foods with a high glycemic index.

Athletes may have impaired muscle glycogen synthesis after unaccustomed exercise that results in muscle damage and delayed onset muscle soreness.[42] The muscular responses to such damaging exercise appear to decrease both the rate of muscle glycogen synthesis and the total muscle glycogen content. Although a diet providing 8 to 10 g of carbohydrate/kg will usually replace muscle glycogen stores within 24 hours, the damaging effects of unaccustomed exercise significantly delay muscle glycogen repletion. Also, Sherman notes that even the normalization of muscle glycogen stores does not guarantee normal muscle function after unaccustomed exercise.[42]

CARBOHYDRATE-BASHING REVISITED

A popular sports nutrition dietary fad revolves around the myth that high-carbohydrate diets impair athletic performance and make athletes fat. Proponents of this dietary regimen believe that food has a tremendous impact on the complex hormonal systems that help control physiologic processes within the body—processes such as cellular oxygen transfer, maintenance of blood glucose, and regulation of body fat.

Athletes must supposedly eat the perfect ratio of protein, carbohydrate, and fat at each meal and snack to control these hormonal systems and reach their maximum athletic performance. This "perfect ratio" consists of 40% carbohydrate, 30% protein, and 30% fat. Proponents claim that this diet promotes optimal athletic performance and health by altering the production of eicosanoids so that the body makes more "good" eicosanoids than "bad" ones. Supposedly, eicosanoids are the most powerful of all hormone systems and have ultimate control over all physiologic functions.

Eicosanoids are the biologically active, hormonelike compounds known as prostaglandins, thromboxanes, and leukotrienes. A balanced production of eicosanoids regulates the local tissue response to stimulatory events such as infection, trauma, allergy, or toxin exposure.[43] Prostaglandin E_1 is a good eicosanoid because it inhibits platelet aggregation, promotes vasodilation, and is anti-inflammatory. Prostaglandin E_2, thromboxanes, and leukotrienes are bad eicosanoids because they promote platelet aggregation and vasoconstriction, and are pro-inflammatory.

The protein-to-carbohydrate ratio of the diet allegedly maintains the proper balance between the hormones insulin and glucagon. The correct insulin–glucagon balance, in turn, supposedly increases the production of good eicosanoids that improve athletic performance. Proponents of the diet recommend limiting carbohydrate to keep the body from producing too much insulin, because high insulin levels allegedly increase the production of bad eicosanoids. Bad eicosanoids purportedly impair athletic performance by reducing oxygen transfer to the cells, lowering blood glucose levels, and interfering with body fat utilization.

The protein content of the diet supposedly increases glucagon levels, thereby maintaining the appropriate balance between insulin and glucagon. Proponents claim that glucagon helps to increase the production of good eicosanoids by opposing the effect of insulin. This glucagon-favorable diet supposedly maintains blood glucose, increases endurance by increasing fatty acid utilization, and reduces body fat by increasing the utilization of stored fat.

Athletes may be impressed and intimidated by such scientific-sounding information. However, the scientific basis for this diet can be faulted on many fronts,[44–46] beginning with the claim that high carbohydrate diets increase insulin levels, thereby causing low blood glucose and suppressing fat mobilization.

During exercise, serum glucose levels increase while serum insulin levels decrease. This occurs because of the exercise-induced increase in the catecholamines and growth hormone, which inhibit the release of insulin from the pancreas. This enhances liver glucose output by making the liver more sensitive to the effects of glucagon and epinephrine. The hormonal changes that occur during exercise prompt greater fat mobilization and oxidation.

Carbohydrate feedings 30 to 60 minutes before exercise do increase insulin levels and decrease blood glucose, but these responses are temporary and will not harm performance.[20] This insulin response does not impair fat mobilization or cause accelerated glycogen depletion.[24] In fact, consuming carbohydrate an hour before exercise has been shown to improve performance.[21] Carbohydrate feedings 3 to 4 hours before exercise also enhance performance by "topping off" muscle and liver glycogen stores.[25] Lastly, carbohydrate feedings during exercise improve performance[26,27] and improve glycogen repletion after exercise.[36,37]

The claim that a high carbohydrate diet promotes greater body fat storage is also unfounded. Insulin is not a "bad" hormone; it is required for the transport of glucose into the cells. Insulin-mediated glucose uptake is also necessary for muscle and liver glycogen synthesis— the primary fuel for most sports. Furthermore, endurance training appears to increase tissue insulin sensitivity, resulting in lower plasma insulin levels for these tasks. Carbohydrates will only promote greater fat storage if they are eaten in excess of calorie requirements. However, when compared to dietary fat, dietary carbohydrate is more likely to be burned for energy than stored as fat.[47]

Carbohydrate, not fat, is the preferred energy source during exercise at or above 70% of VO_{2max}—the intensity at which most athletes train and compete.[1] Fat becomes available for fuel only after about 20 minutes of exercise and most athletes do not usually work out long enough to burn significant amounts of fat during exercise. Rather, it is the caloric deficit resulting from the exercise session that promotes body fat utilization. Athletes do not need this diet to increase fat utilization, because endurance training already creates a metabolic milieu favorable for fat metabolism.[1]

The metabolic pathways that supposedly connect diet, insulin–glucagon, and eicosanoids do not exist in standard nutrition or biochemistry texts.[43,48] The idea that this diet (or any diet) completely controls the secretion of insulin and glucagon is not supported by the relationship between nutrition and endocrinology.[43] Next, the notion that the insulin–glucagon axis controls the production of eicosanoids is not supported by biochemistry.[48] And finally, the belief that eicosanoids control all physiologic functions (including athletic performance) is not only unfounded, it is an appalling over-simplification of complex physiologic processes.[43,48]

Nutrition professionals should not advocate this diet for athletes because nutrition recommendations must be supported by scientific research.[49] In science, no hypothesis is presumed to be true until it has been clearly demonstrated. Current nutrition recommendations are based on double-blind, placebo-controlled, peer-reviewed published research. This dietary regimen, however, is based on case histories, testimonials, and unpublished, poorly controlled studies. Although many athletes seek "the magic bullet," a dietary panacea does not exist.[49] Following the diet may actually impair athletic performance because of inadequate dietary carbohydrate intake, and possibly, calorie intake.[44–46]

Sports bars with the same macronutrient content as this diet are currently heavily marketed to athletes. Manufacturers of these bars boast that their product promotes endurance by increasing fat burning during exercise. There isn't any research support for these claims. Eating a sports bar containing 40% carbohydrate, 30% fat, and 30% protein will not improve fat metabolism or endurance performance. In fact, performance may actually decline. Because these sports bars are lower in carbohydrate, they do not increase blood glucose levels as well as sports bars that are higher in carbohydrate. They also take longer to digest because they are higher in fat.

Case Study

T.G. was a distance runner who wanted to carbohydrate load for a marathon in Southern California whose course would include many hills. He had not tried to carbohydrate load for previous marathons. T.G. was 5 ft, 6 in tall and weighed 132 lb (60 kg). I counseled T.G. on both the training and diet portions of the revised carbohydrate-loading regimen.

Six days before competition, T.G. ran at 70% of aerobic capacity for 90 minutes. On that day and the next 2 days, he followed a diet that provided carbohydrate at 4 g/kg of body weight. On the 2nd and 3rd days, he ran 40 minutes at 70% of aerobic capacity. On the next 2 days, he followed a diet that provided 10 g/kg of body weight and ran 20 minutes at 70% of aerobic capacity. On the last day, he rested and maintained the high-carbohydrate diet.

T.G.'s diet for the first 3 days of the regimen provided about 240 g of carbohydrate, 96 g of protein, and 90 g of fat for a total intake of 2154 calories. On the last 3 days of the regimen, T.G.'s diet provided about 600 g of carbohydrate, 84 g of protein, and 72 g of fat for a total intake of 3384 calories.

A high-carbohydrate supplement was used during the "loading phase" to help increase T.G.'s carbohydrate intake. The supplement was 20% carbohydrate and provided 70 g of carbohydrate per 12 oz. T.G. drank three 12-oz glasses between meals. His carbohydrate intake was approximately 390 g from food and 210 g from the supplement.

Marathon day was unseasonably hot under clear skies with low humidity. T.G. completed the marathon in 3 hours and 28 minutes. This was only 10 minutes off the personal record that he had established on a flat course during a cool, cloudy day. After the race, he noted that he had never felt so good for so long during a marathon. T.G. now always uses the revised carbohydrate-loading regimen while preparing for marathons.

REFERENCES

1. Gollnick PD. Energy metabolism and prolonged exercise. In: Lamb DR, Murray R, eds. *Perspectives in Exercise Science and Sports Medicine. Volume 1: Prolonged Exercise.* Indianapolis, IN: Benchmark Press; 1989;1–36.
2. Sherman WM, Landers N. Fat loading: the next magic bullet? *Int J Sport Nutr.* 1995; suppl 5:S1-S12.
3. Costill DL, Bowers R, Branam G, Sparks K. Muscle glycogen utilization during prolonged exercise on successive days. *J Appl Physiol.* 1971;31:834–838.
4. Costill DL, Sherman WM, Fink WJ, Maresh C, Whitten M, Miller, JM. The role of dietary carbohydrate in muscle glycogen resynthesis after strenuous running. *Am J Clin Nutr.* 1981;34:1831–1836.
5. Fallowfield JL, Williams C. Carbohydrate intake and recovery from prolonged exercise. *Int J Sport Nutr.* 1993;3:150–164.
6. Costill DL, Flynn MJ, Kirwan JP, et al. Effect of repeated days of intensified training on muscle glycogen and swimming performance. *Med Sci Sports Exerc.* 1988;20:249–254.
7. Sherman WM, Wimer GS. Insufficient dietary carbohydrate during training: does it impair athletic performance? *Int J Sport Nutr.* 1991;1:28–44.
8. Walberg-Rankin J. Dietary carbohydrate as an ergogenic aid for prolonged and brief competitions in sport. *Int J Sport Nutr.* 1995; suppl 5:S13–S28.
9. Saris WHM, van Erp-Baart MA, Brouns F, Westerterp KR, ten Hoor F. Study of food intake and energy expenditure during extreme sustained exercise: the Tour de France. *Int J Sports Med.* 1989; suppl 10:26–31.
10. Brouns F, Saris WHM, Stroecken J, et al. Eating, drinking, and cycling: a controlled Tour de France simulation study, part I. *Int J Sports Med.* 1989;suppl 10:S32–S40.
11. Brouns F, Saris WHM, Stroecken J, et al. Eating, drinking, and cycling: a controlled Tour de France simulation study, part II. Effect of diet manipulation. *Int J Sports Med.* 1989;suppl 10:S41–S48.
12. US Department of Agriculture and Department of Health and Human Services. *Nutrition and Your Health: Dietary Guidelines for Americans.* 4th ed. Washington, DC: US Government Printing Office; 1995.

13. US Department of Agriculture and US Department of Health and Human Services. *Food Guide Pyramid: A Guide to Daily Food Choices.* Washington, DC: US Government Printing Office; 1992.

14. Coleman E. Update on carbohydrate: solid versus liquid. *Int J Sport Nutr.* 1994;4:80–88.

15. American Diabetes Association. Nutrition recommendations and principles for people with diabetes mellitus: 1986. ADA position statement. *Diabetes Care.* 1987; 10:126–132.

16. Bergstrom J, Hermansen L, Saltin B. Diet, muscle glycogen, and physical performance. *Acta Physiol Scand.* 1967;71:140–150.

17. Sherman WM, Costill DL, Fink WJ, Miller JM. The effect of exercise and diet manipulation on muscle glycogen and its subsequent use during performance. *Int J Sports Med.* 1981;2:114–118.

18. Karlsson J, Saltin B. Diet, muscle glycogen, and endurance performance. *J Appl Physiol.* 1971;31:203–206.

19. Foster C, Costill DL, Fink WJ. Effects of pre-exercise feedings on endurance performance. *Med Sci Sports Exerc.* 1979;11:1–5.

20. Hargreaves M, Costill DL, Fink WJ, King DS, Fielding RA. Effects of pre-exercise carbohydrate feedings on endurance cycling performance. *Med Sci Sports Exerc.* 1987;19:33–36.

21. Sherman WM, Peden MC, Wright DA. Carbohydrate feedings 1 hr before exercise improves cycling performance. *Am J Clin Nutr.* 1991;54:866–870.

22. Thomas DE, Brotherhood JR, Brand JC. Carbohydrate feeding before exercise: effect of glycemic index. *Int J Sports Med.* 1991;12:180–186.

23. Neufer PD, Costill DL, Flynn MG, Kirwan JP, Mitchell JB, Houmard J. Improvements in exercise performance: effects of carbohydrate feedings and diet. *J Appl Physiol.* 1987;62(3):983–988.

24. Coggan AR, Swanson SC. Nutritional manipulations before and during exercise: effects on performance. *Med Sci Sports Exerc.* 1992; suppl 24:S331–S335.

25. Sherman WM, Brodowicz G, Wright DA, Allen WK, Simonsen J, Dernbach A. Effects of 4 hr preexercise carbohydrate feedings on cycling performance. *Med Sci Sports Exerc.* 1989;12:598–604.

26. Coyle EF, Hagberg JM, Hurley BF, Martin WH, Ehsani AA, Holloszy JO. Carbohydrate feeding during prolonged strenuous exercise can delay fatigue. *J Appl Physiol.* 1983;55:230–235.

27. Coyle EF, Coggan AR, Hemmert WK, Ivy JL. Muscle glycogen utilization during prolonged strenuous exercise when fed carbohydrate. *J Appl Physiol.* 1986; 61:165–172.

28. Millard-Stafford ML, Sparling PB, Rosskopf LB, Hinson BT, Dicarlo LJ. Carbohydrate-electrolyte replacement improves distance running performance in the heat. *Med Sci Sports Exerc.* 1992;24:934–940.

29. Wilber RL, Moffatt RJ. Influence of carbohydrate ingestion on blood glucose and performance in runners. *Int J Sports Nutr.* 1994;2:317–327.

30. American College of Sports Medicine. Position stand: exercise and fluid replacement. *Med Sci Sports Exerc.* 1996;28:i–vii.

31. Below PR, Coyle EF. Fluid and carbohydrate ingestion independently improve performance during 1 hr of intense exercise. *Med Sci Sports Exerc.* 1995;27:200–210.

32. Coyle EF, Montain SJ. Benefits of fluid replacement with carbohydrate during exercise. *Med Sci Sports Exerc.* 1992; suppl 24:S324–S330.

33. Lugo M, Sherman WM, Wimer GS, Garleb K. Metabolic responses when different forms of carbohydrate energy are consumed during cycling. *Int J Sport Nutr.* 1993;3:398–407.

34. Wright DA, Sherman WM, Dernbach AR. Carbohydrate feedings before, during, or in combination improve cycling performance. *J Appl Physiol.* 1991; 71:1082–1088.

35. Murray R, Paul GL, Seifert JG, Eddy DE, Halby GA. The effects of glucose, fructose, and sucrose ingestion during exercise. *Med Sci Sports Exerc.* 1989;21:275–282.

36. Ivy JL, Katz AL, Cutler CL, Sherman WM, Coyle EF. Muscle glycogen synthesis after exercise: effect of time of carbohydrate ingestion. *J Appl Physiol.* 1988;6:1480–1485.

37. Ivy JL, Lee MC, Broznick JT, Reed MJ. Muscle glycogen storage after different amounts of carbohydrate ingestion. *J Appl Physiol.* 1988;65:2018–2023.

38. Blom PCS, Hostmark AT, Vaage O, Kardel KR, Maehlum S. Effect of different post-exercise sugar diets on the rate of muscle glycogen synthesis. *Med Sci Sports Exerc.* 1987;19:471–496.

39. Roberts KM, Noble EG, Hayden DB, Taylor AW. Simple and complex carbohydrate-rich diets and muscle glycogen content of marathon runners. *Eur J Appl Physiol.* 1988;57:70–74.

40. Reed MJ, Brozinick JT, Lee MC, Ivy JL. Muscle glycogen storage postexercise: effect of mode of carbohydrate administration. *J Appl Physiol.* 1989:66:720–726.

41. Burke LM, Collier GR, Hargreaves M. Muscle glycogen storage after prolonged exercise: effect of glycemic index. *J Appl Physiol.* 1993;75:1019–1023.

42. Sherman WM. Recovery from endurance exercise. *Med Sci Sports Exerc.* 1992; suppl 24:S336–S339.

43. Zeman FJ. *Clinical Nutrition and Dietetics.* 2nd ed. New York: Macmillan Publishing Company; 1991.

44. Coleman E. Debunking the "eicotec" myth. *Sports Med Dig.* 1993;15:6–7.

45. Coleman E. The BioZone nutrition system: a dietary panacea? *Int J Sport Nutr.* 1996;6:69–71.
46. Coleman E. Carbohydrate unloading. *Phys Sportsmed.* 1998;25:97–98.
47. Sims EAH, Danforth E. Expenditure and storage of energy in man. *J Clin Invest.* 1987;79:1019–1025.
48. Mayes PA. Metabolism of unsaturated fatty acids & eicosanoids. In: *Harper's Biochemistry.* 23rd ed. Norwalk, CT: Appleton & Lange; 1993.
49. Position of the American Dietetic Association. Food and nutrition misinformation. *J Am Diet Assoc.* 1995; 95:705–707.

CHAPTER 3

Protein Requirements of Athletes

Ann C. Snyder and Jay Naik

Historically, many athletes believed that consuming large quantities of protein was the key to successful athletic performance. Athletes consuming raw eggs and/or a steak before competition was commonplace. Most likely, the high-protein consumption of all types of athletes was due to the results of research done in the 1800s that showed that protein was the major fuel during exercise. Subsequent research indicated that carbohydrates and fats actually provide the majority of the fuel during exercise. Consequently, little attention has been paid to the role of protein in exercise metabolism and performance.

To examine an athlete's need for protein, we must first discuss protein metabolism. In general, amino acids (of which there are 21 different types, Table 3–1) are the building blocks of proteins, and once absorbed into the body, they enter the body's small amino acid pool. As the body tries to maintain homeostasis, protein is replaced using amino acids from this pool when it is degraded. When protein intake is insufficient, protein degradation will surpass protein synthesis, muscle size and strength will be lost, and exercise performance and health will be affected. Conversely, if excess protein is consumed, once the amino acid pool has its full complement, excess amino acids will be converted to carbohydrates or fat once the nitrogen of the amino acid is detached. When amino acids are converted to

Table 3–1 Essential and Nonessential Amino Acids

Essential Amino Acids—must be consumed in your diet as the body cannot produce them.

Isoleucine	Methionine	Tryptophan
Leucine	Phenylalanine	Valine
Lysine	Threonine	

Nonessential Amino Acids—can be produced by the body.

Alanine	Cysteine	Glycine
Arginine	Cystine	Histidine*
Asparagine	Glutamic acid	Proline
Aspartic acid	Glutamine	Serine
Tyrosine		

*Histidine is an essential amino acid for infants, but a nonessential amino acid for adults.

carbohydrates or fat, and when amino acids are broken down, the nitrogen of the amino acid is removed, converted to urea, and excreted from the body primarily in the urine. Thus, whereas lack of protein intake can directly lead to decrements in athletic performance, excess protein intake leads to increased fat stores and a number of other health issues.

Beginning in the late 1970s, research investigations began to show that athletes might require a greater protein intake than their sedentary counterparts. More recently, information has become available that the protein requirements of athletes may depend on the type of physical activity they do and that athletes participating in different activities need this enhanced protein intake for varying reasons. That is, the protein requirements for an athlete who participates in primarily muscular strength activities (very high-intensity activities with few repetitions, shorter than 10 seconds) probably will be different from the requirements of those who participate in primarily muscular endurance activities (high-intensity activities lasting 0.25 to 2.0 minutes), which again will be different from the requirements of those who participate in aerobic endurance activities (low-intensity activities lasting longer than 15 minutes). In this review, we will first discuss the methods available for quantifying protein utilization, then the factors that affect protein utilization, and finally the protein needs of the different athletes.

METHODS USED TO QUANTIFY PROTEIN UTILIZATION

As with those in many other fields that examine the functioning of the body, investigators analyzing protein metabolism during rest and exercise use both whole body and artificial environment (that is, test tube) experimental methodologies. Whereas the in vitro experiments allowed for tight control and precise measurements, the in vivo studies allowed for a description of what was actually occurring within the body. Thus, mainly the in vivo studies will be discussed in this review. Numerous types of in vivo methods have been used to examine protein metabolism; these include the following: nitrogen balance, urinary excretion of urea, examination of N-methylhistidine (N-MH) (an amino acid formed during breakdown of myofibrillar proteins), and radiolabeled tracer investigations.

Nitrogen balance (or, more appropriately, nitrogen status) studies involve the quantification of all sources of nitrogen consumed (that is, dietary consumption) and excreted (that is, from urine, feces, sweat, etc). A positive nitrogen balance occurs when the nitrogen obtained with protein intake is greater than that lost; thus, growth and/or maintenance of protein status can occur. Conversely, a negative nitrogen balance occurs when nitrogen loss is greater than that consumed as protein. Overall nitrogen balance studies are labor-intensive to do, and difficulties can arise in quantifying all sources of nitrogen intake and loss, especially loss through sweat. Thus, results from nitrogen balance studies require that care be taken when they are interpreted.

Although not a complete account of nitrogen intake and loss, measurement of urinary urea excretion has been used to assess protein metabolism, because it is simpler and easier for both the subjects and the investigators. Approximately 85% of the nitrogen is excreted as urea in the urine; thus, examination of urinary urea can be an indicator of protein utilization. Because excess protein is stored as carbohydrates or fat once the nitrogen is removed, as discussed previously, the point at which urea production increases disproportionately to protein intake may help define protein requirements.

N-MH has also been used to assess muscle protein catabolism. During protein synthesis, a methyl group is donated to the amino acid histidine creating N-MH. N-MH is a component of the contractile proteins of skeletal muscle and is found in skeletal muscle in 100 times the amount found in any other tissue. As skeletal muscle is broken down, N-MH is released into the bloodstream and finally is excreted into the urine. Because N-MH is not re-utilized or further degraded by the body, measurement of it in the urine gives an accurate indication of muscle protein metabolism. Although most N-MH is located in the skeletal muscle, some N-MH is found in the gastrointestinal (GI) tract and skin, and these can contribute to N-MH excretion at rest and during exercise.

The measurement of urea, nitrogen balance, and N-MH requires the analysis of a substance in urine. With most exercise, but especially prolonged exercise in a hot and humid environment, blood flow is modified to allow for sufficient blood to the active musculature and to the skin for the removal of excess body heat. Therefore, blood flow to the kidneys necessarily decreases during exercise, and thus the results obtained must be interpreted while considering this.

The most recent and sensitive method of determining protein metabolism is through the use of exogenous metabolic tracers (that is, radioactive or stable isotopes, such as ^{14}C, ^{13}C, ^{15}N, etc). The advantage of using tracers rather than the other techniques to determine protein metabolism is that the fate of individual amino acids can be quantified. Thus, the point at which amino acid oxidation exponentially increases and/or protein synthesis plateaus may be indicative of the protein requirements of the person. There are several drawbacks to these techniques, however, which include expense, invasive nature of process, and whether the process is valid under exercising conditions. In addition, the assumption is made that the amino acid examined in the study (for example, leucine or lysine) responds similarly to other amino acids. When using the metabolic tracer technique, as well as the other techniques discussed previously, care should be taken to control for energy intake and expenditure, muscle glycogen levels, and the amount of exercise done before and/or during the testing session.

FACTORS THAT AFFECT PROTEIN TURNOVER

Because nitrogen balance may be affected by the intensity and duration of exercise, energy content of the diet, and the training level of the subject, care should be taken to control these variables when designing an experimental protocol. Gender has also been shown to affect the substrate used for energy production during exercise, and thus nutrient requirements may be different for male and female athletes.

Exercise Intensity

Exercise intensity has been shown to influence the activation of the rate-limiting enzyme branched-chain keto acid dehydrogenase and thus increase amino acid oxidation.[1] Lemon et al observed that the rate of leucine oxidation was higher during 1 hour of treadmill exercise at 80% VO_{2max} than during exercise at 40% VO_{2max}.[2] Lemon et al also examined urea nitrogen production before, during, and 2 days after a 1-hour treadmill exercise bout at intensities ranging from 42% to 67% VO_{2max}.[3] Urea production was shown to be related to the intensity of the exercise. Exercise done at 42% VO_{2max} did not increase urea production; however, when exercise intensity was greater than 55% VO_{2max}, nitrogen excretion increased to greater than 4.5 g/72 hr (Figure 3–1). Conversely, Carraro et al failed to find any effect of treadmill running on the rate of urea production at either 40% VO_{2max} for 3 hours or 70% VO_{2max} for 1 hour[4] (Figure 3–2).

Exercise Duration

The duration of exercise has also been proposed to affect the magnitude of protein utilization. An increase in blood urea concentration during intense, prolonged exercise has been shown after 60 to 70 minutes of activity.[5] The increase in blood urea is presumed to be the result of an increase in amino acid oxidation, rather than a decreased removal rate caused by reduced kidney function during exercise. Protein is not the preferred source of energy during exercise, but may serve as an alternative during intense exercise if carbohydrate stores become depleted as exercise continues. For example, persons who cycle for 60 minutes in a glycogen-

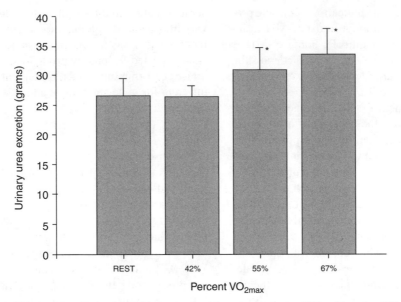

Figure 3–1 Urinary Urea Excretion with Increasing Exercise Intensity [*Significantly different from rest (P < .05)]. *Source:* Data from P. Lemon, D. Dolny, and K. Yarasheski, Effect of Intensity on Protein Utilization During Prolonged Exercise, *Medical Science Sports Exercise*, Vol. 16, pp. 151–152, © 1984.

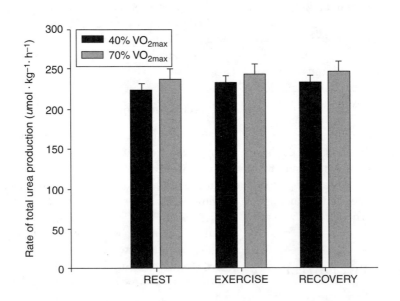

Figure 3–2 Rate of Total Urea Production During and after Exercise at Either 40% or 70% VO_{2max}. *Source:* Data from F. Carraro, T. Kimbrough, and R. Wolfe, Urea Kinetics in Humans at Two Levels of Exercise Intensity, *Journal of Applied Physiology*, Vol. 75, pp. 1180–1185, © 1993.

depleted state may use as much as 2.4 times as much protein as those with high initial muscle glycogen levels.[5]

Training State

Endurance training has been found to increase leucine oxidation both at rest and during exercise. Henderson et al found that the oxidation of continuously infused [^{14}C] leucine was significantly greater in trained than in untrained rats both at rest and during exercise, and although the relative role of the amino acids as an energy source decreased with exercise, the absolute rate of leucine oxidation increased.[6] The effect of exercise training may also depend on the time elapsed between initiation of an exercise program and sample collection. Nitrogen balance is reduced with the initiation of an exercise program and returns to levels before exercise soon after the initiation of exercise training, with a zero nitrogen balance reached in most subjects after approximately 2 weeks of training.[7,8] The mechanism for such a short-term effect of exercise and exercise training on nitrogen balance is unclear, but such an effect could affect interpretation of experimental results.

Energy Consumed

Another factor affecting the evaluation of the protein requirements of persons is the amount of energy consumed. For a given protein intake, nitrogen balance will improve as energy intake increases; thus, less protein will be needed as energy intake increases to remain in nitrogen balance. As stated previously, amino acids can be used to supply glucose; therefore, increased availability of glucose through carbohydrates necessarily reduces the oxidation of amino acids to glucose. Millward et al used continuous infusion of [^{13}C] leucine to study oxidation when a subject is at rest and during submaximal exercise and found that leucine oxidation during exercise was two times that during rest, but glucose ingestion rapidly reduced the oxidation of leucine.[9] Many investigators have shown that there

is a protein-sparing effect of energy intake on protein utilization and that this effect may be related to the initial energy balance of the person at the initiation of an exercise program. When initial energy intake was high, the source of energy deficit did not affect the magnitude of the decline in nitrogen balance. When initial energy intake was low, exercise resulted in half the decline in nitrogen balance as that found with decreased energy intake. When energy intake is high, the magnitude of the response of nitrogen balance to changes in energy balance is great, but when initial energy intake is low or marginal, the body appears to minimize its response to changes in energy balance.

Gender

Gender may also play a role in determining the protein requirements of a person. Tarnopolsky et al observed that during moderate-intensity, long-duration exercise, females demonstrate greater lipid (26.9 g vs 47.6 g) and less carbohydrate (239 g vs 137 g) utilization than equally trained males.[10] In addition, the males excreted significantly more urinary nitrogen over 4 hours than did the females. Exercise was not shown to affect urea nitrogen production for either gender. However, the males excreted significantly more urea nitrogen during the exercise than at rest. Phillips et al, using continuous infusion of [^{13}C] leucine, demonstrated that exercise resulted in a significant increase in leucine oxidation in both males and females, and that male athletes oxidized a greater amount of leucine than females.[11] During 90 minutes of treadmill exercise at 65% VO_{2max}, the males also used significantly more carbohydrates (127 g vs 71.5 g) and protein (8.3 g vs 4.4 g) than did the females.

PROTEIN USAGE AND ATHLETIC PERFORMANCE

The current recommended daily allowance (RDA) for protein of 0.8 g protein/kg body weight/day was based on studies of sedentary men and has not been adjusted for possible increased protein requirements necessary to meet the demands of regular physical activity. Many investigators have proposed that habitual exercise may increase the daily requirements for dietary protein.

Muscular Strength and Resistance Training

Resistance training generally results in an increase in muscle mass and thus muscle strength (a single maximal contraction). However, for muscle mass to be enhanced, the athlete must be in a state of positive nitrogen balance. Thus, to maximize protein synthesis, sufficient amounts of amino acids must be made available to the muscle. More specifically, regular heavy resistance training, in combination with increased protein intake, has been shown to enhance muscle mass development more than just resistance training or enhanced protein intake alone.

Fern et al, when using metabolic tracer techniques, found an increased body mass and a coincident increase in protein synthesis in a group of subjects consuming 3.3 g protein/kg body weight/day when compared to a comparably trained group consuming 1.3 g protein/kg body weight/day. Because amino acid oxidation in the group of subjects consuming 3.3 g protein/kg body weight/day was increased only 150%, Fern et al hypothesized that the amount of protein necessary to maximize muscle mass gains had been exceeded.[12] Tarnopolsky et al found that whole body protein synthesis was increased in strength athletes consuming 1.4 g protein/kg body weight/day (the MP diet) when compared to those consuming 0.9 g protein/kg body weight/day (the LP diet). When intake was increased to 2.4 g protein/kg body weight/day (the HP diet) protein synthesis did not increase above that which was achieved when consuming the MP diet; however, leucine oxidation was increased on the HP diet indicating a nutrient overload.[13] Therefore, the RDA for protein would seem to be insufficient for those persons who are developing muscular mass and strength using a heavy resistance training program. A more appropriate intake for these persons would seem to be 1.7 to 1.8 g protein/kg body weight/day. Further, no evidence could be found for consuming greater than 2.0 g protein/kg body weight/day.

Although the recommended protein intake for persons participating in a heavy resistance training program is greater than that of the current RDA, more than likely it is less than what most persons currently consume. A typical person who weighs 80 kg (175 lb) consuming a total of 4000 kcal daily, of which 15% are protein, would be consuming 150 g of protein or 1.9 g protein/kg body weight/day, or greater than the recommended intake. Sample menus to supply 150 g of protein in a day are found in Exhibits 3–1 and 3–2.

Various individual amino acids have been shown to effect the secretion of the following hormones: human growth hormone, insulin, and somatomedins, all of which are anabolic in nature and lead to protein synthesis.[14,15] Accordingly, supplemental amino acids were produced so that enhancing amino acid intake could be accomplished easily. To that end, the marketing of amino acid supplements has increased considerably. In June 1997, the World Wide Web offered more than 200,000 sites about amino acids, most of them offering the opportunity to purchase amino acid supplements at anywhere between $0.10 and $3.50 per supplement. However, no well-designed research study has ever shown positive effects of the consumption of amino acids, especially arginine, lysine, tyrosine, and ornithine, when total protein consumption is greater than 2.0 g protein/kg body weight/day.[16] Conversely, the most important factors in determining protein needs seem to be total energy intake and carbohydrate consumption, as long as protein intake is within the 1.7 to 1.8 g protein/ kg body weight/day suggested range. With sufficient energy, protein consumed can be devoted solely to protein synthesis within the body and is not used for energy; also, sufficient carbohydrate consumption can lead to increased insulin levels and enhanced muscle synthesis. Thus, the

Exhibit 3–1 Sample Menu Based on a ~3000 kcal/Day Diet (protein intake = 1.6 g/kg twice a day weight, body weight = 70 kg)

Food Item	Serving Size	Protein (grams)
Breakfast		
1 plain bagel	3.5"	7.5
Oatmeal cereal	2 cups	12.0
Peach	1 medium	0.6
Orange juice	8 fl oz	1.6
Lunch		
Green tossed salad	22 oz	9.0
Caesar dressing	2 tbsp	0.0
French roll	1 medium	3.3
Butter	2 tsp	0.0
Skim milk	2 cups	16.0
Snack		
Gaterlode carbohydrate drink	6 fl oz	0.0
Dinner		
Lentils	1 cup	18.0
Long grain enriched rice	3 cups	12.0
Pasta	3.5 cups	23.0
Plums	2 medium	0.0
Skim milk	2 cups	16.0

greatest amount of muscle growth seems to occur when protein intake is 1.7 to 1.8 g protein/kg body weight/day (10% to 15% of nutrient intake), energy intake is sufficient (that is, weight is not lost), and carbohydrate intake is high (60% to 65% of nutrient intake). In fact, resting levels of the hormone testosterone have been shown to be greatest when the ratio of protein to carbohydrate intake is 1:4, or, as recommended previously, 15%:60%, and anything that increases the ratio (that is, increases protein intake and/or decreases carbohydrate intake) reduces testosterone levels.[17] Similarly, as was previously seen with carbohydrate resynthesis,[18] recent information seems to indicate that carbohydrate consumption (1 g/kg or approximately 300 kcal for the person weighing 80 kg), not protein, within the 1st hour after heavy resistance exercise decreases the breakdown of muscle protein and results in a positive protein balance.[19]

The literature describes two problems pertaining to protein intake, heavy resistance training, and development of muscle mass and strength. The first problem is that most studies have been done using males who were of college age; therefore, the influence of protein intake and heavy resistance training on females and younger and older populations is not well-known and is mainly extrapolated from the information on males who are of college age. Likewise, little information is available that actually shows benefits to exercise performance. Thus, further work in these areas should be done.

Muscular Endurance, Exercise Performance, and Training Ability

Muscular endurance activities are high-intensity exercises that generally last from 10 to 120 seconds. Because muscular strength is related to

Exhibit 3–2 Sample Menu Based on a ~4000 kcal/Day Diet (protein intake = 1.9 g/kg twice a day weight, body weight = 80 kg)

Food Item	Serving Size	Protein (grams)
Breakfast		
1% milk	0.25 cups	2.0
Oatmeal cereal	3 cups	18.0
Peach	1 medium	0.0
Orange juice	8 fl oz	1.6
Lunch		
Green tossed salad	22 oz	9.0
Caesar dressing	2 tbsp	0.0
Turkey club submarine sandwich	6 in	23.0
Pasta	3 cups	20.0
Apple	1 medium	0.0
1% milk	1.5 cups	12.0
Snack		
Chocolate powerbar	1	10.0
Dinner		
Roasted chicken breast (no skin)	1.6 oz	16.0
Pasta	5 cups	33.5
Boiled broccoli	5 oz	4.0
French roll	2 medium	6.6
Marinara spaghetti sauce	2 oz	1.0
Butter	2 tsp	0.0
Plum	2 medium	0.0

muscular endurance, enhancing muscle size will, to some extent, enhance performance in muscular endurance activities; thus, those training for muscular endurance activities need to follow the recommendations given for muscular strength. However, other protein needs, specifically that of creatine, are specific to muscular endurance performance. Creatine is found in skeletal muscle primarily in the form of creatine phosphate (CP). CP is used to restore adenosine triphosphate (ATP), the immediate energy source for muscle. The amount of ATP stored in the muscle is small and would be used during muscular strength activities. Once ATP is used, it must be restored or fatigue will occur and exercise performance will have to decrease intensity or cease. For muscular endurance activities

to continue, ATP must be re-synthesized rapidly using creatine phosphate as follows:

$$ATP \rightarrow ADP + Pi$$
$$CP + ADP \rightarrow ATP + C$$

During high-intensity activities, lactate is also produced as an end product of the breakdown of carbohydrates to produce ATP and accumulates in the muscle. The hydrogen ions, which accumulate along with the lactate, cause muscle pH to decrease, which ultimately will cause fatigue. CP also acts as a buffer to minimize changes in pH as follows:

$$CP^{2-} + ADP^{3-} + H^+ \rightarrow ADP^{4-} + C$$

Thus, CP has the following two direct roles in the performance of muscular endurance activities: 1) as an energy source to replenish ATP, and 2) as a buffer to maintain muscle pH. Unfortunately, the stores of CP are limited and thus any means that can increase CP within the muscle should theoretically enhance muscular endurance exercise.

Creatine (or methylguanidine-acetic acid) is synthesized from two amino acids, arginine and glycine. Creatine can be produced in the body by the liver and pancreas, but is primarily produced in the kidney. Creatine can also be consumed in the diet through the intake of meats and fish. Because creatine was first introduced in the early 1990s as a supplement that could enhance exercise performance, some research has been done. The results of these limited investigations would seem to indicate the following:

- Muscle creatine phosphate levels can be increased with 4 to 6 days of intake of supplemental creatine of approximately 20 to 30 g/day.[20,21]
- After a supplemental regimen to increase muscle CP levels, increased levels remain for several weeks.[22]
- Increased levels of muscle CP seem to most enhance performance of repeated bouts of high-intensity exercise with minimal recovery periods.[21,23–25]
- Shorter periods of supplementation and/or exercise did not seem to enhance exercise performance.[26]
- There is little available information about whether enhanced exercise ability from creatine supplementation leads to enhanced training adaptations. Likewise, there is little information about whether longer duration exercise is enhanced with creatine supplementation.
- Although there appear to be no adverse side effects of acute doses of high creatine supplementation (lasting 4 to 6 days), no information is currently available on the effects of longer periods of supplementation. Much more research needs to take place before specific recommendations about the use of creatine and adaptations in exercise

performance and training can occur. This research should address the issues raised previously and many more (for example, Do males and females respond similarly to supplemental creatine?)

Aerobic Endurance Performance and Training

Although the possible need for a greater protein intake is more obvious in persons who are resistance-trained because of their desire to obtain large increases in muscle mass and thus muscle strength, athletes who participate in aerobic endurance activities probably also need increased protein intake. As is obvious from the physical stature of aerobic endurance athletes, muscle mass is not enhanced greatly; however, other mechanisms exist, such as increased amino acid oxidation and increased mitochondrial protein content, that require increased protein intake.

Skeletal muscle is able to oxidize amino acids, especially the branched-chain amino acids (BCAA) (that is, leucine, isoleucine, and valine). However, most of the energy required for a single bout of exercise comes from the breakdown of fats and carbohydrates. Increased amino acid oxidation has been shown to occur during prolonged exercise and could contribute 5% to 10% of the energy needs. Lemon et al found that the oxidation of labeled leucine increased with exercise in previously sedentary rats and that the increase was greatest when the animals exercised at 80% of VO_{2max} when compared to that at 40% VO_{2max}. Leucine oxidation returned to resting values by 5 hours after exercise.[27] Increased leucine oxidation with exercise has also been shown in humans.[28] Similarly, Delvin et al observed an increase in whole body protein degradation during 2 hours of 75% VO_{2max} exercise, returning to baseline levels within 2 hours after the exercise.[29] The difference in recovery times for the two investigations could be due to the amino acids examined; Wolf has calculated different rates of whole body protein synthesis and breakdown with the use of different amino acids.[30]

Another indicator that endurance athletes may require a higher protein intake than the recommended intake is that muscle contractile proteins have been shown to be broken down during prolonged exercise. N-MH has been found to be increased in urine after aerobic endurance exercise.[31–33] Thus, aerobic endurance athletes may require a protein intake substantially higher than the RDA.

Recently, it has been proposed and discussed that ingestion of BCAA might delay fatigue during prolonged aerobic endurance exercise, through delaying central fatigue.[34] The central fatigue hypothesis involves the decrease or lack of adequate central nervous system (CNS) drive to the working muscles that may occur during prolonged periods of exercise. Serotonin (5-HT) has been proposed as a potential mediator of central fatigue. The hypothesis states that during exercise, increased concentrations of brain 5-HT can impair CNS function. Increased brain 5-HT occurs because of increased levels of an amino acid precursor tryptophan (TRP). The transportation of free tryptophan (f-TRP) across the blood brain barrier is shared with the BCAA. Thus, brain 5-HT concentration increases as the ratio of plasma f-TRP:BCAA increases. With prolonged exercise, oxidation of BCAA is increased, thus reducing BCAA levels, whereas increased free fatty acid levels increase the concentration of f-TRP. Field studies using BCAA supplementation with runners, soccer players, and cross-country skiers have shown beneficial effects on performance.[35,36] However, more controlled laboratory studies have shown no beneficial effects of BCAA supplementation on aerobic endurance performance.[37,38] Amino acid oxidation has been shown to increase when muscle glycogen content is low, as would occur during prolonged aerobic endurance exercise, which would result in an increase in the f-TRP:BCAA ratio. BCAA supplement[37] and/or carbohydrate supplementation[39] may suppress endogenous muscle protein breakdown during exercise and result in a reduced ratio. Davis et al investigated the effects of ingesting either water or 6% or 12% carbohydrate-electrolyte drink while cycling at 70% VO_{2max}. When subjects consumed either of the carbohydrate-electrolyte drinks, the increase in f-TRP was reduced, the time to fatigue was increased by approximately 60 minutes as f-TRP greatly decreased, and BCAA slightly decreased, thereby reducing the ratio. However, the effects of glucose ingestion on central and peripheral fatigue cannot be distinguished with these results.[39]

Taken together, it would appear that aerobic endurance athletes would require slightly more protein in their diet than the RDA. Aerobic endurance athletes should consume about 1.2 to 1.4 g protein/kg body weight/day (150%-175% of the current RDA). As was seen with persons undergoing resistance training, more than likely this greater protein intake is already being consumed as part of the normal nutrient intake. A person weighing 70 kg (154 lb) consuming 3000 kcal, 15% of which come from protein sources, would be consuming 113 g of protein or 1.6 g protein/kg body weight/day, which is more than the recommended amount. Thus, this person should be consuming only 91 g of protein (1.3 g protein/kg body weight/day) or 8% of his or her diet as protein.

PROTEIN CONSUMPTION WITH A VEGETARIAN INTAKE

Dietary protein can be obtained from foods of animal and plant origin. When considering protein needs of a person, both the amino acid content and the digestibility of the foods consumed need to be considered. In general, proteins from a plant-based diet are about 85% digestible, whereas proteins from a mixed animal and plant diet are approximately 95% digestible. One of the reasons for lower digestibility in vegetarian diets is that fiber tends to decrease the digestion of proteins. Thus the proteins in dried beans and ready-to-eat cereals are about 75% digestible; whole wheat with rice approximately 88% digestible; and meat, poultry, fish, eggs, and milk 95% digestible. Because of the difference in digestibility, people who consume diets that contain no animal products probably require about 10% more protein or have an adjusted RDA of 0.9 g protein/kg body weight/day.

Plant proteins generally lack one or more of the essential amino acids. The two most deficient essential amino acids in plant foods are methionine and lysine. Methionine is generally found in small amounts in vegetables and legumes, whereas lysine is found in small amounts in grains, nuts, and seeds. Thus, grains and legumes should be combined, and vegetables and nuts and/or seeds should be combined. Adding milk and eggs to the diet complements the plant proteins and ensures that the essential amino acids are consumed.

DANGERS OF EXCESS PROTEIN INTAKE

Excess protein intake should be avoided because it can be detrimental to normal physiologic functioning and, therefore, health. The breakdown of protein requires more water than the breakdown of either fat or carbohydrate because of the increased water loss with the excretion of nitrogen. Therefore, as protein metabolism increases, so does the risk of dehydration, and excess fluids should be consumed to prevent dehydration.

Likewise, excess breakdown and thus excretion of protein have been shown to increase urinary calcium loss.[40] Females who are already prone to bone disease (that is, osteoporosis) due to low bone density could be compromising their bone health by consuming a diet too high in protein.

Certain high-protein diets may also put one at increased risk for coronary artery disease. Protein foods are often associated with high-fat intake, and thus are considered atherogenic. However, because of the strong association among animal protein, fat, and cholesterol, if one chooses protein sources from nonanimal sources, the atherogenic role associated with protein intake can be mediated.

Another concern about protein is the consumption of large quantities of supplemental amino acids. Serious complications ranging from metabolic imbalances and absorption problems to toxicity can result from excess supplementation of amino acids. Thus, until amino acid supplements can be shown to have a positive influence on muscle growth, strength, and protein oxidation, limited use is recommended.

Finally, excess protein intake is generally associated with possible kidney malfunction. Limited information is available in this area, especially for persons who have a normally functioning renal system. In fact, the only controlled study in this area used animals that were on a high-protein diet for more than half of their life and found that no serious adverse effects on the kidneys occurred.[41]

Although not a primary energy source during most exercise bouts, protein consumption is still important for the athlete (see Table 3–2). The RDA for protein for the sedentary person is 0.8 g protein/kg body weight/day. Persons who are trying to increase muscle mass and muscle strength through resistance training require greater rates of protein synthesis and thus require greater intake of protein than the sedentary person (1.7 to 1.8 g protein/kg body weight/day). Athletes participating in muscular endurance activities may enhance performance by consuming creatine, which is found in the body as CP and used to restore the immediate energy source of the muscles. Little information is currently known about creatine intake,

Table 3–2 Protein Requirements of Different Individuals

Type of Individual	Protein Requirements
Sedentary	0.8 g protein/kg body weight
Strength Athlete	1.7–1.8 g protein/kg body weight
Endurance Athlete	1.2–1.4 g protein/kg body weight
Vegetarian	0.9 g protein/kg body weight

but it appears that muscle creatine phosphate stores can be increased with 4 to 5 days of supplementation. Intake of supplemental creatine of approximately 20 to 30 g/day can enhance performance of repeated bouts of high-intensity exercise done with minimal recovery periods. Athletes participating in aerobic endurance activities should also benefit from slightly higher intake of protein (1.2 to 1.4 g protein/kg body weight/day.) Increased protein in endurance athletes may be beneficial in delaying fatigue. In general, athletes using resistance training and/or aerobic endurance training regularly consume protein within the enhanced recommendation. Protein can be obtained from both animal and plant foods. However, excess protein (greater than 2.0 g protein/kg body weight/day) does not lead to enhanced performance and can be detrimental to health by enhancing calcium loss, increasing the risk of cardiovascular disease, and/or enhancing the probability of dehydration occurring.

REFERENCES

1. Kasperek G, Dohm G, Snider R. Activation of branched-chain keto acid dehydrogenase by exercise. *Am J Physiol.* 1985;248:R166–R171.
2. Lemon P, Nagle F, Mullin J, Benevenga N. In vivo leucine oxidation at rest and during two intensities of exercise. *J Appl Physiol.* 1982;53:947–954.
3. Lemon P, Dolny D, Yarasheski K. Effect of intensity on protein utilization during prolonged exercise. *Med Sci Sports Exerc.* 1984;16:151–152.
4. Carraro F, Kimbrough T, Wolfe R. Urea kinetics in humans at two levels of exercise intensity. *J Appl Physiol.* 1993;75:1180–1185.
5. Lemon P, Mullin J. Effect of initial muscle glycogen level on protein catabolism during exercise. *J Appl Physiol.* 1980;48:624–629.
6. Henderson S, Black A, Brooks G. Leucine turnover and oxidation in trained rats during exercise. *Am J Physiol.* 1985;249:E137–E144.
7. Butterfield G. Whole-body protein utilization in humans. *Med Sci Sports Exerc.* 1987;19:S157–S165.
8. Gontzea I, Sutzescu P, Dumitrache S. The influence of adaptation of physical effort on nitrogen balance in man. *Nutri Rep Int.* 1975;11:231–234.
9. Millward D, Davis C, Halliday D, Wolman S, Mattews D, Rennie M. Effects of exercise on protein metabolism in humans as explored with stable isotopes. *Fed Proc.* 1982;41:2686–2691.
10. Tarnopolsky L, MacDougall J, Atkinson S, Tarnopolsky M, Sutton J. Gender differences in substrate for endurance exercise. *J Appl Physiol.* 1990;68:302–308.
11. Phillips S, Atkinson S, Tarnopolsky M, MacDougall J. Gender differences in leucine kinetics and nitrogen balance in endurance athletes. *J Appl Physiol.* 1993; 75:2134–2141.
12. Fern E, Bielinski R, Schutz Y. Effects of exaggerated amino acid and protein supply in man. *Experientia.* 1991;47:168–172.
13. Tarnopolsky M, Atkinson S, MacDougall J, Chesley A, Phillips S, Schwarcz H. Evaluation of protein requirements for trained strength athletes. *J Appl Physiol.* 1992;73:1986–1995.
14. Chandler R, Byrne H, Patterson J, Ivy J. Dietary supplements affect the anabolic hormones after weight-training exercise. *J Appl Physiol.* 1994;76:839–845.
15. Kreider R, Miriel V, Bertun E. Amino acid supplementation and exercise performance. *Sports Med.* 1993;16:190–209.
16. Williams M. Nutritional supplements for strength trained athletes. *Sports Science Exchange.* 1993;6:1–12.
17. Volek J, Kraemer W, Bush J, Incledon T, Boetes M. Testosterone and cortisol in relationship to dietary nutrients and resistance exercise. *J Appl Physiol.* 1997; 82:49–54.
18. Ivy J, Lee M, Brozinick J, Reed M. Muscle glycogen storage after different amounts of carbohydrate ingestion. *J Appl Physiol.* 1988;65:2018–2023.
19. Roy B, Tarnopolsky M, MacDougall J, Fowles J, Yarasheski K. Effect of glucose supplement timing on protein metabolism after resistance training. *J Appl Physiol.* 1997;82:1882–1888.
20. Greenhaff P, Bodin K, Soderlund K. The effect of oral creatine supplementation on skeletal muscle phosphocreatine resynthesis. *Am J Physiol.* 1994;266(5, pt 1):E725–E730.
21. Harris R, Soderlund K, Hultman E. Elevation of creatine in resting and exercised muscle of normal subjects by creatine supplementation. *Clin Sci.* 1992;83:367–374.
22. Maughan R. Creatine supplementation and exercise performance. *Int J Sport Nutr.* 1995;5:94–101.
23. Balsom P, Ekblom B, Soderlund K, Sjodin B, Hultman E. Creatine supplementation and dynamic high-intensity intermittent exercise. *Scan J Med Sci Sports.* 1993; 3:143–149.

24. Brannon T, Adams G, Conniff C, Baldwin K. Effects of creatine loading and training on running performance and biochemical properties of rat skeletal muscle. *Med Sci Sports Exerc*. 1997;29:489–495.

25. Greenhaff P, Casey A, Short A, Harris R, Soderlund K, Hultman E. Influence of oral creatine supplementation on muscle torque during repeated bouts of maximal voluntary exercise in man. *Clin Sci*. 1993;84:565–571.

26. Odland L, MacDougall J, Tarnopolsky M, Elorriaga A, Borgmann A. Effect of oral creatine supplementation on muscle [PCr] and short-term maximum power output. *Med Sci Sports Exerc*. 1997;29:216 219.

27. Lemon P, Tarnopolsky M, MacDougall D, Atkinson S. Protein requirements and muscle mass/strength changes during intensive training in novice bodybuilders. *J Appl Physiol*. 1992;73:767–775.

28. Knapik J, Meredith C, Jones B, Fielding R, Young V, Evans W. Leucine metabolism during fasting and exercise. *J Appl Physiol*. 1991;70:43–47.

29. Delvin J, Brodsky I, Scrimgeour A, Fuller S, Bier D. Amino acid metabolism after intense exercise. *Am J Physiol*. 1990;258:E249–E255.

30. Wolf R. Does exercise stimulate protein breakdown in humans? Isotopic approaches to the problem. *Med Sci Sports Exerc*. 1987;19:S172–S178.

31. Carraro F, Stuart C, Hartl W, Rosenblatt J, Wolfe R. Effect of exercise and recovery on muscle protein synthesis in human subjects. *Am J Physiol*. 1990;259:E470–E476.

32. Dohm G, Tapscott E, Kasperek G. Protein degradation during endurance exercise and recovery. *Med Sci Sports Exerc*. 1987;19:S166–S171.

33. Snyder A, Lamb D, Salm C, Judge M, Aberle E, Mills E. Myofibrillar protein degradation after eccentric exercise. *Experientia*. 1984;40:69–70.

34. Davis J. Carbohydrate, branched-chain amino acids and endurance: the central fatigue hypothesis. *Sports Science Exchange*. 1996;9:1–10.

35. Blomstrand E, Hassmen P, Ekblom B, Newsholme E. Administration of branched-chain amino acids during sustained exercise—effects on performance and plasma concentration of some amino acids. *Eur J Appl Physiol*. 1991;83:83–88.

36. Blomstrand E, Hassmen P, Newsholme E. Effect of branched-chain amino acid supplementation on mental performance. *Acta Physiologica Scandinavica*. 1991;136:473–481.

37. Varnier M, Sarto P, Martines D, et al. Effect of infusing branched-chain amino acids during incremental exercise with reduced muscle glycogen content. *Eur J Appl Physiol*. 1994;69:26–31.

38. Verger P, Aymard P, Cynobert L, Anton G, Luigi R. Effects of administration of branched-chain amino acids vs. glucose during acute exercise in the rat. *Physiol Behav*. 1994;55:523–526.

39. Davis J, Bailey S, Jackson D, Strasner A. Effects of carbohydrate feedings on plasma free-tryptophan and branched-chain amino acids during prolonged cycling. *Eur J Appl Physiol*. 1992;65:513–519.

40. Allen L, Oddoye E, Margen S. Protein-induced hypercalciuria: a longer term study. *Am J Clin Nutr*. 1979;32:741–749.

41. Zaragoza R, Renau-Piqueis J, Portoles M. Rats fed prolonged high protein diets show an increase in nitrogen metabolism and liver megamitochondria. *Arch Biochem Biophys*. 1987;258:426–435.

CHAPTER 4

Fat as a Fuel During Exercise

Asker E. Jeukendrup and Wim H. M. Saris

Carbohydrates and fats are the two main fuels that are metabolized in the muscle to provide energy [adenosine triphosphate (ATP)] for muscular contraction. Both fuels are oxidized simultaneously and the relative contribution of fat and carbohydrates to energy expenditure during exercise is dependent on several factors including the exercise intensity and duration, the diet before exercise, and training. During prolonged exercise for more than 2 hours, fat is the major fuel. Several studies demonstrated the importance of fat as an energy source during prolonged exercise showing that the contribution of fat to energy expenditure may even exceed 90% in extreme circumstances.[1] Also, people who are able to oxidize more fat at a certain workload or speed (endurance-trained athletes) can exercise longer and at a higher intensity, indicating that the capacity to oxidize fat is a major determinant of endurance exercise performance.

Yet, fat in the diet, especially fat in the athlete's diet, is usually regarded as undesirable and unhealthy. It is generally believed that fat impairs performance and increases body weight. This chapter will discuss the role of fat in energy metabolism during exercise and the effects of high-fat diets and fat supplementation during exercise.

HISTORICAL OVERVIEW

Man has always been intrigued by the questions: "Which fuels are used during exercise?" and "How can nutrition improve exercise performance?" Evidence exists that suggests the ancient Greeks and Romans were concerned with finding the best food for optimal performance. In as early as 1842, Von Liebig[2] stated that muscle protein was used during exercise, and he recommended that during periods of heavy physical exercise, large quantities of meat should be eaten to replenish the protein loss. This view changed when, in 1896, Chauveau[3] stated that carbohydrates were the only fuel that could be oxidized by skeletal muscle. In the following years, others supported this concept.[4,5] However, based on his work in exercising military cadets, Zuntz[6,7] did not agree with this view and suggested that both carbohydrates and fat served as a fuel during exercise. In a classic study, Krogh and Lindhard[8] investigated gas exchange in the lungs during exercise (Figure 4–1). Based on the fact that carbohydrates produce an equal amount of CO_2 as O_2 needed for oxidation, whereas fat produces only 0.7 L of CO_2 for each liter of O_2 oxidized, Krogh and Lindhard showed, by measuring VO_2 and VCO_2 in expiratory gases, that fat is an important substrate during endurance exercise. The ratio VCO_2/VO_2 in expired air, the respiratory exchange ratio (R), will be 0.69–0.73 when only fat is oxidized (dependent on the length of the carbon chain of the fatty acid oxidized) and 1.0 when only glucose is oxidized. Krogh and Lindhard[8] demonstrated that after several days of a low-carbohydrate, high-fat diet (one with "very fat bacon, butter, cream, eggs, and cabbage") the average R during 2 hours of cycling exercise was reduced to ~0.80 as compared to 0.85–0.90 when a normal mixed diet was consumed. Conversely, when subjects ate a high-carbohydrate, low-fat diet (potatoes, flour, bread, cake, marmalade, and sugar) R was increased to ~0.95. The subjective feelings of the subjects reported in that study are also very interesting. After the high-fat diet, the exercise was judged more difficult and subjects felt more tired afterwards (Figure 4–1).

Several years later, in 1939, Christensen and Hansen[9] studied the effect of diet on the relative importance of carbohydrates and fat as a fuel at rest and during exercise. They observed that R was significantly lower after a high-fat diet both at rest and during exercise and time to exhaustion was drastically reduced while subjects followed this diet. In 1934 Edwards et al[1] studied a runner who ran 6 hours on a treadmill and saw that as exercise duration progressed the relative importance of fat increased and even exceeded 90% of total energy delivery after 6

hours. These studies indicated that fat was indeed an important fuel during endurance exercise. Subsequent studies were aimed at determining the source of the fatty acids oxidized. Over the years, it was found that oxidizable lipid fuels include free fatty acids (FFAs), circulating plasma triglycerides (TGs), very low density lipoproteins (VLDLs), and intramuscular triglycerides (IMTGs) (Figure 4–2).

Also, fat-derived compounds such as ketone bodies (acetoacetate and β-hydroxybutyrate) can serve as fuel whereas glycerol can be converted into glucose during gluconeogenesis and subsequently be oxidized. After World War II, radioactive materials became available, and it was possible to investigate the kinetics of substrate mobilization and utilization.[10] In the late 1960s the muscle biopsy technique was redeveloped by Bergström and Hultman.[11–13] These new techniques made it possible to quantify substrate fluxes and tissue substrate concentrations. In biomedical research, radioactive isotopes are

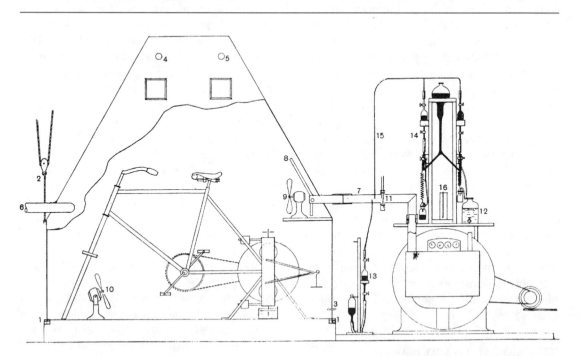

Figure 4–1 A Schematical Presentation of the Respiratory Chamber in which Krogh and Lindhard Conducted Their Experiments. *Source:* Reprinted with permission from A. Krogh and J. Lindhard, The Relative Value of Fat and Carbohydrates as Sources of Muscular Energy, *Biochemical Journal*, Vol. 14, pp. 290–363, © 1920, The Biochemical Society and Portland Press, Ltd.

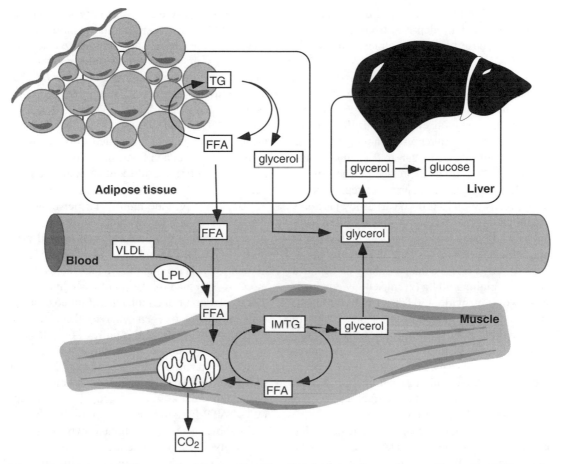

Figure 4–2 Sources of Fat as a Fuel During Exercise. Lipolysis in adipose tissue will provide FFAs to the bloodstream, FFAs may be hydrolyzed from VLDL by lipoprotein lipase (LPL), and intramuscular lipolysis may provide additional FFAs for oxidation. Also, FFAs can be reesterified after lipolysis, while glycerol will be released in the bloodstream.

now more frequently replaced by stable isotopes. More recent developments in the role of fat during exercise are discussed in the following sections.

FATS VERSUS CARBOHYDRATES

Before discussing fat metabolism in more detail, it is important to define the term *fat* and compare fat to the other important source of fuel during exercise: carbohydrates. Fats have several biochemical and physical properties that distinguish them from carbohydrates and, in many cases, make them the substrate of choice.

One of these properties is that fat contains more than twice as much energy per gram than carbohydrates [39 kJ per gram for fats (9 kcal/g) versus 18 kJ per gram (4 kcal/g) for carbohydrates]. Furthermore, carbohydrates are stored in the presence of water, whereas fat is stored in an almost anhydrous atmosphere (1 g of glycogen binds about 3 g of water).[14] This makes fat a much more efficient fuel per unit of weight. If all the fat in our body would be replaced by an equicaloric amount of carbohydrates, our weight would double. Fat, therefore, appears to be the ideal fuel for long-lasting exercise in situations when the provision of food is limited; certain animal species, like migratory birds who have to fly for days and are deprived from food, are an example. These birds store almost exclusively fat as fuel.[15]

In humans, both fat and carbohydrate are stored, although the carbohydrate stores are relatively small. The total amount of muscle glycogen of a man weighing 80 kg is about 400 g (Table 4–1). Liver glycogen represents about 100 g. The total amount of plasma substrates (glucose and lactate) is about 20 g. Expressed in terms of energy, the body carbohydrate stores represent approximately 8000 kJ (2000 kcal). Body fat stores are much larger. The largest quantity of fat is located in adipose tissue (mainly subcutaneous and deep visceral adipose tissue). The amount of energy stored as fat for a man weighing 80 kg and a woman weighing 60 kg (average body composition) would provide 450,000 kJ (110,000 kcal) and 550,000 kJ (135,000 kcal), respectively. In other words, if only fat or only carbohydrates could be used as fuel, the carbohydrate stores would deliver energy for no more than 90 minutes of marathon running, and energy derived from fat stores would be satisfactory for 119 hours of marathon running.[16]

The storage of fat is dynamic, which means that in case of a negative energy balance, the size of the individual fat cells will decrease, whereas with a positive balance, the excess of fatty acids will be converted into triglycerides, and hypertrophy of fat cells will result. Although adipose tissue is by far the most important site of storage, fat is also stored within the muscle. The size of this fat pool is difficult to determine, but muscle biopsy estimates have been between 7 and 40 mol/kg ww^{-1}.[17–20] The total amount of fat stored in all muscle cells has been estimated to be approximately 300 g.[21] Type I fibers have been shown to have a higher triglyceride content than type II fibers.[18]

Fatty acids provide more ATP per molecule than glucose. A glucose molecule produces 38 ATP, whereas a molecule of stearic acid produces 147 ATP. However, to produce the same amount of ATP, oxidation of fatty acids needs more oxygen than oxidation of carbohydrates.[22] The oxidation of one molecule of glucose needs 6 molecules of oxygen whereas the complete oxidation of stearic acid requires 26 molecules of oxygen. Per unit of time, more ATP can be derived from carbohydrates (glucose) than from the oxidation of fatty acids.[22] When blood-borne fatty acids are oxidized, the maximum rate of ATP formation is ~0.40 mol/min^{-1} while the aerobic or anaerobic breakdown of endogenous glycogen can generate ~1.0 to 2.4 mol/min^{-1}.[23] This is one of the reasons why carbohy-

Table 4–1 The Energy Stores of an 80 kg Man

Substrate		Weight (kg)	Energy (kJ)
Carbohydrates	Plasma glucose	0.02	320
	Liver glycogen	0.1	1600
	Muscle glycogen	0.4	6400
	Total (±)	0.52	8320
Fat	Plasma FFAs	0.0004	16
	Plasma triglycerides	0.004	160
	Adipose tissue	12	404,000
	Intramuscular triglycerides	0.3	10,800
	Total (±)	12.3	414,976

Note: The values given are estimates for a normal man weighing 80 kg. The amount of protein in the body is not mentioned but would be approximately 10 kg (160,000 kJ), mainly located in the muscle.

Source: Adapted from E.A. Newsholme and A.R. Leech, *Biochemistry for the Medical Sciences*, p. 337, © 1983, John Wiley & Sons, Ltd. Reproduced with permission.

drates play such an important role during exercise of higher intensity. At higher exercise intensities, the rate of ATP hydrolysis is too high to be matched by ATP formation from FFA oxidation, and carbohydrates become the substrate of choice. The factors that limit the rate of ATP production from the oxidation of fat are not completely understood. Possible limitations will be discussed in the following sections.

FAT METABOLISM DURING EXERCISE

Mobilization of Fatty Acids

Before fatty acids can be oxidized, they have to be mobilized and transported to the site of oxidation. Adipose tissue triglycerides are mobi-

lized during exercise when the enzyme hormone-sensitive lipase (HSL) is stimulated (Figure 4–3).

This stimulation is mainly through the sympathetic nervous system and circulating epinephrine, whereas insulin is probably the most important counterregulatory hormone. The process that splits a triglyceride molecule into one molecule of glycerol and three molecules of FFAs is known as lipolysis. The glycerol released by this reaction diffuses freely into the blood. The adipocyte cannot reuse it because the enzyme glycerokinase, which is required to reesterify the glycerol to FFA, is present in only very low concentrations. Therefore, all the glycerol produced by lipolysis is released into the plasma, and the

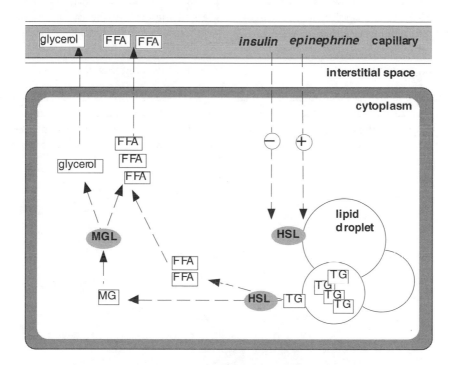

Figure 4–3 Mobilization of Fatty Acids from Adipose Tissue. Triglycerides are transported from the lipid droplet to the cytoplasm of the adipocyte. This triglyceride is subjected to cleavage by the enzyme hormone-sensitive lipase. A monoglyceride is formed and fatty acids can diffuse into the circulation. The remaining monoglyceride is split by the enzyme monoglyceride lipase (MGL) into glycerol and another fatty acid that can also diffuse into the circulation. The rate-limiting step in this mobilization of fatty acids from the lipid droplet is the HSL. This enzyme is stimulated by the sympathetic nervous system via α-adrenergic receptors, which stimulate cAMP and protein kinase, which in turn activates HSL. *Source:* Adapted with permission from A. E. Jeukendrup, *Aspects of Carbohydrates and Fat Metabolism During Exercise*, p. 29, © 1997, Uitgeverij De Vrieseborch.

measurement of glycerol appearance in the blood is believed to be a convenient and reliable measure of lipolysis. FFAs released by lipolysis can either be reesterified within the adipocyte or transported into the bloodstream, where they are bound to albumin. At rest, approximately 70% of all FFAs are reesterified.[24] However, during exercise, reesterification is suppressed and, at the same time, the rate of lipolysis is accelerated. As a result, there is a massive appearance of FFAs in the blood.[24,25]

FFAs are transported through the cytoplasm of the adipocyte bound to a fatty acid binding protein (FABP), and when they are released into the blood they are bound to albumin. These binding proteins (FABP and albumin) are needed to make the FFA soluble in an aqueous environment. The FFAs may be released from albumin in the muscle where they are transported into the sarcoplasm and again bound to FABP.

Intramuscular Triglycerides

The IMTG stores are another source of FFAs. IMTG stores, usually adjacent to the mitochondria as lipid droplets, have been recognized as an important energy source during exercise. Stud-

ies in which muscle samples were examined under a microscope revealed that these lipid droplets were smaller after exercise. Like adipose tissue, muscle contains an HSL that is activated by epinephrine and inhibited by insulin. FFAs liberated from IMTGs may be released into the blood or oxidized within the muscle. During exercise at 25%VO_{2max} most of the fat oxidized is derived from plasma FFAs and only a little comes from IMTGs (Figure 4–4).[25] However, during moderate exercise intensity (65% VO_{2max}) the contribution of plasma FFAs declined whereas contribution of IMTGs increased and provided half of the FFAs for total fat oxidation.[25] Training also decreased the contribution of plasma FFAs despite a dramatic increase of total fatty acid oxidation.[26] This decrease in plasma FFA oxidation was accounted for by a marked increase in the contribution of muscle triglycerides to energy expenditure.

Plasma Lipoproteins

Triglycerides bound to lipoproteins (VLDLs and chylomicrons) are another potential source of fatty acids.[27] The enzyme lipoprotein lipase (LPL) in the vascular wall will hydrolyze some

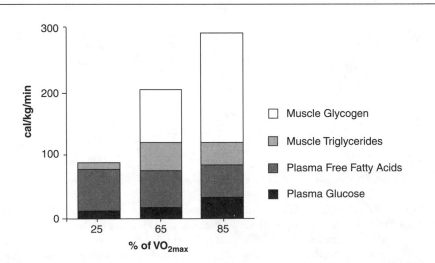

Figure 4–4 Substrate Utilization at Different Exercise Intensities. *Source:* Data from J. A. Romijn et al., Regulation of Endogenous Fat and Carbohydrate Metabolism in Relation to Exercise Intensity, *American Journal of Physiology*, Vol. 265, pp. E380–E391, © 1993.

of the triglycerides in circulating lipoproteins passing through the capillary bed. As a result, FFAs will be released that the muscle can use for oxidation. However, the FFA uptake from plasma lipoprotein triglycerides occurs slowly and accounts for fewer than 5% of the FFA-derived CO_2 during prolonged exercise.[27,28] Therefore, it is generally believed that plasma triglycerides contribute only minimally to energy production during exercise. However, there are some interesting observations that need further investigation. For instance, LPL activity is significantly increased after training[29] and after a high-fat diet[30]; in both situations, fat oxidation is markedly increased. In addition, acute exercise also stimulates LPL activity. Therefore, additional research is needed to elucidate the role of LPL and the role of VLDL as an energy source.

FFAs in the cytoplasm may be activated by acyl-CoA synthase to form an acyl-CoA complex (often referred to as an activated fatty acid). This acyl-CoA complex can be used for the synthesis of IMTGs, or it can be bound to carnitine under the influence of the enzyme carnitineacyltransferase I (CAT I), which is located at the outside of the outer mitochondrial membrane. The bond between carnitine and the activated fatty acid is the first step of the transport of fatty acyl-CoA into the mitochondria. The fatty acyl-CoA carnitine complex is transported with a translocase and reconverted into fatty acyl-CoA at the matrix side of the inner mitochondrial membrane by the enzyme carnitineacyltransferase II (CAT II; Figure 4–5).

Fatty acyl carnitine crosses the inner membrane in a 1:1 exchange with a molecule of free carnitine.[23,31] Although it is often believed that short-chain fatty acids (SCFAs) and medium-chain fatty acids (MCFAs) can more freely diffuse into the mitochondrial matrix, carrier proteins with a specific maximum affinity for short- or medium-chain acyl-CoA transport at least some of these fatty acids.[32,33] Once in the mitochondrial matrix, the fatty acyl-CoA is subjected to β-oxidation, a series of reactions that splits a two-carbon acetyl-CoA molecule of the multiple carbon fatty acid chain. The acetyl-CoA is then oxidized in the tricarboxylic acid (TCA) cycle. The complete oxidation of fatty acids in the mitochondria is dependent on several factors [for example, the activity of β-oxidation enzymes, TCA-cycle intermediates and enzymes (that is TCA-cycle activity), and the presence of oxygen].

FAT UTILIZATION DURING EXERCISE

When exercise is initiated, the rate of lipolysis and the rate of FFA release from adipose tissue are increased. During the first 15 minutes of exercise, plasma FFA concentrations usually decrease because the rate of FFA uptake by the muscle exceeds the rate of FFA appearance from lipolysis. Thereafter, the rate of appearance is in excess of the utilization by muscle, and plasma FFA concentrations increase. Fat oxidation increases as the exercise duration increases. Relatively fat oxidation will be maximal at low intensities whereas during high exercise intensities, carbohydrates are the major fuel. In absolute terms, however, fatty acids will be oxidized most at an exercise intensity between 60% and 70% of the maximal aerobic work capacity.[25] Edwards et al[1] reported fat oxidation rates of over 1.0 g/min[-1]. Christensen and Hansen[9] observed that the contribution of fat could even increase to levels as high as 90% of energy expenditure when a fatty meal was consumed, leading to fat oxidation rates of 1.5 g/min[-1]. Comparable results were found when subjects were adapted to a high-fat diet and exercised at submaximal intensities (60% VO_{2max}).[34–36] At high exercise intensities (80% VO_{2max} and higher) both the absolute and the relative contribution of fatty acids to energy expenditure are decreased.[25]

TRAINING AND FATTY ACID OXIDATION

Endurance training affects both substrate utilization and exercise capacity. A large number of studies involving both animals and humans has established a marked adaptive increase in oxidative potential in response to an increased

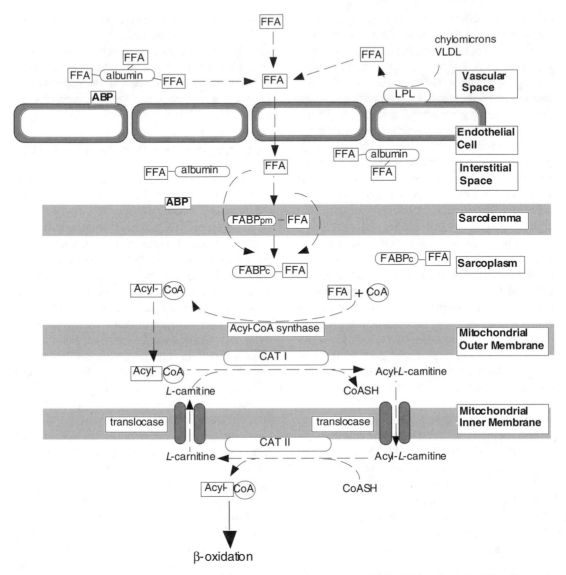

Figure 4–5 A Schematic Presentation of the Transport of Free Fatty Acids (FFAs) from the Blood into the Mitochondria. The transport involves several fatty acid binding proteins (FABPs). The transport through the sarcolemma is at least partially mediated by a plasma membrane FABP (FABPpm). The FABP in the cytoplasm of the cell is a specific FABPc. The FFA is then bound to a CoA to form a fatty acyl-CoA, which can be transported into the mitochondria through the carnitine acyl transferase transport system (VLDL=very low density lipoprotein; ABP=albumin-binding protein; LPL=lipoprotein lipase; CAT I=carnitineacyltransferase I; CAT II=carnitineacyltransferase II). *Source:* Adapted with permission from A.E. Jeukendrup, *Aspects of Carbohydrates and Fat Metabolism During Exercise*, p. 33, © 1997, Uitgeverij De Vrieseborch.

physical activity.[37,38] A notable consequence and probably contributing factor to the enhanced exercise capacity after endurance training is the shift of metabolism to a greater use of fat and a concomitant sparing of the glycogen stores.[17,19,37–45] The contribution of fat to total energy expenditure increases after training at both the same relative and absolute exercise intensity.[19,46–49] This is of utmost importance during prolonged exercise of moderate to high intensity (50% to 90% VO_{2max}) because carbohydrates are required to maintain those levels of exercise. As soon as glycogen stores become depleted and carbohydrate oxidation decreases below a critical level, the exercise intensity has to be reduced because the required ATP production rate cannot be maintained when carbohydrates are lacking.[50] Although the advantages of increased fat oxidation during exercise are obvious, the cellular and molecular mechanisms underlying this beneficial effect of training are incompletely understood. Several adaptations may contribute to a stimulation of fat oxidation in subjects who train, including the following:

1. an increase in the number of oxidative enzymes
2. increased mitochondrial content in trained muscle
3. increased muscle triglyceride oxidation
4. increased FFA uptake
5. alterations in mobilization of FFAs from adipose tissue

It seems unlikely that other training adaptations, such as an increased maximal cardiac output, will be major factors in explaining the shift from carbohydrate to fat metabolism in the trained skeletal muscle.[41]

FAT SUPPLEMENTATION DURING EXERCISE

Ingestion of Long-Chain Triglycerides

Nutritional fats include triglycerides (mostly C16 and C18), phospholipids, and cholesterol, of which only triglycerides can contribute to any extent to energy provision during exercise. In contrast to carbohydrates, nutritional fats reach the circulation slowly because they are potent inhibitors of gastric emptying.[51] Furthermore, the digestion in the gut and absorption of fat are

also rather slow processes compared to the digestion and absorption of carbohydrates. Bile salts, produced by the liver, and lipase, secreted by the pancreas, are needed to split the long-chain triglycerides (LCTs) into glycerol and three long-chain fatty acids (LCFAs) or monoacylglycerol and two fatty acids (Figure 4–6). The fatty acids diffuse into the intestinal mucosa cells and are reesterified in the cytoplasm to form LCTs. These LCTs will be encaptured by a coat of proteins (chylomicrons) to make them water-soluble. These chylomicrons are then released in the lymphatic system, which ultimately drains in the systemic circulation. Exogenous LCTs enter the systemic circulation much slower than carbohydrates, which are absorbed as glucose (or to minor extents as fructose or galactose) and directly enter the main circulation through the portal vein. Long-chain dietary fatty acids typically enter the blood 3 to 4 hours after ingestion.

The fact that these LCFAs enter the circulation in chylomicrons is also important, and it is generally believed that the rate of breakdown of chylomicron-bound triglycerides by muscle is relatively low. It has been suggested that the primary role of these triglycerides in chylomicrons is the replenishment of IMTG stores after exercise.[52]

In summary, LCT ingestion during exercise is not desirable because of the following reasons:

1. It slows gastric emptying.
2. The LCTs only slowly appear in the systemic circulation.
3. LCTs enter the systemic circulation in chylomicrons, which are believed to be an insignificant fuel source during exercise.

Ingestion of Medium-Chain Triglycerides

Although fat in general is slowly hydrolyzed and absorbed, this process also depends on the chain length of the fatty acids. In contrast to the LCTs, short-chain triglycerides (SCTs) and medium-chain triglycerides (MCTs) are more rap-

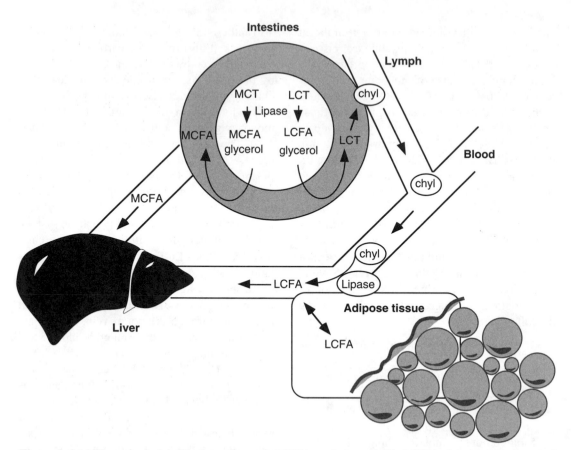

Figure 4–6 MCTs are hydrolyzed in the gut lumen to MCFAs and glycerol. The MCFAs then cross the intestinal mucosa, enter the bloodstream, and are transported to the liver through the portal vein. LCTs are hydrolyzed in the gut lumen, pass the intestinal mucosa, are reesterified to LCTs, and are incorporated in chylomicrons (chyl). These chylomicrons follow the lymph system and enter the bloodstream 3 to 4 hours after ingestion. LCFA may be split from chylomicrons by the enzyme lipase by different tissues including adipose tissue and muscle.

idly absorbed, and they are not transported by chylomicrons but directly enter the systemic circulation through the portal vein (Figure 4–6).

With the introduction of MCFAs in liquid enteral and parenteral nutrition, their possible role in sports nutrition became subject to investigation. MCFAs contain 6, 8, or 10 carbons, whereas LCFAs contain 12 or more carbons. Unlike most LCTs, MCTs are liquid at room temperature. This is, in part, the result of the small molecular size of MCTs. MCTs are also better soluble in water. This greater water solubility and smaller molecular size have consequences in all levels of their metabolism. MCTs are more rapidly digested and absorbed in the

intestines than LCTs. Furthermore, MCFAs follow the portal venous system and enter the liver directly, whereas LCFAs follow the slow lymphatic system. It has been suggested that MCTs may be a valuable exogenous energy source during exercise in addition to carbohydrates.[53] Also, it has been suggested that MCT ingestion may improve exercise performance by increasing plasma FFA levels and sparing muscle glycogen[54] because it has been observed that increased availability of plasma FFA reduced the rate of muscle glycogen breakdown and delayed the onset of exhaustion.[46,55–58]

MCT added to carbohydrate drinks did not inhibit gastric emptying.[59] In fact, the drinks with

MCTs emptied faster from the stomach than an isocaloric carbohydrate drink. In a subsequent study, the oxidation rates of orally ingested MCT were investigated.[53] Eight well-trained athletes cycled four times 180 min at 50% W_{max} (57% VO_{2max}). Subjects ingested either carbohydrates, carbohydrates + MCT, or MCT. During the second hour (60- to 120-minute period) the amount of MCTs oxidized was 72% of the amount ingested with carbohydrates + MCTs, whereas during the MCT trial, only 33% was oxidized. It was concluded that more MCTs, were oxidized when ingested in combination with carbohydrates. Data confirmed the hypothesis that oral MCTs might serve as an energy source in addition to glucose during exercise because the metabolic availability of MCTs was high during the last hour of exercise with oxidation rates being as high as 70% of the ingestion rate. However, the maximal amount of oral MCTs (trioctanoate) that could be tolerated in the gastrointestinal (GI) tract was small (about 30 g),[53,60] and this limited the contribution of oral MCTs to total energy expenditure to values between 3% and 7% (Figure 4–7).

It has also been suggested that MCT supplements may be especially effective during extreme endurance exercise when the reliance on blood substrates is maximal. To test this hypothesis, MCT oxidation in carbohydrates + MCT supplements was studied in a glycogen-depleted state.[61] Subjects exercised to exhaustion the evening before the experiment in which MCT oxidation was determined during exercise at 57% VO_{2max}. Although total fat oxidation was markedly increased, MCT oxidation increased only marginally. The contribution of MCT to total energy expenditure was still small (about 6%–8%).[61]

In theory, MCT could be a way to elevate plasma FFA levels, which may lead to glycogen sparing.[46,55] However, well-trained athletes who ingested carbohydrates or carbohydrates with 30 g MCTs during exercise displayed no significant differences in glycogen breakdown between the trials nor in the respiratory exchange ratio during exercise.[62] However, there may be large individual variations in the tolerance of MCTs. Van Zeyl et al[54] fed their subjects 86 g MCTs in combination with carbohydrates during prolonged cycling exercise and observed small increases in fat oxidation and improvements in time trial performance. When Jeukendrup et al fed subjects 85 g MCTs in a

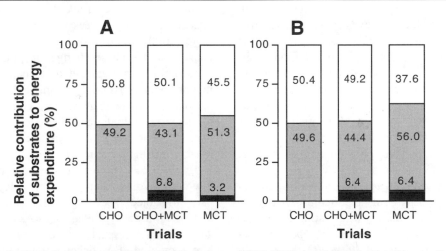

Figure 4–7 The Relative Contribution of Carbohydrates (CHO; White) and Fat (Gray) to Energy Expenditure during Exercise (A: 0–60 minutes; B: 60–120 minutes) and the Relatively Small Contribution of Ingested Medium-Chain Triglycerides (MCTs; Black). *Source:* Data from A. E. Jeukendrup et al., Metabolic Availability of Medium Chain Triglycerides Coingested with Carbohydrates During Prolonged Exercise, *Journal of Applied Physiology*, Vol. 79, pp. 756–762, © 1995.

similar experiment, subjects developed gastrointestinal problems, no increases in fat oxidation were observed, and there was no effect of carbohydrate + MCT ingestion on performance.[63] In fact, when subjects received MCTs without carbohydrates, performance was decreased compared to water (placebo) ingestion.

In conclusion, MCTs were rapidly emptied from the stomach, absorbed, and oxidized, and the oxidation of exogenous MCTs was enhanced when coingested with carbohydrate. Ingestion of 30g MCTs did not affect muscle-glycogen breakdown and contributed only a little to energy expenditure (7%). Ingestion of larger amounts of MCT resulted in GI distress.

EFFECT OF DIET ON FAT METABOLISM AND PERFORMANCE

Fasting

Fasting has been proposed as a way to increase fat utilization, spare muscle glycogen, and improve exercise performance. In rats, short-term fasting increases plasma epinephrine and norepinephrine concentrations, stimulates lipolysis, and increases the concentration of circulating plasma FFAs. This, in turn, increases fat oxidation and spares muscle glycogen, leading to a similar,[64] or even increased, running time to exhaustion in rats.[65] In humans, fasting also results in an increased concentration of circulating catecholamines, increased lipolysis, increased concentration of plasma FFAs,[66] and a decreased glucose turnover.[67] Muscle-glycogen concentrations, however, were unaffected by fasting.[67,68] Although it has been reported that fasting had no effect on endurance capacity at low exercise intensities (45% VO_{2max}),[67] Zinker et al[69] observed a 38% decreased performance at 50% VO_{2max}, Loy et al[68] reported a 15% to 63% decreased performance with fasting at 79% to 86% VO_{2max}, and Gleeson et al[70] reported a decreased performance at 100% VO_{2max}. The observed decreased performance was not reversible by carbohydrate ingestion during exercise.[71]

It has been argued that the effects observed in most of these studies may be due to the fact that in the control situation the last meal was provided 3 hours before the exercise to exhaustion. The effects, therefore, may have been an effect of the feeding before exercise improving endurance capacity instead of decreased performance after fasting. However, the studies comparing a prolonged fast (greater than 24 hours) to a 12-hour fast show decreased performance,[67,69] and thus it seems justified to conclude that fasting decreases endurance capacity.

In summary, fasting increases the availability of lipid substrates resulting in increased oxidation of fatty acids at rest and during exercise. However, since the glycogen stores are not maintained, fatigue resistance and exercise performance are impaired.

Effects of a Short-Term High-Fat Diet

Short-term exposure to a high-fat diet may lead to impaired fatigue resistance as shown already in 1939 by Christensen and Hansen.[9] Many years later, when muscle biopsy techniques were redeveloped, it was discovered that a high-fat, low-carbohydrate diet resulted in decreased muscle glycogen levels, and this was the main factor causing lack of fatigue resistance during prolonged exercise.[11–13,72] Plasma FFA concentrations are increased at rest and increase more rapidly when a low-carbohydrate diet is consumed.[73–75] These changes in plasma FFA concentrations are attributed to changes in the rate of lipolysis. Not only plasma FFAs but also plasma glycerol concentrations are increased after a low-carbohydrate diet.[65–69,76] Jansson and Kaijser[77] reported that the uptake of FFAs by muscle during 25 minutes of cycling at 65% VO_{2max} was 82% higher in subjects receiving a low-carbohydrate diet (5%) for 5 days, compared to subjects receiving a high-carbohydrate diet (75%) for 5 days. Plasma FFAs contributed 24% and 14% respectively to energy expenditure. Increased FFA concentrations in the blood after a period of carbohydrate restriction will lead to an increased ketogenesis. After a few days of high-fat feeding, the ketone body production increases fivefold,[78] and the arterial concentration of ketone bodies may increase ten- to twentyfold.[78] During the first phase of light to moderate exercise, ketone body concentrations usually decline, and after 30 to 90 minutes they will increase again.[67,69,78] However, the observed concentrations under those conditions are still higher after a high-fat diet compared to those associated with low-fat diets. Carbohydrate-restricted diets may also lead to an increased breakdown of muscle triglycerides.[48,73,79]

In summary, short-term, high-fat diets increase the availability of lipid substrates but reduce the storage of glycogen. As a result, although fat oxidation may be increased during exercise, fatigue resistance and exercise performance are decreased.

Effects of a Long-Term High-Fat Diet

It has been suggested that a 5- to 7-day alteration in the dietary composition is an insufficient time to induce an adaptive response to the changed diet. Jansson and Kaijser[48] concluded that a high-fat diet over a prolonged period resulted in a decreased utilization of carbohydrates and that this relative shortage of carbohydrates was compensated by an increased contribution of fat to energy metabolism.[77,80] In rats, it has been shown that adaptation to a high-fat diet leads to considerable improvements in endurance capacity.[76,81] These adaptations can be attributed to the number of oxidative enzymes and a decreased degradation of liver glycogen during exercise.[81] The results suggest that after adaptation to a high-fat diet, the capacity to oxidize fatty acids instead of carbohydrates is increased, because of an adaptation of the oxidative enzymes in the muscle cell. Only a few studies looked at the effect of long-term, high-fat diets on fat metabolism and exercise performance.

Phinney et al[34] investigated exercise performance in subjects who were obese, after these subjects followed a high-fat diet (90% of energy intake from fat) for 6 weeks. Before and after the diet, subjects exercised at 75% VO_{2max} until exhaustion. Subjects were able to exercise as long

while following the high-fat diet as they did while following their normal diet, but after the high-fat diet, fat became the main substrate. Results of this study, however, may have been influenced by the fact that these subjects were not in energy balance and lost 11 kg of body weight. So, although there were no differences in the absolute VO_{2max} before and after the dietary period, there were considerable differences in the relative intensity.

The observed improvement in performance may have been an artifact rather than a positive effect of the adaptation period. Therefore, Phinney et al[35,36] conducted a follow-up study in which trained subjects were studied before and after a 4-week high-fat diet (less than 20 g of carbohydrates per day). The diet drastically reduced the muscle glycogen concentration that appeared before exercise (143 ± 10 versus 76 ± 4 mmol glucose/kg wet weight muscle). However, no difference in the average time to exhaustion at 62% to 64%VO_{2max} before and after the diet was found. However, the results are difficult to interpret because of the large variability of the subjects' performance times (times to exhaustion). One subject exercised 57% longer whereas other subjects showed no improvement or even decreased times to exhaustion. Also, the exercise intensity was relatively low, and subjects' reliance on carbohydrates during exercise at 62% to 64% VO_{2max} was low. In such a situation, reduced carbohydrate stores may not be limiting. It is possible that at higher exercise intensities performance would have been impaired. The results of the study of Phinney may be supportive of this view because the subjects with the highest R values (higher rates of carbohydrate oxidation) showed a decreased performance whereas the subjects with the lowest R values displayed an increased time to exhaustion.

Nevertheless, it is remarkable that performance was not reduced in all subjects even though muscle glycogen levels that appeared before exercise were decreased by almost 50% and fat oxidation during exercise was markedly increased. These observations have been attributed to enzymatic adaptations [including 44%

increase of acyl-carnitine palmitoyl transferase (CPT) activity, and a 46% decrease of the hexokinase activity].[36]

Lambert et al[82] fed five cyclists who were endurance-trained a somewhat less extreme high-fat diet or high-carbohydrate diet for 14 days. The high-fat diet contained 67% fat and 7% carbohydrate, whereas the high-carbohydrate diet contained 74% carbohydrate and 12% fat. To evaluate exercise performance, the following three different exercise tests were done:

1. a Wingate test (sprint exercise)
2. a cycling time-to-exhaustion test at a high intensity (90% VO_{2max})
3. an exhaustion test at a moderate intensity (60% VO_{2max})

Muscle glycogen concentrations were 44% lower after the high-fat diet was consumed. No differences were found in sprint performance and time to exhaustion during high-intensity exercise. However, time-to-exhaustion during the moderate-intensity exercise test was significantly longer (80±8 minutes versus 43±7 minutes) after the high-fat diet. The high-fat diet also resulted in increased fat-oxidation rates during exercise. In the studies of Lambert et al[82] and Phinney et al,[36] maintained or improved performance was seen at relatively low exercise intensities (60% to 65% VO_{2max}), which are far below intensities during competition. So, it is unclear how these results translate into practical applications in training and competition.

From a health perspective, eating large amounts of fat has been associated with the development of obesity and cardiovascular disease. It has not yet been determined if this is also true for athletes. To our knowledge, there are no studies available at the current time describing the effects of high-fat diets on cardiovascular risk factors in athletes who train regularly. Pendergast et al[83] reported no changes in plasma low-density lipoprotein, high-density lipoprotein, and total cholesterol levels in male and female runners with diets in the range of 17%–40% fat. Although it is generally accepted that the risk of obesity and cardiovascular diseases increases with the consumption of high-fat diets in sedentary people, regular exercise or endurance training seems to attenuate these risks.[84] Exposure to high-fat diets has also been associated with insulin resistance and recently has been linked to an effect of the intramuscular triacylglycerol pools on glucose uptake.[85] However, this observation was made in obese subjects, and it is not clear whether these results can be extrapolated to athletes, especially since athletes seem to have larger IMTG stores and increased insulin sensitivity. Because there is little information about the negative effects of high-fat diets for athletes and the effects of those diets on performance are unclear, we suggest that caution should be exercised when recommending high-fat diets to athletes.

In conclusion, although the hypothesis that chronic high-fat diets may increase the capacity to oxidize fat and improve exercise performance during competition is attractive, there are only few indications that this may indeed be the case. The available positive studies are done at exercise intensities lower than intensity during competition. Therefore, more well-controlled studies are needed to clarify the importance of the effect of dietary carbohydrate and fat content on athletic performance and, at this time, because there is little information about the negative effects of high-fat diets for athletes, we again suggest that caution be exercised when recommending a high-fat diet to athletes.

DIETARY FISH OIL

Guezennec et al[86] suggested that by increasing the fraction of polyunsaturated fatty acid in the phospholipids of erythrocyte membranes, membrane fluidity would be improved and red blood cell deformability would be increased, resulting in improved peripheral oxygen supply. They conducted a study in which 14 male subjects were divided into two groups, one group receiving a normal diet and the second group receiving a diet rich in fish oil for 6 weeks. Gas liquid chromatography showed that the fraction of n-3 fatty acids increased in erythrocyte membranes. However, no change in red blood cell deformability was seen under resting conditions. During hypobaric exercise, red blood cell deformability decreased less with the fish oil feeding. However, only six subjects participated in this study, although it is known that there is a large variation in day-by-day VO_{2max}. Therefore, the observed increased VO_{2max} might have been an artifact rather than a real effect of n-3 supplementation. This is supported by the fact that no change in maximal workload (W_{max}) was seen. The same W_{max} with an increased VO_{2max} would mean a decreased efficiency of motion. Brilla and Landerholm[87] studied the effects of fish oil feeding and exercise in 32 sedentary males. It was found that exercise led to an increased VO_{2max}, whereas fish oil supplementation had no effect on VO_{2max}. It has been shown that physical training improves red blood cell deformability and changes the fatty acid composition of membranes toward a higher percentage of unsaturated fatty acids so that the enhanced fluidity under resting conditions could be masked by physical training.[88] The enhanced membrane fluidity may be especially important when the uptake of oxygen becomes limiting as with exercise under hypoxic conditions. However, the physiologic consequences, especially the physiologic importance, are still hypothetical, and further studies are necessary to evaluate the possible effects of PUFA on hemorrheologic changes during exercise.

CONCLUSION

In contrast to carbohydrate stores, fat stores are large in humans and can be regarded as practically unlimited. The stores of fat are mainly located in adipose tissue but also in IMTGs. During exercise, plasma FFAs (liberated from adipose tissue) and IMTGs are the most important lipid substrates. IMTG stores are especially important during moderate-intensity exercise and for well-trained athletes. Total fat oxidation is also maximal at moderate exercise intensities.

Ingestion of LCTs during exercise may reduce the gastric emptying rate, and LCTs will appear in the plasma only slowly. MCTs do not have these disadvantages; they are rapidly oxidized. However, the contribution of MCTs to energy expenditure is only small because they can be ingested only in small amounts without causing GI distress. Therefore, at present, fat supplementation (either LCTs or MCTs) during exercise cannot be recommended.

High-fat diets and fasting have been suggested to increase FFA availability and spare muscle glycogen, resulting in improved performance. Both fasting and short-term high-fat diets will decrease muscle glycogen content and reduce fatigue resistance. Chronic high-fat diets may provoke adaptive responses, preventing the decremental effects on exercise performance. Because there is little information about the negative effects of high-fat diets for athletes and the effects of those diets on performance are unclear, we suggest that caution should be exercised when recommending high-fat diets to athletes.

REFERENCES

1. Edwards HT, Margaria R, Dill DB. Metabolic rate, blood sugar and the utilization of carbohydrate. *Am J Physiol.* 1934;108:203–209.

2. Von Liebig J. *Animal Chemistry or Organic Chemistry in its Application to Physiology and Pathology.* London: Taylor and Walton; 1842.

3. Chauveau A. Source et nature du potentiel directment utilise dans le travail musculaire d'apres les exchanges respiratoires, chez l'homme en etat d'abstinance. *C R Acad Sci (Paris).* 1896;122:1163–1221.

4. Meyerhof O. *Chemical Dynamics of Life Phenomena.* Philadelphia: Lippincott; 1924.

5. Hill AV. *Muscular Activity*. Baltimore: Williams & Wilkins; 1926.

6. Zuntz N. Über die Bedeutung der verschiedene Nahrstoffe als Erzeuber der Muskelkraft. *Pflüglers Arch*. 1901;83:557–571.

7. Zuntz N. Über die Rolle des Zuckers in thierischen Stoffwechsel. *Arch Physiol*. 1896;538–577.

8. Krogh A, Lindhard J. The relative value of fat and carbohydrate as sources of muscular energy. *Bioch J*. 1920;14:290–363.

9. Christensen EH, Hansen O. Arbeitsfähigkeit und ernährung. *Scand Arch Physiol*. 1939;81:160–171.

10. Paul P. *Effects of Long Lasting Physical Exercise and Training on Lipid Metabolism. Metabolic Adaptation to Prolonged Physical Exercise*. Basel, Switzerland: Birkhauser Verlag; 1975:156–193.

11. Bergström J, Hultman E. Muscle glycogen synthesis after exercise: an enhancing factor localized in muscle cells in man. *Nature*. 1966;210:309–310.

12. Bergström J, Hermansen L, Hultman E, Saltin B. Diet, muscle glycogen and physical performance. *Acta Physiol Scand*. 1967;71:140–150.

13. Hultman E. Physiological role of muscle glycogen in man, with special reference to exercise. *Circ Res*. 1967;10:I-99–I-114.

14. Holloszy JO. *Utilization of Fatty Acids During Exercise. Exerc Sport Sci Rev*. Champaign, IL: Human Kinetics; 1988:319–327.

15. George JC, Jyoti D. Histological features of the breast and leg muscles of bird and bat and their physiological and evolutionary significance. *Evolution*. 1955:31–36.

16. Newsholme EA, Leech AR. *Biochemistry for the Medical Sciences*. Chichester, England: John Wiley & Sons; 1990.

17. Saltin B, Gollnick PD. *Skeletal Muscle Adaptability: Significance For Metabolism And Performance. Handbook Of Physiology*. Baltimore: Williams & Wilkins; 1983:555–661.

18. Essen B. Intramuscular substrate utilization during prolonged exercise. *Ann N Y Acad Sci*. 1977;301:30–44.

19. Hurley BF, Nemeth PM, Martin III WH, Hagberg JM, Dalsky GP, Holloszy JO. Muscle triglyceride utilization during exercise: effect of training. *J Appl Physiol*. 1986;60:562–567.

20. Brouns F, Saris WHM, Beckers E, et al. Metabolic changes induced by sustained exhaustive cycling and diet manipulation. *Int J Sports Med*. 1989;10:S49–S62.

21. Bjorkman O. *Fuel Utilization During Exercise. Biochemical Aspects of Physical Exercise*. Amsterdam: Elsevier; 1986:245–260.

22. McGilvery RW. *The Use Of Fuels For Muscular Work. Metabolic Adaptation To Prolonged Physical Exercise*. Basel, Switzerland: Birkhauser Verlag; 1975:12–30.

23. Van der Vusse GJ, Reneman RS. *Lipid Metabolism In Muscle. Handbook Of Physiology, Section 12: Exercise: Regulation and Integration of Multiple Systems*. New York: Oxford Press; 1996: 952–994.

24. Wolfe RR, Klein S, Carraro F, Weber J-M. Role of triglyceride-fatty acid cycle in controlling fat metabolism in humans during and after exercise. *Am J Physiol*. 1990;258:E382–E389.

25. Romijn JA, Coyle EF, Sidossis LS, Gastaldelli A, Horowitz JF, Endert E, Wolfe RR. Regulation of endogenous fat and carbohydrate metabolism in relation to exercise intensity. *Am J Physiol*. 1993;265:E380–E391.

26. Martin III WH, Dalsky GP, Hurley BF, Matthews DE, Bier DM, Hagberg JM, Rogers MA, King DS, Holloszy JO. Effect of endurance training on plasma free fatty acid turnover and oxidation during exercise. *Am J Physiol*. 1993;265:E708–E714.

27. Havel RJ, Pernow B, Jones NL. Uptake and release of free fatty acids and other metabolites in the legs of exercising men. *J Appl Physiol*. 1967;23:90–99.

28. Issekutz B, Miller HI, Paul P, Rodahl K. Source of fat in exercising dogs. *Am J Physiol*. 1964;207:583–589.

29. Kiens B, Lithell H. Lipoprotein metabolism influenced by training induced changes in human skeletal muscle. *J Clin Invest*. 1989;83:558–564.

30. Kiens B, Essen-Gustavsson B, Gad P, Lithell H. Lipoprotein lipase activity and intramuscular triglyceride stores after long-term high-fat and high-carbohydrate diets in physically trained men. *Clin Physiol*. 1987;7: 1–9.

31. Numa S. *Fatty Acid Metabolism And Its Regulation*. Amsterdam: Elsevier; 1984.

32. Saggerson ED, Carpenter CA. Carnitine palmitoyltransferase and carnitine octanoyltransferase activities in liver, kidney cortex, adipocyte, lactating mammary gland, skeletal muscle and heart. *FEBS Letter*. 1981;129:229–232.

33. Groot PHE, Hülsmann WE. The activation and oxidation of octanoate and palmitate by rat skeletal muscle mitochondria. *Biochim Biophys Acta*. 1973;316:124–135.

34. Phinney SD, Horton ES, Sims EAH, Hanson JS, Danforth E, LaGrange BM. Capacity for moderate exercise in obese subjects after adaptation to a hypocaloric, ketogenic diet. *J Clin Invest*. 1980;66:1152–1161.

35. Phinney SD, Bistrain BR, Wolfe RR, Blackburn GL. The human metabolic response to chronic ketosis without caloric restriction: physical and biochemical adaptation. *Metabolism*. 1983;32:757–768.

36. Phinney SD, Bistrian BR, Evans WJ, Gervino E, Blackburn GL. The human metabolic response to chronic ketosis without caloric restriction: preservation of submaximal exercise capability with reduced carbohydrate oxidation. *Metabolism*. 1983;32:769–776.

37. Holloszy JO, Booth W. Biochemical adaptations to endurance exercise in muscle. *Ann Rev Physiol.* 1976;38:273–291.

38. Holloszy JO, Coyle EF. Adaptations of skeletal muscle to endurance exercise and their metabolic consequences. *J Appl Physiol.* 1984;56:831–838.

39. Baldwin KM, Klinkerfuss GH, Terjung RL, Mole PA, Holloszy JO. Respiratory capacity of white, red, and intermediate muscle: adaptative response to exercise. *Am J Physiol.* 1972;222:373–378.

40. Gollnick PD, Saltin B. Significance of skeletal muscle oxidative enzyme enhancement with endurance training. *Clin Phys.* 1982;2:1–12.

41. Gollnick PD, Saltin B. *Fuel For Muscular Exercise. Exercise, Nutrition and Energy Metabolism.* New York: Macmillan Publishing Company; 1988:71–88.

42. Holloszy JO, Dalsky GP, Nemeth PM, Hurley BF, Martin III WH, Hagberg JM. *Utilization of Fat as Substrate During Exercise: Effect of Training. Biochemistry of Exercise VI.* Champaign, IL: Human Kinetics; 1986: 183–190.

43. Saltin B, Åstrand P-O. Free fatty acids and exercise. *Am J Clin Nutr.* 1993;57:752S–758S.

44. Coggan AR, Williams BD. *Metabolic Adaptations to Endurance Training: Substrate Metabolism during Exercise. Exercise metabolism.* Champaign, IL: Human Kinetics Publishers; 1995:41–71.

45. Coggan AR, Kohrt WM, Spina RJ, Bier DM, Holloszy JO. Endurance training decreases plasma glucose turnover and oxidation during moderate-intensity exercise in man. *J Appl Physiol.* 1990;68:990–996.

46. Costill DL, Coyle EF, Dalsky G, Evans W, Fink W, Hoopes D. Effects of elevated plasma FFA and insulin on muscle glycogen usage during exercise. *J Appl Physiol.* 1977;43:695–699.

47. Henriksson J. Training induced adaptation of skeletal muscle and metabolism during submaximal exercise. *J Physiol.* 1977;270:661–675.

48. Jansson E, Kaijser L. Substrate utilization and enzymes in skeletal muscle of extremely endurance-trained men. *J Appl Physiol.* 1987;62:999–1005.

49. Jeukendrup AE, Mensink M, Saris WHM, Wagenmakers AJM. Exogenous glucose oxidation during exercise in endurance-trained and untrained subjects. *J Appl Physiol.* 1997;82:835–840.

50. Newsholme EA. *Metabolic Causes of Fatigue in Track Events and the Marathon. Advances in Myochemistry.* Montrouge, France: John Libbey Eurotext Ltd.; 1989: 263–271.

51. Hunt JN, Knox MT. *Regulation of Gastric Emptying. Handbook of Physiology.* Bethesda, MD: American Physiological Society; 1968:1917–1935.

52. Oscai LB, Essig DA, Palmer WK. Lipase regulation of muscle triglyceride hydrolysis. *J Appl Physiol.* 1990;69:1571–1577.

53. Jeukendrup AE, Saris WHM, Schrauwen P, Brouns F, Wagenmakers AJM. Metabolic availability of medium chain triglycerides co-ingested with carbohydrates during prolonged exercise. *J Appl Physiol.* 1995;79:756–762.

54. Van Zeyl CG, Lambert EV, Hawley JA, Noakes TD, Dennis SC. Effects of medium-chain triglyceride ingestion on carbohydrate metabolism and cycling performance. *J Appl Physiol.* 1996;80:2217–2225.

55. Vukovich MD, Costill DL, Hickey MS, Trappe SW, Cole KJ, Fink WJ. Effect of fat emulsion infusion and fat feeding on muscle glycogen utilization during cycle exercise. *J Appl Physiol.* 1993;75:1513–1518.

56. Issekutz B, Miller HI, Rodahl K. Lipid and carbohydrate metabolism during exercise. *Fed Proc.* 1966;25:1415 1420.

57. Hickson RC, Rennie MJ, Conlee RK, Winder WW, Holloszy JO. Effect of increased plasma fatty acids on glycogen utilization and endurance. *J Appl Physiol.* 1977;43:829–833.

58. Rennie MJ, Winder WW. A sparing effect of increased plasma fatty acids on muscle and liver glycogen content in the exercising rat. *Biochem J.* 1976;156:647–655.

59. Beckers EJ, Jeukendrup AE, Brouns F, Wagenmakers AJM, Saris WHM. Gastric emptying of carbohydrate-medium chain triglyceride suspensions at rest. *Int J Sports Med.* 1992;13:581–584.

60. Ivy JL, Costill DL, Fink WJ, Maglischo E. Contribution of medium and long chain triglyceride intake to energy metabolism during prolonged exercise. *Int J Sports Med.* 1980;1:15–20.

61. Jeukendrup AE, Saris WHM, Van Diesen R, Brouns F, Wagenmakers AJM. Effect of endogenous carbohydrate availability on oral medium-chain triglyceride oxidation during prolonged exercise. *J Appl Physiol.* 1996; 80:949 954.

62. Jeukendrup AE, Wagenmakers AJM, Brouns F, Halliday D, Saris WHM. Effects of carbohydrate (CHO) and fat supplementation on CHO metabolism during prolonged exercise. *Metabolism.* 1996;45:915–921.

63. Jeukendrup AE, Thielen JJHC, Wagenmakers AJM, Brouns F, Saris WHM. Effect of MCT and carbohydrate ingestion on substrate utilization and cycling performance. *Am J Clin Nutr.* 1998; in press.

64. Koubi HE, Desplanches D, Gabrielle C, Cottet-Emard JM, Sempore B, Favier RJ. Exercise endurance and fuel utilization: a reevaluation of the effects of fasting. *J Appl Physiol.* 1991;70:1337–1343.

65. Dohm GL, Tapscott EB, Barakat HA, Kasperek GJ. Influence of fasting on glycogen depletion in rats during exercise. *J Appl Physiol.* 1983;55:830–833.

66. Dohm GL, Beeker RT, Israel RG, Tapscott EB. Metabolic responses after fasting. *J Appl Physiol.* 1986;61:1363–1368.

67. Knapik JJ, Meredith CN, Jones BH, Suek L, Young VR, Evans WJ. Influence of fasting on carbohydrate and fat metabolism during rest and exercise in men. *J Appl Physiol.* 1988;64:1923–1929.

68. Loy SF, Conlee RK, Winder WW, Nelson AG, Arnall DA, Fisher AG. Effect of 24-hour fast on cycling endurance time at two different intensities. *J Appl Physiol.* 1986;61:654–659.

69. Zinker BA, Britz K, Brooks GA. Effects of a 36-hour fast on human endurance and substrate utilization. *J Appl Physiol.* 1990;69:1849–1855.

70. Gleeson M, Greenhaff PL, Maughan RJ. Influence of a 24 h fast on high intensity cycle exercise performance in man. *Eur J Appl Physiol.* 1988;57:653–659.

71. Riley ML, Israel RG, Holbert D, Tapscott EB, Dohm GL. Effect of carbohydrate ingestion on exercise endurance and metabolism after 1-day fast. *Int J Sports Med.* 1988;9:320–324.

72. Hultman E, Bergstrom J. Muscle glycogen synthesis in relation to diet studied in normal subjects. *Acta Med Scand.* 1967;182:109–117.

73. Conlee RK, Hammer RL, Winder WW, Bracken ML, Nelson AG, Barnett DW. Glycogen repletion and exercise endurance in rats adapted to a high fat diet. *Metabolism.* 1990;39:289–294.

74. Martin B, Robinson S, Robertshaw D. Influence of diet on leg uptake of glucose during heavy exercise. *Am J Clin Nutr.* 1978;31:62–67.

75. Maughan RJ, Williams C, Campbell DM, Hepburn D. Fat and carbohydrate metabolism during low intensity exercise: effects of the availability of muscle glycogen. *Eur J Appl Physiol.* 1978;39:7–16.

76. Miller WC, Bryce R, Conlee RK. Adaptations to a high-fat diet that increase exercise endurance in male rats. *J Appl Physiol.* 1984;56:78–83.

77. Jansson E, Kaijser L. Effect of diet on the utilization of blood-borne and intramuscular substrates during exercise in man. *Acta Physiol Scand.* 1982;115:19–30.

78. Fery F, Balasse EO. Ketone body turnover during and after exercise in overnight-fasted and starved humans. *Am J Physiol.* 1983;245:E18–E25.

79. Stankiewicz-Choroszucha B, Gorski J. Effect of decreased availability of substrates on intramuscular triglyceride utilization during exercise. *Eur J Appl Physiol.* 1978;40:27–35.

80. Jansson E. Diet and muscle metabolism in man. *Acta Physiol Scand.* 1980;487:1–24.

81. Simi B, Sempore B, Mayet M-H, Favier RJ. Additive effects of training and high-fat diet on energy metabolism during exercise. *J Appl Physiol.* 1991;71:197–203.

82. Lambert EV, Speechly DP, Dennis SC, Noakes TD. Enhanced endurance in trained cyclists during moderate intensity exercise following 2 weeks adaptation to a high fat diet. *Eur J Appl Physiol.* 1994;69:287–293.

83. Pendergast DR, Horvath PJ, Leddy JJ, Venkatraman JT. The role of dietary fat on performance, metabolism and health. *Am J Sports Med.* 1996;24:S53–S58.

84. Sarna S, Kaprio J. Life expectancy of former elite athletes. *Sports Med.* 1994;17:49–51.

85. Pan DA, Lillioja S, Kriketos AD, Milner MR, Baur LA, Bogardus C, Jenkins AB, Storlien LH. Skeletal muscle triglyceride levels are inversely related to insulin action. *Diabetes.* 1997;46:983–988.

86. Guezennec CY, Nadaud JF, Satabin P, Léger F, Lafargue P. Influence of polyunsaturated fatty acid diet on the hemorrheological response to physical exercise in hypoxia. *Int J Sports Med.* 1989;10:286–291.

87. Brilla LR, Landerholm LR. Effect of fish oil supplementation on serum lipids and aerobic fitness. *J Sports Med Phys Fitness.* 1990;30:173–180.

88. Kamada T, Tokuda S, Aozaki S-I, Otsuji S. Higher levels of erythrocyte membrane fluidity in sprinters and long-distance runners. *J Appl Physiol.* 1993;74:354–358.

CHAPTER 5

Minerals and Trace Minerals

Emily M. Haymes and Priscilla M. Clarkson

Recognition that dietary mineral sources were essential to health began in the latter part of the 19th century.[1] However, use of mineral salts (for example, magnesium) for therapeutic purposes dates back at least two centuries.[2] Recommended dietary allowances (RDA) have been established for only the following seven minerals: calcium, phosphorus, magnesium, iron, zinc, selenium, and iodine.[3] Additionally, estimated safe and adequate daily dietary intake (ESADDI) has been established for five other trace minerals. See Table 5–1 for the RDA and ESADDIs of minerals discussed in this chapter.

Minerals are inorganic chemical elements commonly found in the foods we consume. Approximately 4% of the human body mass is composed of 21 minerals that are essential for life. Those minerals found in larger quantities (more than 5 g) in humans are classified as macrominerals whereas those found in smaller quantities (less than 5 g) are known as trace minerals. Macrominerals include (in descending order of magnitude) calcium, phosphorus, potassium, sulfur, sodium, chlorine, and magnesium. The following (also in descending order of magnitude) are included among the trace minerals:

Table 5–1 Recommended Dietary Allowances (RDA) and Estimated Safe and Adequate Daily Dietary Intake (ESADDI) for Minerals, 1989

| | RDA | | | | | | ESADDI | |
| | Males | | | Females | | | | |
Mineral	15–18	19–24	25–50	15–18	19–24	25–50	Adolescents	Adults
Calcium, mg/d	1200	1200	800	1200	1200	800		
Phosphorus, mg/d	1200	1200	800	1200	1200	800		
Magnesium, mg/d	400	350	350	300	280	280		
Iron, mg/d	12	12	10	15	15	15		
Zinc, mg/d	15	15	15	12	12	12		
Selenium, µg/d	50	70	70	50	55	55		
Copper, mg/d							1.5–2.5	1.5–3.0
Chromium, µg/d							50–200	50–200

Source: Adapted with permission from *Recommended Dietary Allowances*, 10th ed., © 1989, National Academy Press.

iron, fluoride, zinc, copper, silicon, vanadium, tin, nickel, selenium, manganese, iodine, molybdenum, chromium, and cobalt.

Use of mineral supplements by athletes is common in the United States. In one study of Ironman triathletes, the four most widely used mineral supplements were, in descending order, iron, zinc, calcium, and selenium.[4] Daily mineral supplement use by marathon runners was reported as the following: calcium, 7%, zinc, 4%, and iron, 2.3%.[5] In another study of elite female marathon runners, 21% took zinc supplements and 18% took copper supplements.[6] In this chapter, we will examine the effects of exercise on mineral requirements and homeostasis, dietary intakes by athletes, and effects of supplementation for three macrominerals (calcium, phosphorus, and magnesium) and five trace minerals (iron, zinc, copper, chromium, and selenium).

CALCIUM

The mineral found in the largest quantity in the body is calcium, making up 1.5% to 2.0% of the body weight. Most of the calcium (99%) is found in the skeleton where it forms salts primarily with phosphorus. Much of the remaining 1% is found in the extracellular fluids where it plays important roles in neuromuscular transmission and blood coagulation. A small, but significant amount is found inside muscle fibers where its release from the sarcoplasmic reticulum initiates the muscle contraction process. Plasma calcium concentration is maintained within a narrow range (2.2 to 2.5 mmol/L) by two hormones, parathyroid hormone (PTH) and calcitonin. PTH release is stimulated when plasma calcium decreases to below normal. PTH then stimulates 1) bone resorption, which increases the release of calcium from bones, 2) tubular reabsorption of calcium from the filtrate in the kidneys, and 3) activation of vitamin D $(1,25(OH)_2D_3)$, which facilitates increased absorption of calcium in the small intestine. The result is restoration of the plasma calcium concentration. Calcitonin release, stimulated by increased plasma calcium concentration, restores plasma calcium by stimulating increased calcium uptake for bone formation.

Because bone serves as a calcium reservoir, inadequate dietary calcium intake may have a negative effect on bone mass. This is especially true during growth when bones are increasing in length as well as mass. Adequate intake for calcium is greatest (1300 mg/d) during adolescence (ages 9 to 18 years). Adults (19 years old and older) have an adequate intake for calcium of 1000 mg/d. The age at which peak bone mass is achieved varies according to the bone site measured. Cross-sectional studies suggest bone mineral density (BMD) at the proximal femur and lumbar vertebrae reaches its peak at age 18 years,[7] and peak trabecular and cortical BMD of the distal forearm is reached at 15 and 16.5 years, respectively, in females.[8] However, longitudinal research suggests peak BMD in the lumbar vertebrae and forearm bones is reached at 29.5 and 28.3 years, respectively.[9]

Calcium Balance and Physical Activity

Calcium balance is the relationship between calcium intake and calcium loss. If the intake of calcium exceeds the amount lost, the person is in positive calcium balance. Negative calcium balance occurs when calcium losses exceed calcium intake. Positive calcium balance is required for bone growth whereas negative calcium balance leads to loss of BMD and bone mass. Calcium loss is the sum of the calcium excreted in the feces, urine, and sweat. In most studies of calcium balance, only fecal and urinary calcium are actually measured whereas the dermal calcium is estimated as 60 mg/d.[10] Unfortunately, this may lead to an underestimation of actual calcium loss because of incomplete collection of excreta and dermal loss estimates that are too low. One study has reported sweat calcium losses during exercise of 57 mg/h.[11]

Calcium balance studies of subjects from infancy through age 30 years were undertaken to determine the threshold calcium intake (calcium intake above which calcium retention is not enhanced by increasing calcium intake).[12] Threshold calcium intake was estimated to be 1090 mg/d for infants (0 to 1 years old), 1390 mg/d for children (2 to 8 years old) 1480 mg/d for adolescents (9 to 17 years old), and 957 mg/d for young adults (18 to 30 years old). Adolescents with calcium intakes in the lowest quartile (below 682 mg/d) were in negative calcium balance whereas young adults with calcium intakes in the first and second quartiles (below 963 mg/d) were also in negative calcium balance.[10]

There is considerable evidence that both calcium intake and physical activity affect bone density of female adults. Bone mineral content (BMC) and BMD of the radius at distal and midshaft sites are significantly greater in women who are premenopausal (20 to 50 years) who have lifetime calcium intakes greater than 500 mg/d compared to women with lower lifetime calcium intakes.[13] Women with high levels of lifetime physical activity (longer than 45 min/d, 4 to 7 d/wk of moderate to strenuous activities) also have significantly greater radial BMC and greater BMD at the distal site than women with moderate or low lifetime physical activity. Other studies have also reported significant associations between current or lifetime calcium intake and BMD.[14–17] Two studies found vertebral BMD was significantly associated with physical activity in young adult females.[9,15] In other studies, calcaneal BMD was reported to be significantly higher in young women who were very active as children, and radial BMD was found to be higher in young adult females who had participated in sports at age 12 years.[14,18] Weight-bearing activity was significantly related to change in BMD of boys ages 8 to 16 years and girls before adolescence, but not adolescent girls.[8] However, two other studies found no significant relationships between either current calcium intake or physical activity of young adult females and BMD at several sites.[18,19]

Calcium Intake

Many females consume diets that contain less calcium than the RDA of 1200 mg/d. Dietary intake data collected during the third National Health and Nutrition Examination Survey (NHANES III) indicated that adolescent females (16 to 19 years) had a mean calcium intake of 822 mg/d, young adult females (20 to 29 years) had a mean intake of 778 mg/d, and females age 30 years and older had mean intakes less than 760 mg/d.[20] In contrast, adolescent males (16 to 19 years) had a mean calcium intake of 1274 mg/d, slightly above the RDA. Studies conducted on the dietary intake of athletes have also found some adolescent females, especially gymnasts,[21,22] ballet dancers (Benson et al),[23] and distance runners,[24] have calcium intakes well below the RDA. However, not all adolescent athletes have low calcium intakes, as has been shown by other studies of swimmers and soccer players.[25,26] Low dietary calcium intake is also common among female collegiate athletes (Table 5–2).[27–31] Most male athletes consume adequate calcium because of their greater energy intake.[29,32] Despite calcium intakes below the RDA, female college gymnasts were found to have significantly higher lumbar, proximal femur, and whole body BMDs than matched controls,[30] and a significant increase in lumbar BMD of female collegiate gymnasts was found after 6 months of training.[33]

Inadequate calcium intake in female athletes is of concern not only because peak adult bone mass may not be achieved but also because lower bone density increases the risk of stress fractures. Lower lumbar and femoral BMDs have been found more frequently in female and male athletes who experienced stress fractures in the lower extremities than in uninjured athletic control subjects who were matched for body weight and training distance.[34] Intake of calcium and dairy products was significantly lower in the athletes who had stress fractures. Female athletes with stress fractures were also more likely to have irregular menstrual cycles. Female ballet dancers who had experienced stress fractures were less likely to consume dairy products than dancers without stress fractures, but there was no significant difference in calcium intake between the two groups.[35] In older adults, the inci-

Table 5–2 Calcium Intakes of Selected North American Athletes

Sport	Age (yrs)	Level	Sex	Calcium Intake (mg/d)	Reference
Ballet	14.6	Adolescent	F	933	23
Gymnastics	15.2	High school	F	707	21
Gymnastics	11–14	Elite juniors	F	867	22
Running	17.1	High school	F	812	24
Soccer	15.3	High school	F	1316	26
	15.3	High school	M	1372	26
Swimming	15.5	High school	F	1623	26
	15.0	High school	M	1901	26
Swimming	15.0	Elite juniors	F	1235	25
	16.0	Elite juniors	M	1634	25
Ballet	24.4	Elite	F	821	27
	26.0	Elite	M	1031	27
Basketball	19.6	College	F	816	28
		College	M	2116	29
Gymnastics	19.7	College	F	747	30
		College	M	1041	29
Lacrosse		College	F	798	29
		College	M	1805	29
Running, marathon	29.1	Elite	F	1227	31
Skiing, Nordic	20.0	Elite	F	1188	32
	22.0	Elite	M	1966	32
Swimming	18.4	College	F	1087	28
Volleyball	19.6	College	F	865	28

dence of hip fractures was lower in females and males who had higher lifetime calcium intakes (more than 800 mg/d) than in females and males with low lifetime calcium intakes.[16]

There are numerous reports of low BMD among female athletes who are amenorrheic.[36–39] Resumption of normal menstrual cycles by athletes was accompanied by an increase in vertebral BMD, but it was also reported that most of these athletes had increased their calcium intake as well.[40] Another study examined the effects of calcium (1200 mg/d) and vitamin D (400 IU/d) supplements on lumbar BMD of adolescent runners with amenorrhea and eumenorrhea. Even though the calcium intake of the runners with amenorrhea was significantly higher, lumbar BMD decreased in two of the runners with amenorrhea over 1 year. Runners with amenorrhea experience more running-related injuries than runners with eumenorrhea,[41] and an in-

creased incidence of stress fractures.[42] Recent evidence suggests a relationship between disordered eating, amenorrhea, and osteoporosis (that is, female athlete triad). Elite female athletes with the eating disorder anorexia nervosa were found to have a very low mean calcium intake of 373 mg/d whereas those classified as anorexia athletica also had a low mean calcium intake of 983 mg/d.[43]

Calcium Supplementation

Numerous studies have examined the effects of calcium supplementation on increasing bone mass and density during growth as well as its effect of decreasing the rate of bone loss in females who are postmenopausal. Children who were prepubertal and who received 300 mg of calcium carbonate/d for 18 months increased the BMC of the distal radius at a significantly faster rate than children who received a placebo; however, there was no difference in height gain between groups.[44] In pairs of identical twins who received either 1000 mg of calcium citrate malate per day or a placebo, the twins who were prepubertal and who received the calcium supplement for 3 years had significantly greater increases in radial and lumbar BMD than their placebo twin.[45] However, there were no significant differences in BMD increases at any site between twin pairs who were pubertal and postpubertal who received calcium supplementation and those who received a placebo. The investigators suggested calcium supplementation was more beneficial before than during puberty because sex hormones were the primary stimulators of bone growth during puberty.[45]

The diets of adolescent females (age 14 years) were supplemented with calcium carbonate or milk (900 mg calcium/d) for 2 years.[46] Although forearm and vertebral BMD increased, there were no significant differences between the treatment and control groups. Several other studies examined the effects of calcium citrate malate supplements on BMC and BMD of adolescent females. Female subjects (x = 11.4 years) received either 500 or 1000 mg/d of calcium citrate malate or a placebo for 6 months.[47] Total BMC increased in all subjects, but the subjects who received 1000 mg/d gained significantly more BMC than the placebo group. After 18 months of a calcium citrate malate supplement (500 mg calcium/d), lumbar and total BMD increases were significantly greater in the adolescent females (x = 12 years) who received calcium supplements than in the placebo groups.[48] One possible explanation for the differences in results among the studies could be the variation in age of the subjects. It has been found that calcium absorption is significantly higher in females in early puberty (x = 10.9 years) than in females who are prepubertal (x = 7.7 years) and those in puberty (x = 15.2 years).[49] Furthermore, calcium retention was significantly higher in females in early puberty and those who are prepubertal than in females who are in late puberty. Calcium supplements appear to be more effective in increasing BMD in children before puberty, and in females in early puberty than in those who are in the latter stages of puberty.

Results of calcium supplementation studies of women who are postmenopausal are equivocal. For the first 5 years after the onset of menopause, calcium supplements appear to have little effect in reducing the rate at which bone mass is lost.[50-53] However, there is some evidence that women who are postmenopausal who take calcium carbonate supplements (1500 mg/d) have reduced rates of bone loss[54] and a lower risk of vertebral fractures.[55] Calcium supplements may be more beneficial when combined with estrogen replacement therapy in slowing the loss in bone mass.[50] In older women (more than 5 years since menopause onset), supplementing the dietary calcium intake appears more effective in reducing bone loss. In older women who are postmenopausal (age = 60 years), a milk supplement (831 mg/d) taken for 1 year significantly increased the BMD at the proximal femur but not at lumbar or radial sites whereas a walking program slightly increased lumbar BMD.[56] Use of a 500-mg calcium supplement (calcium citrate malate) significantly reduced the decrease in BMD of the lumbar vertebrae, proximal femur, and radius over 2 years in older women who are postmenopausal (x = 60 years).[53] The investigators also observed that the calcium citrate malate supplement was more effective than calcium carbonate in reducing bone loss. Finally, use of a 1000-mg calcium supplement over 4 years significantly reduced the rate of total body BMD decline as well as the decline in BMD at the lumbar vertebrae and proximal femur in women who are postmenopausal (x = 58 years).[57] Women in the placebo group experienced significantly more fractures (hip, forearm, and vertebral) than women who took calcium supplements during the 4-year period.

It is recommended that most forms of calcium supplements be ingested in small quantities (500 mg or less per dose) between meals to enhance their absorption.[58] The exception is calcium carbonate, which requires gastric acid for optimal absorption. Consumption of some calcium supplements will also inhibit the absorption of nonheme iron from food.[59] This could lead to a reduction in iron stores and possibly anemia. Calcium supplements that contain citrate enhance rather than inhibit iron absorption.[58]

Summary

Both calcium intake and physical activity are important factors influencing peak bone mass in young adults. However, not all female athletes consume the recommended dietary intake for calcium of 1200 mg/d. Because low dietary calcium intake is associated with an increased risk of stress fractures, athletes should consume diets that contain adequate calcium. Dairy products are primary sources of calcium in the diet.[3] Other good sources of calcium include green leafy vegetables (for example, broccoli, turnip greens), tofu, canned fish, and calcium-fortified foods (for example, orange juice, fruit drinks).[58] Calcium supplementation appears to be more beneficial in preventing bone loss when women are 60 years and older than immediately after menopause.

MAGNESIUM

Magnesium plays a role in a wide variety of biochemical and physiologic processes that are important to exercise performance. It is involved in excitation contraction coupling, serves as a modulator of many rate-limiting enzymes, is an essential co-factor in enzymes in carbohydrate metabolism, and is involved in muscle and nerve excitability by maintaining electrical potentials at the membrane.[3,60,61] Numerous ATP-dependent reactions use magnesium as a co-factor.[61]

The body contains about 10 to 28 g of magnesium with a distribution of about 60% in bones, 26% in muscle, 6% to 7% in other cells, and about 1% in the extracellular fluid.[60,62] During exercise, there appears to be a shift in the distribution whereby magnesium levels change in the blood. It is not clear why this occurs, but it is thought that magnesium is released from storage into the blood so that it can be made available for other tissues.

The RDA for adults older than 19 years is 350 mg/d for males and 280 mg/d for females, and for ages 15 to 18 years, the recommended values are 400 mg and 300 mg, respectively.[3] Green leafy vegetables, unrefined grains, nuts, and legumes are rich in magnesium.[60,61] For the general population, NHANES III data[20] showed that white teenage boys and girls had low intakes, and adult men had adequate intake, but not adult women. Minority groups, especially non-Hispanic blacks, had low intakes of magnesium.

Because magnesium functions in many processes necessary for exercise, it is important that athletes have adequate status. Magnesium status could be compromised if athletes are not ingesting sufficient amounts of magnesium, and/or exercise causes a loss in magnesium. However, when magnesium intake is very low, urinary excretion of magnesium is reduced within 4 to 6 days.[63] Also, absorption appears to be inversely related to the amount of magnesium in the diet. The interactions among exercise, magnesium intake, and magnesium excretion are not known. For example, the body may be able to account for any loss of magnesium due to exercise by increasing absorption even if inadequate amounts of magnesium are ingested. For more information on magnesium and exercise, Brilla and Lombardi[64] have presented a detailed review of this topic.

Dietary Intake and Status of Athletes

Based on self-reported dietary records, the intake of magnesium for most athlete groups is at least two thirds the RDA or above.[31,65–71] Athletes who may not be ingesting sufficient amounts are those attempting to maintain low body weights, such as dancers, gymnasts, light-weight crew, wrestlers, and jockeys. For example, 41% of adolescent gymnasts[72] and 43.4% of adolescent ballet dancers did not ingest two thirds of the RDA. Fifty-two percent of wrestlers during the mid-season and about 30% before and after the season ingested less than two thirds the RDA for magnesium.[73] There is a positive correlation between magnesium intake and energy (caloric) intake so that athletes who are obtaining sufficient energy in their diets should be getting sufficient magnesium.[74] However, athletes who are restricting caloric intake may be concerned that their magnesium ingestion is suboptimal.

An athlete's magnesium status is determined from plasma or erythrocyte concentrations. These methods are questioned because they may not reflect magnesium levels in tissues. Extracellular magnesium represents only approximately 1% of the total body magnesium, and several factors, including acute exercise or stress, can alter these levels.[61] To accurately determine magnesium status, it is recommended that renal magnesium excretion be assessed after administration of an intravenous (IV) magnesium load.[62,63] A decrease in excretion would indicate impaired status.[61] Intracellular measures of magnesium from muscle biopsy samples may also provide accurate information about tissue status.[63] Thus, levels of magnesium in the blood do not accurately reflect tissue stores, but may provide an estimate of magnesium nutriture.

Most studies report that athletes have resting serum magnesium levels within the normal range,[67,75–80] but low serum magnesium levels, especially with overtraining, have also been found.[81] Kleiner et al[82] found that for male and female body builders, the males had serum magnesium levels above the normal range, but females had slightly lower than normal levels despite the fact that their intake was higher than the RDA. Data for athletes maintaining low body weights do not exist. One report[76] showed that 14% of Finnish athletes did not ingest adequate magnesium in their diet but blood magnesium levels were adequate. Whether this reflects the body's ability to maintain status under less than advantageous magnesium intake or that blood magnesium is simply too gross a measure of status is not known. Trained runners had lower blood magnesium levels than sedentary subjects, and it was suggested that these athletes could suffer from magnesium deficiency.[64,75] The implication of low blood magnesium levels in some athletes remains to be determined.

Effects of Exercise

Evidence exists that exercise could lower magnesium status.[83] Some studies have shown that urinary excretion of magnesium increases as a result of exercise,[84–86] and there may be a very small loss of magnesium in the sweat.[87] The reason for the increased excretion of magnesium is not clear but may be related to the redistribution of magnesium during exercise.[74] Once released from stores, magnesium is either used or lost in the urine. Also, hormones [aldosterone and antidiuretic hormone (ADH)] that regulate magnesium handling by the kidneys are increased by strenuous exercise.[74]

Plasma magnesium levels during a 2-hour run on a treadmill at 60% to 65% of VO_{2max} were found to decline throughout the exercise with the lowest value occurring at the end of the exercise.[88] Values approached resting level 1 hour after exercise. Blood levels of magnesium were significantly lower than baseline after 30 minutes of swimming in well-trained swimmers,[89,90] a 120-km hike[91] in well-trained young men, a marathon race,[92,93] high-intensity anaerobic treadmill running,[84] a 40-minute run,[94,95] a 140-minute volleyball practice,[95] 12 minutes of cycling at 80% anaerobic threshold,[96] and during a 20-day road race.[97]

The reason for the decline in magnesium levels in the blood with exercise is unclear. Erythrocytes are known to take up magnesium.[64,84,98] However, both plasma and erythrocyte magnesium were found to decrease after a marathon.[85] Although adipocytes[92] were thought to take up magnesium during exercise to stimulate free fatty acid (FFA) release, when FFA release was suppressed, the decrease in magnesium was not prevented.[88] Magnesium may be needed for muscle during exercise to assist with metabolic processes.[64]

High-intensity anaerobic exercise results in increased magnesium levels in the blood, but this could, in part, be attributed to changes in plasma volume.[64] One study[90] reported that after an exercise causing muscle damage, magnesium levels in the blood were increased for up to 24 hours, perhaps indicating a release from damaged muscle cells. An increase in plasma magnesium levels was found immediately after a 100-km race, and this increase correlated with plasma creatinine levels, which could indicate a transient renal failure during prolonged endurance exercise.[99] Because an increase in plasma creatine kinase activity (an enzyme released from damaged muscle) was also found, increased magnesium in the blood may be due to release from damaged muscle fibers.

During exercise, magnesium excretion appears to be reduced but then increases after exercise.[85] Magnesium levels were higher in the 24-hour urine samples taken the day subjects participated in high-intensity, anaerobic exercise.[84] Although these data show an increased urinary excretion, at this time we cannot state with any certainty that exercise causes a net loss in magnesium from the body. Also, although one study reported an increase in urinary excretion of magnesium at the start of an exercise program, after 5 weeks of training, the levels began to return to values that appeared before training.[86] Nor can we say that if exercise does result in some loss, that it is not made up by dietary intake.

No magnesium balance studies have been done with athletes. Data on magnesium status on athletes have been obtained only from blood samples that provide an estimation. Furthermore, in a study in which plasma and erythrocyte magnesium levels were assessed after 1 month of daily prolonged training, there was no significant change in these levels.[96] Training results in a decrease in red-blood-cell magnesium, which could suggest a redistribution of magnesium into muscle or plasma with training.[100] Although resistance training resulted in increased urinary excretion of magnesium in 4 weeks of training, excretion rates returned to initial values during the last 4 weeks of training.[86] These data suggest an adaptation to conserve the body's magnesium.

A few reports show that low magnesium status may have negative consequences. A female tennis player with low blood magnesium levels suffered carpopedal spasms that were reversed by magnesium supplements.[101] One study found that the decrease in serum magnesium levels during a 100-mile cycling race was related to the incidence of muscle cramps.[102] Cramps that miners experience by working in a hot environment may be due to magnesium loss because there is a relationship between sweat magnesium loss and the incidence of cramps.[74] Bodybuilders use magnesium supplements to prevent muscle cramps.[64]

In a case study report, a 23-year-old well-trained man, not acclimatized to heat, displayed epileptic-type convulsions immediately after 4 hours of continuous exercise in the heat.[103] Before this, he completed the identical exercise test but at room temperature with no symptoms. Before the exercise began, his serum magnesium level was abnormally low. The decrease in serum magnesium during exercise has been found to be greater in the heat for persons who are not acclimatized. The 23-year-old patient began the exercise test (that resulted in convulsions) with a low serum magnesium level and he was not acclimatized so that the decrease during exercise produced dangerously low magnesium levels. After supplementation with magnesium as well as acclimatization to the heat, the subject repeated the same exercise with no problem.

Although these case reports are interesting, at present there is not sufficient reason to be concerned that athletes in general have any magnesium deficiency. Certainly, some persons may appear to be susceptible. If athletes chronically experience muscle spasms or cramps, it is advisable to have their blood levels of magnesium checked before supplementing with magnesium.

Magnesium Supplementation

If future research shows that persons are not ingesting sufficient magnesium to account for any loss due to exercise and there is no adaptation to conserve magnesium, there may be reason to believe that magnesium supplements are warranted. However, this appears to be unlikely. Furthermore, few studies suggest that magnesium status is related to performance. Although one study[104] demonstrated a relationship between plasma magnesium and VO_{2max}, the relationship was found for athletes but not for nonathletes, with no apparent reason for the difference.

Fourteen days of magnesium supplementation (15 mmol magnesium-L-aspartate-hydrochloride) in nine healthy males resulted in an 8% increase in plasma magnesium content and a 27% increase in erythrocyte magnesium content.[105] Rather than an expected increase in urinary output, the resting urinary magnesium excretion was unchanged over the course of supplementation. These findings may suggest that the supplement resulted in increased magnesium storage. Magnesium supplementation (250 mg/day) for 12 weeks produced an increase in plasma magnesium in a group who trained with both anaerobic and aerobic exercise, but there was no change in a group who participated only in aerobic exercise during the 12-week period.[100] Thus, the type of training may influence magnesium needs.

When subjects ingested 14.8 mmol/d of magnesium or a placebo for 1 month, plasma and erythrocyte magnesium were higher after exercise in the group who received supplements compared with the placebo group.[94] It was suggested that the decrease in plasma magnesium with exercise could be counteracted by adequate magnesium supplementation. Because we do not know the reason for the exercise-induced decrease in plasma magnesium, the significance of these results is unclear.

Magnesium-L-aspartate-hydrochloride administered three times per day (equivalent of 365 mg/d) for 10 weeks did not increase serum or muscle magnesium concentration, had no effect on performance of the marathon, and had no effect on the recovery of muscle damage induced by the marathon.[106] This 10-week period included 4 weeks before the marathon race and 6 weeks after the marathon. Because the runners had adequate magnesium status before the supplementation, the authors concluded that magnesium supplementation would have no beneficial effect on those with adequate status.

Studies have suggested a relationship between strength and magnesium status.[107,108] One study reported that a magnesium oxide supplement that increased magnesium intake, including diet, to 8 mg/kg body weight/d for 7 weeks resulted in greater isokinetic strength of the knee extensors compared to the placebo group.[107] The results of this study should be considered preliminary because magnesium status of the subjects was not assessed, the placebo group had an average magnesium intake that was less than the RDA, the sample size was small, and magnesium oxide has low bioavailability. Although the authors suggested that magnesium may aid protein synthesis, the mechanism to explain this is unclear.

Summary

There is reason to be concerned that strenuous exercise training could result in a net loss of magnesium; however, there are no data at present to confirm this. No magnesium balance studies have been done with athletes. To automatically supplement with magnesium is not recommended because of the interaction that magnesium has with other minerals. For example, magnesium and calcium are antagonistic such that excess magnesium could impair bone calcification,[61] which could have serious consequences for young female athletes. The composition of the diet may also affect magnesium balance because it has been shown that both low and very high protein intakes are associated with impaired magnesium retention.[61] Although a multivitamin mineral supplement containing no more than the RDA may not be harmful, a diet rich in magnesium is recommended.

PHOSPHATE

About 85% (850 g) of the body's phosphorus is found in bone.[109] Phosphorus mostly exists as phosphate esters in soft tissue[3] and has numerous functions. In addition to its structural role in bone and teeth, it is a component of nucleic acids and membranes, and participates in energy metabolism, particularly in the form of high-energy phosphates. Diets are generally adequate in phosphate,[3] because phosphorus is ubiquitously present in foods. The RDA for males and females aged 11 to 24 years is 1200 mg and for those older than 25 years, it is reduced to 800 mg.

Athletes' diets are generally adequate in phosphate and it is unlikely that they would incur a deficiency. Absorbed phosphate by the body is linearly related to both ingested phosphate and urinary phosphate.[61] Thus, the body is well able to adapt to fluctuations in phosphate intake. The interest in phosphate in sports is mainly due to its use in acute high doses (referred to as phosphate loading) to improve performance. High amounts of phosphorus over a long period could decrease intestinal calcium absorption.[109]

Phosphate Loading

Studies that have investigated the effects of phosphate loading are equivocal. Phosphate loading involves ingesting a large amount of phosphate in the form of phosphate salts (usually 4 g/d) for several days before or immediately before a competitive event. One study[110] found that 1 g neutral-buffered sodium phosphate taken four times per day for 3 days resulted in an increase in VO_{2max} and a reduction in the increase in blood lactate compared to the placebo group. Another study[111] had eight trained cyclists ingest 3.6 g sodium phosphate or placebo for 3 days and found that VO_{2max} was significantly higher in the phosphate loading condition.

Two studies from the same laboratory documented beneficial effects from having highly trained athletes ingest 1 g of tribasic sodium phosphate or a placebo four times a day for several days before testing.[112,113] One study found that there was a significant 10.1% increase in maximal oxygen uptake and an 11.8-second nonsignificant reduction in performance time for the 5-mile run in the phosphate loading trial. In a subsequent study, the phosphate loading significantly increased anaerobic threshold and

VO_{2max}. A significant 3.5-minute reduction in the 40-km performance time was also found. The mechanisms to explain the physiologic changes noted after phosphate loading have not been determined.

However, other studies have found no benefit to performance from ingesting a phosphate load.[114–116] A glucose-phosphate drink (129 mmol phosphorus) did not affect oxygen delivery and cardiac output during submaximal exercise.[117] Another study[115] reported that 1.24 g of phosphate salts [200 mg dibasic sodium phosphate (Na_2HPO_4), 186.8 mg monobasic sodium phosphate (NaH_2PO_4), 27.5 mg tribasic potassium phosphate (K_3PO_4), and 30 mg vitamin C] given 1 hour before leg power isokinetic tests and high-intensity treadmill runs or 3.73 g/d of the same formulation ingested for 6 days before the same exercise testing resulted in no significant improvement in leg power test or time-to-fatigue on the treadmill run compared to the placebo.

No ergogenic effects were found in the most recent study of phosphate loading.[116] Six trained cyclists and six untrained persons ingested 22.2 g dibasic calcium phosphate (or a placebo) 90 minutes before a 20-minute cycle ergometer test at 70% VO_{2max}. After a rest, an incremental ride to exhaustion was done. The study found no difference between the phosphate and the placebo trial in several physiologic parameters or performance measures (time to exhaustion or VO_{2max}).

Summary

The results of studies on phosphate loading are equivocal. However, they differ in the type and amounts ingested, the duration of ingestion (just before an exercise versus for several days before), the training level of the subjects, and the modes of exercise used. Also, the studies had small sample sizes. Mechanisms of how phosphate loading could exert an ergogenic effect have not been established. It is difficult to interpret the results of the phosphate loading studies because of several confounding variables. Further, studies with rigorous methodologic controls are warranted to state with any certainty that phosphate loading is effective.[118]

IRON

Iron plays a critical role in the human body even though the total amount of iron in the body is relatively small (3 to 5 g). Two thirds or more of this iron is in hemoglobin molecules found inside red blood cells. Most of the oxygen (O_2) transported in the blood is bonded to the iron in hemoglobin. Smaller quantities of iron are found in the muscles as myoglobin, which serves a similar function as hemoglobin, and inside the mitochondria of cells as cytochromes and other iron-containing proteins involved in aerobic metabolism. The body iron stores are located in the bone marrow, liver, and spleen. Mean iron storage in the adult male is 1000 mg and 300 mg in the adult female.

The amount of iron storage is highly correlated with the plasma ferritin concentration.[119] Plasma ferritin levels below 12 µg/l are a reliable indicator of storage iron depletion, the first stage of iron deficiency. Depletion of bone marrow iron stores leads to impaired synthesis of hemoglobin and, therefore, erythropoiesis. The liver increases the formation of transferrin, an iron transport protein, to deliver more iron to the bone marrow. The second stage of iron deficiency, known as iron-deficient erythropoiesis, is characterized by increased transferrin levels and a reduction in the iron saturation of transferrin (less than 16%). Anemia is the third stage of iron deficiency in which the red blood cells are microcytic (smaller than normal) and hypochromic (low in hemoglobin). Low levels of hemoglobin in the female (less than 12 g/dl) and male (less than 13 g/dl) are used as diagnostic indicators of anemia.

Iron Status and Physical Activity

Approximately one fifth of adult females and one fourth of adolescent females in the United States are reported to have low ferritin (less than 12 µg/l) levels.[120] Several studies of adult female distance runners and collegiate athletes have reported a slightly higher prevalence of low ferritin levels ranging from 25% to 35%.[31,121–124] However, other studies of elite female Nordic skiers from the United States and Canada found similar percentages of low ferritin levels (20% to 21%) to those found in the adult female population.[125,126] Higher percentages of low ferritin levels also have been found among adolescent female swimmers and runners.[127,128] Although several studies found no significant difference in plasma ferritin between female runners and control subjects,[121,123] Fogelholm[129] concluded from his research review that the prevalence of low ferritin levels was significantly greater among female athletes than nonathletes. The prevalence of low ferritin levels in male athletes is less than in female athletes, ranging from 3.5% to 13%.[121,122,125,126,130,131]

In spite of the relatively high incidence of low ferritin levels and, therefore, depleted iron stores, the incidence of iron deficiency anemia does not appear to be greater among female athletes[124,128,132] than the 5% to 6% incidence found among adolescent and adult females in the general U.S. population.[133] Interestingly, two studies of male athletes[121,127] reported the prevalence of anemia was 6.7%, which is somewhat higher than the 2% reported for adolescent and adult males in the U.S. population.[133]

There are several possible causes of low iron status among athletes including inadequate iron intake (which will be discussed in a later section), plasma volume expansion, and increased iron excretion. Expansion of plasma volume, which is known to occur during the early part of training, would dilute the concentration of blood constituents including ferritin and hemoglobin. After 3 weeks of training, plasma volume expanded by 15%.[134] If ferritin and hemoglobin decrease by a similar percentage during training, the decline could be due to hemodilution. Several studies have reported significant decreases in plasma ferritin during sports training,[135–137] as well as fitness programs,[138,139] whereas other studies reported no significant changes after training.[126,140,141] Significant decreases in ferritin ranged from 18% to 50% after sports training and 19% to 40% after fitness programs. Failure to observe a significant decrease in ferritin after training may be due to the timing of the blood sample taken after training. Increased plasma ferritin concentrations have been observed for 48 to 72 hours after prolonged exercise bouts (for example, marathon, triathlon).[140,142] Infection and inflammation are also accompanied by an increase in plasma ferritin. Significant decreases in serum iron after prolonged exercise have also been observed, and it has been suggested that the iron and ferritin changes were part of an acute phase response to inflammation.[142] Such changes could mask low plasma ferritin levels.

Iron Excretion

Increased iron excretion is also a possible contributing factor to depleted iron stores and low ferritin levels. It is estimated that the average adult male loses 0.5 mg of iron from the body per day through the GI tract, 0.1 mg/d through the urinary tract, and 0.24 to 0.33 mg/d from the skin for a total daily iron loss of 0.86 to 0.95 mg/d.[143–145] Estimated average daily iron losses for females are 0.45 mg/d through the GI tract, 0.1 mg/d through the urinary tract, 0.24 mg/d from the skin, and 0.6 mg/d through the menses for a total loss of 1.4 mg/d.[143,145,146] Because of the iron loss through the menses, females from adolescence to menopause have a greater requirement for iron than males. There is considerable variation in the iron loss through the menses with some females losing as much as 2.8 mg/d.[147] In general, females who use oral contraceptives lose less blood and iron through the menses whereas those who use intrauterine devices lose more blood and iron than the average female.

Excessive iron losses during exercise are most likely to occur through the GI tract or sweating. Some athletes experience GI bleeding especially during distance running. Iron loss through GI bleeding can be detected by fecal hemoglobin assays. The percentage of runners who experience GI bleeding ranges from 8%[148] to more than 80%.[149] Iron lost by runners through GI bleeding has been estimated to be 0.75 to 1.1 mg/d,[149,150] approximately two times the average iron loss through the GI tract. Several case studies of female runners with iron-deficiency anemia suggest that GI bleeding contributed to the depletion of iron stores.[151,152]

The iron concentration of sweat during exercise ranges from 0.13 to 0.42 mg/L.[153–155] One recent study observed that the sweat iron concentration was significantly lower during exercise in a hot environment (35°C) than in a thermoneutral environment (25°C).[155] Because sweating was greater in the heat, this resulted in the same amount of sweat iron loss (0.08 mg/m^2/h) during 1 hour of exercise in both environments with male athletes losing three times as much sweat iron (0.12 mg/m^2/h) as female athletes (0.04 mg/m^2/h). Furthermore, sweat iron concentration decreased significantly from 30 to 60 minutes. This suggests that much of the dermal iron is lost in the initial sweat. Use of sweat iron concentrations measured after 30 minutes of exercise to estimate sweat iron loss during prolonged exercise will likely lead to overestimation of iron losses.

Iron Intake

Females, from menarche to menopause (ages 11 to 50 years), have a greater need for iron, which is reflected in the RDA of 15 mg/d. Males have a lower RDA for iron of 10 mg/d except during the rapid adolescent growth spurt, ages 11 to 14 years, when it is 12 mg/d. Older adult females (older than 50 years) and children (ages 1 to 10 years) also have an RDA for iron of 10 mg/d. Mean dietary intake of iron by males in the United States generally exceeds the RDA (15.8 to 19.5 mg/d).[20] However, mean iron intake by adolescent and adult females in the United States falls below the RDA ranging from 11.8 to 12.7 mg/d.[20] Iron intake averages 6 mg/1000 kcal in the diet.

Among athletes, the iron intake of males usually exceeds the RDA, whereas female athletes are more variable in their iron intakes (Table 5–3). Especially in the aesthetic sports (for example, ballet, gymnastics), female athletes tend to consume less iron than the RDA.[21–23,27] Mean iron intakes below the RDA have also been found in other adolescent and young adult female athletes.[24,29,132,135,141] This may be due, in part, to restricted caloric intakes to maintain a lower body weight. Many female athletes with eating disorders, especially anorexia nervosa, also have very low iron intakes.[43]

Absorption of food iron varies according to the form of iron, heme and nonheme, the presence of enhancing and inhibiting factors, and the amount of body iron storage. Heme iron is the more highly absorbable form (23%) found in meats, fish, and poultry. The absorption of nonheme iron varies from 3% to 8% and is enhanced by the presence of meat, fish, poultry, and ascorbic acid. Phytates found in bran and tannins found in tea inhibit the absorption of iron. Persons with depleted iron stores absorb more food iron than those with high iron stores.

Some female athletes with low ferritin levels and depleted iron stores appear to have adequate dietary iron intakes. Female runners who consumed vegetarian diets had lower ferritin levels than those who consumed meat.[156] Another study found that female collegiate distance runners with low ferritin levels consumed significantly less heme iron than sprinters who had significantly higher ferritin levels and consumed the same total amount of food iron.[123] Female distance runners with low ferritin levels were also found to consume fewer servings (7.4) of meat per week than sedentary women (12.3 servings/week).[132] Because a lower percentage of nonheme iron is absorbed, athletes whose iron

Table 5–3 Iron Intakes of Selected U.S. Athletes

Sport	Age (yrs)	Level	Sex	Iron Intake (mg/d)	Reference
Ballet	14.6	Adolescent	F	13.4	23
Gymnastics	11–14	Elite juniors	F	11.0	22
Gymnastics	15.2	High school	F	11.3	21
Running	17.1	High school	F	13.0	24
Swimming	15.0	Elite juniors	F	18.3	25
	16.0	Elite juniors	M	26.4	25
Ballet	24.4	Elite	F	13.5	27
	26.0	Elite	M	41.7	27
Basketball		College	F	16.0	29
		College	M	23.0	29
Field hockey	20.2	College	F	13.0	135
Lacrosse		College	F	14.0	29
		College	M	20.0	29
Running, marathon	29.1	Elite	F	41.7	31
Running, distance	18.8	College	F	15.5	154
	19.4	College	M	22.9	154
Running, distance	29.9	Club	F	11.0	132
Skiing, Nordic	20.0	Elite	F	19.2	32
	22.0	Elite	M	22.9	32
Swimming		College	F	14.0	141
		College	M	20.7	141
Volleyball		College	F	12.0	29

intake is primarily composed of nonheme iron may be at a greater risk of depleting their iron stores.

Food intake data collected during the NHANES II, in 1976 through 1980, suggest that meat, fish, and poultry sources contribute 37% of the iron in U.S. diets.[157] Another major contributor to the dietary iron intake (27% of the total) is breads, cereals, crackers, and other bakery products made from flour that is enriched with iron. Other sources of dietary iron are beans, potatoes, spinach, tomatoes, and coffee.

Iron Supplementation

Iron supplements, especially ferrous sulfate, have been found to be effective in increasing plasma ferritin in female athletes with low iron stores.[158–164] If an athlete has a low hemoglobin concentration (less than 13 g/dL), iron supplementation is beneficial in restoring normal hemoglobin levels.[158,159] The amount of elemental iron ingested in these studies ranged from 60 to 300 mg per day. Supplements containing less iron (18 to 50 mg/d) are beneficial in preventing plasma ferritin levels of female athletes from decreasing during training.[126,139]

Studies with rats have clearly demonstrated that iron deficiency anemia reduces VO_{2max} and endurance and that restoration of hemoglobin concentration to normal levels by transfusion significantly improves VO_{2max} but not endurance.[165,166] Davies and colleagues[167] found that improvements in endurance corresponded to increases in tissue iron levels. Results of the rat studies led to speculation that depleted iron stores may impair endurance performance of athletes. Using repeated phlebotomies to lower the hemoglobin of male athletes to anemic levels, both VO_{2max} and endurance were significantly reduced.[168] Blood transfusions that restored hemoglobin levels also increased VO_{2max} and endurance performance.

Some iron supplement studies with female athletes have found no significant improvements in VO_{2max} or endurance performance after supplementation.[159,160,162] However, a few studies have reported beneficial effects of iron supplements on performance. Four weeks of iron supplementation (300 mg/d) significantly improved endurance of adolescent female runners.[163] Significantly increased VO_{2max} and reduced blood lactate were found after 100 mg iron/d for 8 weeks, but endurance was not significantly increased.[161] Another study reported that female runners had faster 3000-m times and the onset of blood lactate accumulation (OBLA) occurred at higher velocities after iron supplementation.[164] Reductions in blood lactate after iron supplementation could be due to improved oxygen delivery to the muscles.

Although iron supplements are beneficial in replacing iron stores, too much iron in the body may be toxic. Hemochromatosis is a genetic disorder in which excessive iron is stored in the liver and other tissues. Increased ferritin levels in patients with hemochromatosis are associated with increased free radical production, which can lead to tissue damage.[169] There is some evidence linking excessive iron storage with increased risk of both myocardial infarction[170] and cancer.[171] Large dosages of supplemental iron (75 mg and more) should be used only by those persons who have been diagnosed as iron depleted or anemic, and their use curtailed when the iron stores have returned to normal. Some female athletes may need a low dosage iron supplement (15 mg/d) to prevent iron depletion during training.

Summary

The prevalence of low ferritin levels indicative of depleted iron stores is greater in female endurance athletes than among females in the U.S. population. Low ferritin levels have also been observed in some male athletes as well. There are several possible causes of poor iron status in athletes, including increased iron excretion through sweating and GI bleeding during exercise, low dietary iron intake, and consumption of foods with low iron bioavailability. Iron supplementation is beneficial in improving iron stores of athletes who are iron depleted, but the effects on aerobic performance of nonanemic athletes are equivocal. Because large doses of iron (75 mg/d or greater) may be toxic in persons with the genetic disorder hemochromatosis, such supplements should be used only by those diagnosed as iron depleted or anemic. Use of a small dosage iron supplement (15 mg/d) may prevent iron depletion in some female athletes during training.

ZINC

Zinc plays an important role in many metabolic pathways because it is essential for the functioning of many enzymes. Included among the zinc-dependent enzymes are lactate dehydrogenase (LDH), carbonic anhydrase, malate dehydrogenase, and superoxide dismutase. Zinc dependent enzymes are also involved in growth and tissue repair. Bones and muscles are the major storage sites of zinc, about 2 g in adults. Erythrocytes are the primary carriers of zinc in the blood with smaller amounts carried by plasma proteins, albumin and alpha-macroglobulin.

Zinc Status and Physical Activity

There are several reports of hypozincemia (plasma zinc less than 80 µg/dL) in athletes[6,31,172,173]; however, other studies found that athletes had plasma zinc concentrations within the normal range.[67,70,174] Furthermore, plasma zinc concentrations have been observed to decrease during military and endurance training.[175–177] Possible explanations for the decline in plasma zinc with training include 1) expansion of the plasma volume, 2) increased zinc excretion, and 3) redistribution of zinc within the body.

The observed decrease in plasma zinc during training has ranged from 12% to 33%.[175–177] Expansion of the plasma volume is a possible explanation for the decrease in plasma zinc only in the study with the 12% decrease.[176] Increased zinc excretion through the urine and sweat may contribute to the decline in plasma zinc. Urinary

zinc excretion increased 10% to 45% after exercise,[178,179] is increased after training,[176] and is higher in trained athletes than in nonathletes.[180] Sweat zinc losses of 0.65 mg/h in males and 0.4 mg/h in females were observed after 1 hour of moderate-intensity exercise.[181] Because the estimated dermal zinc loss is 0.76 mg/d,[144] excessive zinc may be excreted by persons who lose several liters of sweat during exercise.

Redistribution of zinc after exercise may also contribute to the decrease in plasma zinc observed during training. Significant decreases in plasma zinc have been found 2 to 24 hours after distance runs.[178,179,182] Zinc may be redistributed to the liver and/or the erythrocytes after exercise. During stress, which includes exercise, the liver removes zinc from the plasma for metallothionein formation.[183] Acute phase responses to inflammation that may occur during exercise also reduce the plasma zinc concentration.[175] Erythrocyte zinc concentration increases after training,[184,185] accompanied by increases in carbonic anhydrase I zinc in the erythrocyte and a reduction in the plasma zinc bound to albumin. Both male and female endurance athletes have higher erythrocyte zinc concentrations compared to nonathletes.[6,76] After short, high-intensity exercise, there is an immediate increase in plasma zinc and decreases in erythrocyte zinc and carbonic anhydrase I concentrations, which returns to normal 30 minutes after exercise.[186] The shift in zinc to the plasma after high-intensity exercise is attenuated after endurance training.[184] Another possible explanation for the increased plasma zinc immediately after high-intensity exercise is release of zinc from the muscle due to catabolism. However, no increase in plasma zinc was observed in subjects who complained of muscle soreness after eccentric exercise.[187]

Dietary Intake of Athlete

The RDA for zinc is 15 mg/d for adolescent and adult males and 12 mg/d for adolescent and adult females.[3] Mean zinc intake of adolescent and young adult males in the U.S. population is

16.2 and 15.2 mg/d, respectively, whereas the mean intake of adolescent and young adult females is 9.6 and 9.7 mg/d, respectively.[20,188] Dietary zinc density averages 5 mg/100 kcal.[189] The richest sources of zinc in the diet are meats, eggs, and seafood. Although whole grains contain zinc, the presence of phytate and fiber reduces its bioavailability.

Many female athletes consume diets containing less zinc than the RDA. The mean zinc intake of adolescent ballet dancers was 7.6 mg/d,[23] of adolescent gymnasts was 7.5 mg/d,[21] of college swimmers was 10.4 mg/d,[141] and of highly trained runners was 10.3 mg/d.[180] Although mean zinc intake of elite female marathon runners was 14.2 mg/d, three fourths of the women consumed less zinc than the RDA.[31] Little information is available on the dietary zinc intake of males. Mean zinc intake of male swimmers and skiers exceeded 15 mg/d,[141,174] whereas the mean zinc intake of male marathon runners was below the RDA.[190]

Zinc Supplement

Few studies have examined the effect of zinc supplements on exercise performance in athletes. Significant increases in isometric endurance and isokinetic strength at 180°/s of the knee extensors were reported after two weeks of 135 mg zinc/d supplement, but no changes in the isokinetic strength at slower speeds were observed.[191] However, no effect on VO_{2max} was found after 1 month of receiving 33.6 mg of zinc supplement.[192] Another study found that 50 mg zinc/d for 6 days significantly increased plasma zinc concentration, but had no significant effect on heart rate, plasma lactate, perceived exertion, or time to exhaustion during a run at 75% VO_{2max}.[182] The investigators also observed that zinc supplementation suppressed superoxide anion production and T-lymphocyte activity after exercise. Although suppression of free radical (superoxide anions) production may be a beneficial effect, suppression of lymphocyte activity may increase susceptibility to infections.

Large quantities of zinc in supplements are likely to be detrimental. Significant decreases in

polymorphonuclear leukocyte and lymphocyte activity, and high-density lipoprotein (HDL) cholesterol were reported after 6 weeks of 150 mg zinc/d.[193] Other studies have also reported significant reductions in HDL cholesterol and increases in low-density lipoprotein (LDL) cholesterol after similar quantities of zinc.[194,195] However, supplements containing less than 30 mg zinc/d did not lower HDL cholesterol.[196] For these reasons, the quantity of supplemental zinc consumed should be limited to less than two times the RDA.

Summary

Low plasma zinc concentrations have been observed in some athletes, and reductions in plasma zinc have occurred after endurance training. Decreases in plasma zinc may be due to a redistribution of zinc into erythrocytes or the liver after endurance exercise. Increased excretion of zinc in the sweat and urine has also been observed during exercise. However, plasma zinc increases and erythrocyte zinc decreases after high-intensity exercise. The dietary zinc intake of many female athletes is below the RDA of 12 mg/d. There is little evidence that zinc supplements have a beneficial effect on exercise performance. Large dosages of zinc (150 mg/d) have been found to impair immunity and reduce HDL cholesterol levels. Use of zinc supplements should be limited to those containing no more than 30 mg/d.

COPPER

Copper is another trace mineral that has several important functions in the body. Most of the copper in the plasma is bound to the protein ceruloplasmin, which serves as a catalyst for iron absorption and mobilization. Copper also plays important roles in the formation of collagen, formation of the neurotransmitter norepinephrine, and the release of cholesterol from the liver.[197] Adult humans store approximately 75 mg of copper, with the liver being the major storage site. Two important metalloenzymes, cytochrome oxidase and superoxide dismutase, are copper-containing enzymes. Cytochrome oxidase plays a critical role in aerobic energy production at the last step in the electron transport system. Superoxide dismutase (SOD), an important antioxidant, catalyzes the removal of the superoxide anion in the cytosol. Ceruloplasmin is also an important antioxidant in the plasma.

Copper Metabolism and Physical Activity

Several studies have reported that male athletes have higher plasma copper concentrations than nonathletes,[104,198] another study reported that male distance runners had significantly lower plasma copper,[199] and still another study found no significant difference in plasma copper between male athletes and nonathletes.[200] Female athletes have been found to have significantly higher plasma copper concentrations in comparison to males.[201,202] The effects of training on plasma copper concentration are equivocal. In two studies conducted with competitive swimmers over several months of training, one study reported significant decreases in plasma copper and ceruloplasmin concentrations after training,[203] whereas the other study reported no significant changes in plasma copper and ceruloplasmin but a significant increase in erythrocyte SOD activity.[141] Although plasma copper concentration is frequently used as an indication of copper status, erythrocyte SOD activity appears to be a better indicator in humans.[3]

Plasma copper concentration changes during strenuous exercise. Most studies have reported significant increases in plasma copper immediately after acute exercise with a return to baseline levels 2 hours after exercise.[78,204,205] However, one study found that plasma copper decreases immediately after strenuous exercise.[201] It has been suggested that the increase in plasma copper during exercise might be beneficial in protecting against free radicals because most of the copper is in ceruloplasmin.[206] Only small changes in plasma copper have been observed during prolonged exercise bouts.[178,198]

The primary route of copper excretion is through the GI tract. Copper loss through the

skin is 0.4 mg/d and the sweat copper concentration is 0.1 mg/L in sedentary men.[144] Higher sweat copper concentrations have been observed during exercise.[206] There is, however, little evidence that excessive copper losses during exercise lead to low copper status in athletes.

Copper Intake

There is no RDA for copper; however, the ESADDI of copper is 1.5 to 3 mg for adults and 1.5 to 2.5 mg for adolescents.[3] Dietary data collected between 1988 and 1991 on the U.S. population found that the mean copper intake of adolescent and young adult females was 1.0 and 1.1 mg/d, respectively, which is below the ESADDI, and the mean intake of adolescent and young adult males was 1.3 and 1.6 mg/d, respectively.[20] The best food source of copper is liver. Other good sources of copper are seafood, nuts, and legumes.

Few studies have reported the copper intake of athletes. Mean copper intake of elite female marathon runners was 2.1 mg/d.[6] In a group of male and female ultramarathon athletes, a mean copper intake of 1.8 mg/d was found.[70] Somewhat lower mean copper intakes of female and male college swimmers of 1.3 and 1.6 mg/d, respectively, have also been reported.[141] With the exception of the female college swimmers, most athletes appeared to have dietary copper intakes within the ESADDI.

Summary

Few studies have examined the copper status of athletes. Female athletes have been found to have higher plasma copper levels than males. One study found a significant increase in erythrocyte SOD activity, which may be the best indicator of copper status, after several months of training. Most studies reported plasma copper increases immediately after acute exercise. Based on the limited information available on the dietary copper intake of athletes, it would appear that most athletes are consuming adequate amounts.

SELENIUM

Selenium is a trace mineral that plays an important role as a co-factor for the enzyme glutathione peroxidase.[207] This enzyme serves to reduce tissue damage from free radicals and is, therefore, part of the antioxidant defense system. Glutathione peroxidase and vitamin E are complementary in their role as antioxidants. The RDA for selenium is 70 µg and 55 µg for males and females, respectively, 19 years and older.[3] Food sources of selenium are seafood, liver, muscle meats, and grain if grown in soil containing selenium.

The best index of selenium status is unknown.[63] Commonly, selenium concentrations in the plasma or serum are assessed, but these fluctuate from day to day, unlike whole blood or erythrocyte concentrations that provide an index of long-term status.[63] Also assessed is the activity of glutathione peroxidase; however, this enzyme assay has not been well-standardized.[63]

Selenium is not considered effective as an ergogenic aid, per se. The interest for athletics is due to its role as an antioxidant. Because selenium is necessary to reduce oxidative damage during exercise and aid in the recovery, adequate levels of selenium may allow athletes to train more intensely.

Selenium and Oxidative Stress

Strenuous exercise can produce an increase in free radicals as by-products of metabolism.[208–210] Free radicals are chemical species containing unpaired electrons that make them highly reactive with other cellular components such that damage results. The initial damage from free radicals causes a chain of reactions, called lipid peroxidation, producing additional damage, especially to cell membranes. Free radicals do not act alone; they generate other reactive oxygen species (ROS), such as hydrogen peroxide (H_2O_2). The body has several defenses to deal with the generation of free radicals and ROS. One of these defenses involves the glutathione-peroxidase catalyzed reaction of glutathione and H_2O_2. Glutathione (GSH) will react with H_2O_2 thereby "inactivating" it to produce glutathione disulfide (GSSG) (the oxidized form of glutathione).

$$2GSH + 2H_2O_2 \rightarrow GSSG + 2H_2O$$
$$\text{Glutathione}$$
$$\text{Peroxidase}$$
$$\text{(selenium co-factor)}$$

Dietary Intake and Status of Athletes

Information on selenium intake or selenium status of athletes is limited. Competing wrestlers had adequate levels of plasma and red blood cell (RBC) glutathione peroxidase activity despite repeated bouts of low dietary intake with low selenium intake.[211] There is some indication that training can decrease serum selenium levels by a small amount.[77,175] One study[175] assessed selenium intake and plasma levels before and after a week of sustained exercise, psychologic stress, and lack of sleep in Navy Seals during "Hell Week." Although selenium intake was substantially greater during Hell Week, the plasma selenium values at the end of the week were lower. It was suggested that the lower serum selenium values may reflect a redistribution of selenium to other tissues requiring antioxidant protection.[175]

Athletes in countries where the food content of selenium is adequate, or where food grown in low-selenium soil is fertilized with selenium, generally have adequate status.[77,202] For example, Finland and Sweden both have low soil content of selenium. However, Finland began enriching its fertilizer with selenium in 1984, which increased the selenium content of cereal crops.[202] This is not the case in Sweden, possibly explaining why serum selenium levels of Swedish orienteers were lower than those of Finnish orienteers. In fact, one third of the Swedish athletes had values below the reference level.

Selenium Supplementation and Lipid Peroxidation

Acute ingestion of selenium (150 µg) and 14 days' supplementation of selenium (100 µg) (or placebo) did not prevent or affect the increase in lipid peroxidation from 2 hours of swimming exercise.[212] After 14 days of selenium supplementation, there was a significant decrease in lipid peroxidation compared to the placebo, but only in the group that received the placebo first and then selenium.

A second study by the same laboratory[213] found that a supplement containing selenium, vitamin E, glutathione, and cysteine (concentrations were unspecified) administered to trained cyclists for 3 weeks resulted in a smaller change in lipid peroxidation compared with the placebo. However, this was a cross-over design similar to their first study, and it appeared that the first leg of the cross-over affected the response on the second leg of the cross-over. Both studies appear to have used a cross-over design where the "wash-out" period may not have been long enough.

Two studies from another laboratory reported some benefits of selenium supplements.[214,215] Ten weeks of selenium supplementation (180 μg/day) or placebo during an endurance training program resulted in moderate correlation between erythrocyte glutathione peroxidase activity and VO_{2max} in the supplemented group only.[214] Also, there was an increase in muscle glutathione peroxidase activity in response to acute exercise in the supplemented group only.[215] Although it is tempting to suggest these data indicate that selenium supplementation would enhance antioxidant defense, this is still uncertain.

Summary

From the little information that exists, selenium intake of athletes is probably sufficient, and status may not be compromised by routine exercise training. There are some data to suggest that selenium supplementation could result in improved antioxidant defense, but the results are preliminary. Although excessive amounts of selenium (more than 200 μg/day) could have toxic effects,[207] supplementation with RDA amounts or slightly more than the RDA does not appear

harmful. Little information exists on the long-term effects of selenium ingestion above the RDA. At present, the recommendation for athletes is to eat foods rich in selenium and other antioxidants (vitamins E, A, and C).

CHROMIUM

Chromium, unlike trace minerals iron, zinc, and copper, does not have a function in enzyme systems and is not a component of metalloprotein complexes.[61] The primary function of chromium is to potentiate the effects of insulin in carbohydrate, lipid, and protein metabolism.[61,216] Exactly how chromium exerts its function on insulin is still uncertain. It is thought that chromium may help bind insulin to its receptor.[217] Chromium appears to form a complex with nicotinic acid and glutathione, resulting in an organic compound.[61] This compound is referred to as the glucose tolerance factor (GTF) because of its purported role in transport of glucose into the cell. Chromium is thought to be released from body stores in response to insulin.[61] Often, glucose intolerance is improved after chromium supplementation.[216]

Chromium mostly exists in food in the trivalent form (Cr^{+3}) either present in an inorganic compound that is poorly absorbed or the biologically active organic form (GTF).[61] The body stores about 4 to 6 mg of chromium.[61,63] Little is known about the absorption of chromium, but it is thought that the inorganic form is about 0.5% to 1% and the organic form is higher, possibly 10% to 25%, as has been found in animal studies.[61] It appears that absorption of chromium is enhanced when given in conjunction with vitamin C.[216] Brewer's yeast contains a high amount of the organic form. Mushrooms, prunes, nuts, asparagus, wine, beer, and whole grains are examples of foods rich in chromium. Foods prepared in stainless steel cookware can increase the amount of chromium available because chromium can leach out from the pans by the action of acidic foods.[61]

Because so little is known about the body's need for chromium, the Food and Nutrition

Board was unable to establish an RDA. Instead, a range of chromium values (50 to 200 µg/day), the ESADDI, is recommended.[3] Chromium supplements are available in the following three forms: chromium picolinate, chromium nicotinate, and chromium chloride. Whether one is more effective than another has not been proven.

Dietary Intake and Status of Athletes

Many databases used to assess micronutrient intake do not include chromium; therefore, there is little information about its intake in athletes and even the general population. However, it has been estimated that approximately 50% of the population consume less than the ESADDI.[218] Although this may suggest that athletes, too, are not ingesting sufficient chromium, it should be noted that most athletes are ingesting more calories, so they may have diets adequate in chromium. Athletes who are restricting calories to maintain low body weights may not ingest sufficient chromium; however, this has not been examined.

Little is also known about the chromium status of athletes because there is no accurate means to assess chromium status. Whether serum or plasma levels of chromium reflect tissue chromium levels is not fully known.[63] Although assessment of the increase in chromium response to a glucose load has been used to assess status, the results have not been consistent.[63] However, the latter test appears the best means to assess a marginal deficiency. Because exercise results in an increased urinary excretion of chromium, it has been suggested that those who exercise regularly may require more chromium in the diet. This will be discussed in the next section. Also, more detailed reviews can be found elsewhere.[219–221]

Urinary Chromium Excretion and Exercise

Exercise results in an increase in chromium levels in the blood.[178,222,223] After a 6-mile run, serum chromium levels were increased immediately after exercise, and these levels remained

for 2 hours.[178,222] Twelve minutes of cycling at 80% of anaerobic threshold resulted in increased plasma chromium 12 minutes after the exercise.[223] It is thought that chromium is mobilized from stores into the blood to be carried to a target organ like muscle to enhance insulin function. Once chromium is mobilized into the blood, it cannot be reabsorbed and is lost into the urine.[178] Several studies from the same laboratory showed that exercise increases urinary chromium excretion. In fact, 24-hour chromium losses were twice as high on the day of exercise as on a rest day.[178,218,222]

Because chromium is mobilized in response to insulin, the carbohydrate composition of the diet may influence urinary chromium excretion.[216] The insulinogenic properties of the carbohydrate are positively related to urinary chromium excretion.[216] A high carbohydrate diet was not found to result in increased chromium excretion,[218] but ingestion of glucose and fructose drinks did increase chromium excretion.[224] Whether athletes who ingest high amounts of simple sugars and sports drinks need more chromium is not known.

The consistent finding, albeit from few studies, is that chromium excretion is increased in response to exercise. However, it is not known whether this increased excretion can result in a chromium deficiency such that athletes require greater amounts of chromium in their diet. It is possible that the body can adapt to the increased loss by retaining more that is ingested, although no studies have evaluated this. Moreover, resting urinary excretion of chromium appears to be lower in trained athletes than untrained persons,[225] which may suggest that trained persons are more efficient in chromium usage.

Chromium Supplementation and Lean Body Weight

Perhaps the greatest interest in chromium comes from its purported use to increase lean body mass and decrease fat. The first studies to gain attention in this area[226] showed that chromium supplements enhanced lean muscle mass in resistance-training athletes. Supplemental chromium then gained notoriety as the healthy alternative to anabolic steroids. Chromium is suggested to affect lean body mass by facilitating the transport of amino acids into the muscle cells.

One of the original studies to examine chromium supplementation and exercise[226] found that a group of five subjects who took 200 μg of chromium picolinate for 40 days showed a significantly greater increase in lean body mass over the course of a weight-training class compared to five subjects who took a placebo. A second study from the same laboratory found that 16 football players who took 200 μg chromium picolinate per day for 42 days had greater increases in lean body mass than the 15 players who took a placebo. It should be noted that lean body mass was estimated from skinfold measures, which may not provide an accurate assessment.

Several studies since have failed to confirm the previous findings. A chromium picolinate supplement (200 μg) and a placebo ingested over the course of a 12-week weight-lifting program produced similar changes in skinfolds, circumferences, and strength.[227] The only significant treatment effect was that the female subjects (n = 12) who ingested the chromium supplement gained more total body weight than the other three groups. This could be due to the fact that the women may not have an adequate amount of chromium in their diet or that the amount of chromium ingested was proportionally larger for the women than it was for the men, making the supplements more effective.

In another study,[228] where football players ingested 200 μg of chromium picolinate (n = 9) or a placebo (n − 12) for 9 weeks during spring training, which included a weight-lifting program, there was no difference between groups in the development of strength or lean body mass assessed by hydrostatic weighing. This study also found that the subjects who ingested the chromium supplement had greater urinary chromium losses at the midpoint and at the end of the study, possibly suggesting that chromium levels

were already optimal or near optimal before the supplementation period and the excess was excreted. A near duplicate study to the one previously mentioned[229] also reported no effects of 200 μg chromium picolinate on strength or lean body mass during 12 weeks of resistance training and that chromium excretion was increased in the group that received supplements.

Another study examined the effect of 8 weeks of chromium supplementation (chromium chloride and chromium picolinate) or a placebo in 36 men undergoing weight training. The chromium supplements increased urinary chromium excretion, and there was no effect of the supplements on fat loss, muscle mass gain, or strength.[86] The authors also noted a possible negative effect on iron status in the groups that received chromium supplements such that there was a tendency for a greater decrease in transferrin saturation after chromium supplementation with the largest effect for the picolinate type. It is possible that increases in serum chromium as noted with supplementation may adversely affect iron transport and distribution.

The purpose of the studies discussed previously was to examine the efficacy of chromium in enhancing muscle mass during resistance training. However, the marketing for the product extended these findings to suggest that chromium would be effective as a weight loss product. In one study,[217] ninety-five overweight subjects following an aerobic exercise program were given chromium supplements (400 μg/day of chromium picolinate) or a placebo for 16 weeks. There was no difference between the group receiving supplements and the group receiving a placebo in percent body fat estimated from circumferences measures.

Summary

Chromium supplements do not appear to be effective in enhancing muscle mass gain. Perhaps in those persons who are chromium-deficient there may be a benefit, but this has not been established. Indiscriminate use of chromium supplements should be avoided because chromium can interact with other nutrients, especially iron and zinc.[86,218] One study showed that chromium administration to cultured hamster cells resulted in chromosomal damage.[230] However, this study was criticized because it used supraphysiologic doses in cell cultures rather than oral doses in animals or humans.[231] The levels of ingestion when chromium becomes harmful are not known, but because chromium is slowly excreted from cells, chromium supplementation could cause a detrimental accumulation.[232]

Based on pharmacokinetic models used to quantitate absorption of chromium, it was concluded that 1) the normal dietary intake of chromium may be adequate to maintain a positive chromium balance in most people even at levels of ingestion somewhat below the 50 to 200 μg range, and 2) the long-term use of chromium supplements should be approached with caution.[232] These models did not take into consideration the exercise-induced loss of chromium into the urine. However, it is not known whether the body will adapt to this loss by increasing retention. Chronic under-ingestion of chromium or impaired chromium status could predispose a person to developing glucose intolerance and maturity-onset diabetes. A prudent course of action for athletes would be to ingest foods rich in chromium. A multivitamin and mineral supplement containing chromium could be taken. However, not all supplements contain chromium, so before purchasing, check the label to ensure that it contains chromium at levels between 50 and 200 μg.

CONCLUSION

Because minerals play such an important role in many processes related to energy production, metabolism, oxidative stress, oxygen-carrying capacity, and structure, athletes must be sure that their diets contain sufficient amounts. At present, we cannot say that exercise in itself will increase a person's need for minerals. There are data to show that exercise increases urinary ex-

cretion of chromium, zinc, and magnesium, and several minerals are present in sweat. However, it is not known whether the body can adapt to this loss by increased absorption or retention. Iron stores are low, especially in female athletes, but this, in part, can be attributed to diets low in iron. Calcium and zinc intake of many groups of female athletes is also low. Although a few studies reported that selenium supplementation reduced oxidative stress of exercise, these results are still preliminary. Also, the role that copper plays in protecting against free radical damage remains to be determined.

Chromium and phosphate have been purported to serve as ergogenic aids. Chromium supplements are touted to increase muscle mass and reduce fat, and phosphate in acute large doses is alleged to improve performance. Most studies report that chromium does not increase muscle mass or fat loss, and results about the efficacy of phosphate loading are equivocal.

Although it is tempting to think that a supplement can provide the "winning edge," evidence does not support this. However, one cannot dismiss the placebo effect that these supplements impart to the athletes who strongly believe that the supplements will work. The reason for such belief is the recommendation of other athletes who "swear" by them as well as enticing advertising. Most athletes have not learned to be skeptical of marketing claims. These claims offer hope, such that the supplements often become expensive placebos. Over time, the placebo effect generally wears off, but often after spending a sizable amount in purchases.

The concern about mineral ingestion should be focused on being sure that athletes obtain sufficient amounts from their diet. This will ensure good health and perhaps allow for the ability to train optimally. Many athletes are not ingesting sufficient amounts of minerals because of their bizarre or restrictive diets. Those athletes who restrict energy intake to maintain low body weights are at high risk of not ingesting adequate minerals. Not only do these athletes ingest too little food, the composition of the diet can also be a major problem. As an example, one study reported that the majority of elite body builders had repetitive, monotonous diets with limited selection of vegetables.[82] For each of four meals over the course of a day, one female body builder ate a rice cake, a tomato, 1.5 oz turkey, and 1 tsp of french dressing. Although this is probably an extreme example, many athletes ingest diets that tend to be repetitive and monotonous. Minerals occur in small amounts across a variety of foods, and not all minerals are present in all foods. Therefore, it is important that diets be as varied as possible to ensure that all minerals are ingested in adequate amounts.

We do not know the long-term consequences of taking supplements of any single mineral. Be-

cause most minerals in large amounts can interact with the absorption of another mineral, it is preferred that athletes obtain minerals from foods. However, we realize that this may not always be possible. To account for occasional poor diets, a multivitamin mineral supplement containing no more than the RDA level could be taken. If a deficiency of a mineral is suspected, the athlete should be advised to consult a physician and have his or her status assessed. The most challenging task for nutritionists and health professionals is to convince athletes that a sound nutritional game plan is more effective for optimal training and performance than the latest diet fads and scams.

REFERENCES

1. Todhunter EN. 'Historical landmarks' in nutrition. *Present Knowledge in Nutrition.* 5th ed. Washington, DC: Nutrition Foundation; 1984;871–882.

2. Clarkson PM, Haymes EM. Exercise and mineral status of athletes: calcium, magnesium, phosphorus, and iron. *Med Sci Sports Exerc.* 1995;27:831–843.

3. National Research Council. *Recommended Dietary Allowances.* 10th ed. Washington, DC: National Academy Press; 1989.

4. Khoo C-S, Rqwson NE, Robinson ML, Stevenson RJ. Nutrient intake and eating habits of triathletes. *Ann Sports Med.* 1987;3:144–150.

5. Nieman DC, Gates JR, Butler JV, Pollett LM, Dietrich SJ, Lutz RD. Supplementation patterns in marathon runners. *J Am Diet Assoc.* 1989;89:1615–1619.

6. Singh A, Deuster PA, Moser PB. Zinc and copper status of women by physical activity and menstrual status. *J Sports Med.* 1990;30:29–36.

7. Matkovic V, Jelic T, Wardlaw GM, et al. Timing of peak bone mass in caucasian females and its implications for the prevention of osteoporosis. *J Clin Invest.* 1994;93:799–808.

8. Gunnes M, Lehmann EH. Physical activity and dietary constituents as predictors of forearm cortical and trabecular bone gain in healthy children and adolescents: a prospective study. *Acta Paediatr.* 1996;85:19–25.

9. Recker RR, Davies KM, Hinders SM, Heaney RP, Stegman MR, Kimmel DB. Bone gain in young adult women. *JAMA.* 1992;268:2403–2408.

10. Matkovic V. Calcium metabolism and calcium requirements during skeletal modeling and consolidation of bone mass. *Am J Clin Nutr.* 1991;54:245S–260S.

11. Krebs J, Schneider V, Smith J, Leblanc A, Thornton W, Leach C. Sweat calcium loss during running. *FASEB J.* 1988;2:A1099.

12. Matkovic V, Heaney RP. Calcium balance during human growth: evidence for threshold behavior. *Am J Clin Nutr.* 1992;55:992–996.

13. Halioua L, Anderson JB. Lifetime calcium intake and physical activity habits: independent and combined effects on the radial bone of healthy premenopausal caucasian women. *Am J Clin Nutr.* 1989;49:534–541.

14. Fehily AM, Coles RJ, Evans WD, Elwood PC. Factors affecting bone density in young adults. *Am J Clin Nutr.* 1992;56:579–586.

15. Kanders B, Dempster DW, Lindsay R. Interaction of calcium nutrition and physical activity on bone mass in young women. *J Bone Miner Res.* 1988;3:145–149.

16. Matkovic B, Kostial K, Simonovic I, Buzina R, Brodarec A, Nordin BEC. Bone status and fracture rates in two regions of Yugoslavia. *Am J Clin Nutr.* 1979;32:540–549.

17. Sandler RB, Slemeda CW, Laporte RE, et al. Postmenopausal bone density and milk consumption in childhood and adolescence. *Am J Clin Nutr.* 1985;42:270–274.

18. McCulloch RG, Bailey DA, Houston CS, Dodd BL. Effects of physical activity, dietary calcium intake and selected lifestyle factors on bone density in young women. *Can Med Assoc J.* 1990;142:221–227.

19. Mazess RB, Barden HS. Bone density in premenopausal women: effects of age, dietary intake, physical activity, smoking, and birth-control pills. *Am J Clin Nutr.* 1991;53:132–142.

20. Alaimo K, McDowell MA, Briefel RR, et al. Dietary intake of vitamins, minerals, and fiber of persons age 2

months and over in the United States. *Third National Health and Nutrition Examination Survey, Phase 1, 1988–91. Advance Data from Vital and Health Statistics: no 258.* Hyattsville, MD: National Center for Health Statistics; 1994.

21. Moffatt RJ. Dietary status of elite female high school gymnasts: inadequacy of vitamin and mineral intake. *J Am Diet Assoc.* 1984;84:1361–1363.

22. Benardot D, Schwarz, Heller DW. Nutrient intake in young, highly competitive gymnasts. *J Am Diet Assoc.* 1989;89:401–403.

23. Benson J, Gillien DM, Bourdet K, Loosli AR. Inadequate nutrition and chronic caloric restriction in adolescent ballerinas. *Physician Sportsmed.* 1985;13:79–90.

24. Moen SM, Sanborn CF, Dimarco N. Dietary habits and body composition in adolescent female runners. *Women in Sport & Physical Activity J.* 1992;1:85–95.

25. Berning JR, Troup JP, VanHandel PJ, Daniels J, Daniels N. The nutritional habits of young adolescent swimmers. *Int J Sport Nutr.* 1991;1:240–248.

26. McCulloch RG, Bailey DA, Whalen RL, Houston CS, Faulkner RA, Craven BR. Bone density and bone mineral content of adolescent soccer athletes and competitive swimmers. *Pediat Exer Sci.* 1992;4:319–330.

27. Cohen JL, Patosnak L, Frank O, Baker H. A nutritional and hematologic assessment of elite ballet dancers. *Physician Sportsmed.* 1985;13:43–54.

28. Risser W, Lee E, LeBlanc A, Poindexter HB, Risser JM, Schneider V. Bone density in eumenorrheic female college athletes. *Med Sci Sports Exerc.* 1990;22:570–574.

29. Short SH, Short WR. Four-year study of university athletes' dietary intake. *J Am Diet Assoc.* 1983;83:632–645.

30. Kirchner EM, Lewis RD, O'Connor PJ. Bone mineral density and dietary intake of female college gymnasts. *Med Sci Sports Exerc.* 1995;27:543–549.

31. Deuster PA, Kyle SB, Moser PB, et al. Nutritional survey of highly trained women runners. *Am J Clin Nutr.* 1986;45:954–962.

32. Ellsworth NM, Hewitt BF, Haskell WL. Nutrient intake of elite male and female Nordic skiers. *Physician Sportsmed.* 1985;13:78–92.

33. Nichols DL, Sanborn CF, Bonnick SL, Ben-Ezzra V, Gench B, DiMarco NM. The effects of gymnastics training on bone mineral density. *Med Sci Sports Exerc.* 1994;26:1220–1225.

34. Myburgh KH, Hutchins J, Fataar AB, Hough SF, Noakes TD. Low bone density is an etiologic factor for stress fractures in athletes. *Ann Intern Med.* 1990;113:754–759.

35. Frustajer NT, Dhuper S, Warren MP, Brooks-Gunn J, Fox RP. Nutrition and the incidence of stress fractures in ballet dancers. *Am J Clin Nutr.* 1990;51:779–783.

36. Drinkwater BL, Nilson K, Chesnut CH, Bremner WJ, Shainholtz S, Southworth MB. Bone mineral content of amenorrheic and eumenorrheic athletes. *N Engl J Med.* 1984;311:277–281.

37. Drinkwater BL, Bremner B, Chesnut CH. Menstrual history as a determinant of current bone density in young adults. *JAMA.* 1990;263:545–548.

38. Cann CE, Martin MC, Genant HK, Jaffe RB. Decreased spinal mineral content in amenorrheic women. *JAMA.* 1984;251:626–629.

39. Marcus R, Cann C, Madvig P, et al. Menstrual function and bone mass in elite women distance runners. *Ann Intern Med.* 1985;102:158–163.

40. Drinkwater BL, Nilson K, Ott S, Chesnut CH. Bone mineral density after resumption of menses in amenorrheic athletes. *JAMA.* 1986;256:380–382.

41. Baer JT, Taper J, Gwazdauskas FG, et al. Diet, hormonal, and metabolic factors affecting bone mineral density in adolescent amenorrheic and eumenorrheic female runners. *J Sports Med Phys Fitness.* 1992;32:51–58.

42. Lloyd T, Triantafyllou SJ, Baker ER, et al. Menstrual disturbance in women athletes: association with increased skeletal injuries. *Med Sci Sports Exerc.* 1986;18:374–379.

43. Sundgot-Borgun J. Nutrient intake of female elite athletes suffering from eating disorders. *Int J Sport Nutr.* 1993;3:431–442.

44. Lee WTK, Leung SSF, Wang SH, et al. Double-blind, controlled calcium supplementation and bone mineral accretion in children accustomed to a low-calcium diet. *Am J Clin Nutr.* 1994;60:744–750.

45. Johnston CC, Miller JZ, Slemnda CW, Reister TK, Christian JC, Peacock M. Calcium supplementation and increases in bone mineral density in children. *N Engl J Med.* 1992;327:82–87.

46. Matkovic V, Fontana D, Tomnac C, Goel P, Chesnut CH. Factors that influence peak bone mass formation: a study of calcium balance and the inheritance of bone mass in adolescent females. *Am J Clin Nutr.* 1990;52:878–888.

47. Andon MB, Lloyd T, Matkovic V. Supplementation trial with calcium citrate malate: evidence in favor of increasing the calcium RDA during childhood and adolescence. *J Nutr.* 1994;124:1412S–1417S.

48. Lloyd T, Andon MB, Rollings N, et al. Calcium supplementation and bone mineral density in adolescent girls. *JAMA.* 1993;270:841–844.

49. Abrams SA, Stuff JE. Calcium metabolism in girls: current dietary intakes lead to low rates of calcium absorption and retention during puberty. *Am J Clin Nutr.* 1994;60:739–743.

50. Ettinger B, Genant HK, Cann CE. Postmenopausal bone loss is prevented by treatment with low-dosage estrogen with calcium. *Ann Intern Med.* 1987;106:40–45.

51. Nilas L, Christiansen C, Rodbro P. Calcium supplementation and postmenopausal bone loss. *Br Med J.* 1984;289:1103–1106.

52. Riis B, Thomsen K, Christiansen C. Does calcium supplementation prevent postmenopausal bone loss? *N Engl J Med.* 1987;316:173–177.

53. Dawson-Hughes B, Dallai GE, Krall EA, Sadowski L, Sahyoun N, Tannenbaum S. A controlled trial of the effect of calcium supplementation on bone density in postmenopausal women. *N Engl J Med.* 1990;323:878–883.

54. Recker RR, Saville PD, Heaney RP. Effect of estrogens and calcium carbonate on bone loss in postmenopausal women. *Ann Intern Med.* 1977;87:649–655.

55. Riggs BL, Seeman E, Hodgson SF, Taves DR, O'Fallon WM. Effect of the fluoride/calcium regimen on vertebral fracture occurrence in postmenopausal osteoporosis. *N Engl J Med.* 1982;306:446–450.

56. Nelson ME, Fisher EC, Dilmanian FA, Dallal GE, Evans WJ. A 1-y walking program and increased dietary calcium in postmenopausal women: effects on bone. *Am J Clin Nutr.* 1991;53:1304–1311.

57. Reid IR, Ames RW, Evans MC, Gamble GD, Sharpe SJ. Long-term effects of calcium supplementation on bone loss and fractures in postmenopausal women: a randomized controlled trial. *Am J Med.* 1995;98:331–335.

58. NIH Consensus Development Panel on Optimal Calcium Intake. Optimal calcium intake NIH Consensus Conference. *JAMA.* 1994;272:1942–1948.

59. Monsen ER, Cook JD. Food iron absorption in human subjects. IV. The effects of calcium and phosphate salts on the absorption of nonheme iron. *Am J Clin Nutr.* 1976;29:1142–1148.

60. Mahan LK, Arlin M. *Krause's Food, Nutrition, and Diet Therapy.* 8th ed. Philadelphia: W.B. Saunders Company; 1992;109–140.

61. Hunt SM, Groff JL. *Advance Nutrition and Human Metabolism.* St. Paul, MN: West Publishing Co; 1990:273–281, 310–316.

62. Shils ME, Magnesium. In: Ziegler EE, Filer LJ Jr, eds. *Present Knowledge in Nutrition.* 7th ed. Washington, DC: International Life Sciences Institute; 1996;256–264.

63. Gibson RS. *Principles of Nutritional Assessment.* New York: Oxford Press; 1990:494–510, 511–520, 532–541.

64. Brilla LR, Lombardi VP. Magnesium in sports and performance. In: Kies CV, Driskell JA, eds. *Sports Nutrition: Minerals and Electrolytes.* Boca Raton, FL: CRC Press; 1995:139–178.

65. Bazzarre TL, Scarpino A, Sigmon R, Marquart LF, Wu SL, Izurieta M. Vitamin-mineral supplement use and nutritional status of athletes. *J Am Coll Nutr.* 1993;12:162–169.

66. Chen JD, Wang JF, Li KL, et al. Nutritional problems and measures in elite and amateur athletes. *Am J Clin Nutr.* 1989;49:1084–1089.

67. Fogelholm GM, Himberg J, Alopaeus K, Gref C, Laakso JT, Mussalo-Rauhamaa H. Dietary and biochemical indices of nutritional status in male athletes and controls. *J Am Coll Nutr.* 1992;11:181–191.

68. Peters AJ, Dressendorfer RH, Rimar J, Keen CL. Diet of endurance runners competing in a 20-day road race. *Physician and Sportsmedicine.* 1986;14:63–70.

69. Singh A, Day BA, Debolt JE, Trostmann UH, Bernier LL, Deuster PA. Magnesium, zinc, and copper status of US Navy SEAL trainees. *Am J Clin Nutr.* 1989;49:695–700.

70. Singh A, Evans P, Gallagher KL, Deuster PA. Dietary intakes and biochemical profiles of nutritional status of ultramarathoners. *Med Sci Sports Exerc.* 1993;25:328–334.

71. Steen SN, Mayer K, Brownell KD, Wadden TA. Dietary intake of female collegiate heavyweight rowers. *Int J Sport Nutr.* 1995;5:225–231.

72. Loosli AR, Benson J, Gillien DM, Bourdet K. Nutrition habits and knowledge in competitive adolescent female gymnasts. *Physician and Sportsmedicine.* 1986;14:118–130.

73. Steen SN, McKinney S. Nutritional assessment of college wrestlers. *Physician and Sportsmedicine.* 1986;14:101–116.

74. Rayssiguier Y, Guezennec CY, Durlach J. New experimental and clinical data on the relationship between magnesium and sport. *Magnes Res.* 1990;3:93–102.

75. Casoni I, Gugliemini C, Graziano L, Reali MG. Mazzotta D, Abbasciano V. Changes in magnesium concentrations in endurance athletes. *Int J Sports Med.* 1990;11:234–237.

76. Fogelholm M, Laakso J, Lehto J, Ruokonen I. Dietary intake and indicators of magnesium and zinc status in male athletes. *Nutr Res.* 1991;11:1111–1118.

77. Fogelholm GM, Lahtinen PK. Nutritional evaluation of a sailing crew during a transatlantic race. *Scand J Med Sci Sports.* 1991;1:99–103.

78. Olha AE, Klissouras V, Sullivan JD, Skoryna SC. Effect of exercise on concentration of elements in the serum. *J Sports Med Phys Fitness.* 1982;22:414–425.

79. Telford RD, Catchpole EA, Deakin V, McLeay AC, Plank AW. The effect of 7 to 8 months of vitamin/mineral supplementation on the vitamin and mineral status of athletes. *Int J Sport Nutr.* 1992;2:123–134.

80. Weight LM, Noakes TD, Labadarios D, Graves J, Jacobs P, Berman PA. Vitamins and mineral status of trained athletes including the effects of supplementation. *Am J Clin Nutr.* 1988;47:186–191.

81. Lehman M, Foster C, Keul J. Overtraining in endurance athletes; a brief review. *Med Sci Sports Exerc.* 1993;25:854–862.

82. Kleiner SM, Bazzarre TL, Ainsworth BE. Nutritional status of nationally ranked elite bodybuilders. *Int J Sport Nutr.* 1994;4:54–69.

83. Rowe WJ. Extraordinary unremitting endurance exercise and permanent injury to normal heart. *Lancet.* 1992;340:712–714.

84. Deuster PA, Dolev E, Kyle SB, Anderson RA, Schoomaker EB. Magnesium homeostasis during high-intensity anaerobic exercise in men. *J Appl Physiol.* 1987;62:545–550.

85. Lijnen P, Hespel P, Fagard R, Lysens R, Vanden Eynde E, Amery A. Erythrocyte, plasma and urinary magnesium in men before and after a marathon. *Eur J Appl Physiol.* 1988;58:252–256.

86. Lukaski HC, Bolonchuk WW, Siders WA, Milne DB. Chromium supplementation and resistance training: effects of body composition, strength, and trace element status of men. *Am J Clin Nutr.* 1996;63:954–965.

87. McDonald R, Keen CL. Iron, zinc and magnesium nutrition and athletic performance. *Sports Med.* 1988;5:171–184.

88. Deuster PA, Singh A. Response of plasma magnesium and other cations to fluid replacement during exercise. *J Am Coll Nutr.* 1993;12:286–293.

89. Laires MJ, Alves F, Halpern MJ. Changes in serum and erythrocyte magnesium and blood lipids after distance swimming. *Magnes Res.* 1988;1:219–222.

90. Stendig-Lindberg G, Shapiro Y, Epstein Y, et al. Changes in serum magnesium concentration after strenuous exercise. *J Am Coll Nutr.* 1988;6:35–40.

91. Laires MJ, Alves F. Changes in plasma, erythrocyte, and urinary magnesium with prolonged swimming exercise. *Magnes Res.* 1991;4:119–122.

92. Franz KB, Ruddel H, Todd GL, Dorheim TA, Buell JC, Eliot RS. Physiological changes during a marathon, with special reference to magnesium. *J Am Coll Nutr.* 1985;4:187–194.

93. Rose LI, Carroll DR, Lowe SL, Peterson EW, Cooper KH. Serum electrolyte changes after marathon running. *J Appl Physiol.* 1970;29:449–451.

94. Laires MJ, Madeira F, Sérgio J, et al. Preliminary study of the relationship between plasma and erythrocyte magnesium variation and some circulation pro-oxidant and antioxidant indices in a standardized physical effort. *Magnes Res.* 1993;6:233–238.

95. Laires MJ, Monteiro CP, Sérgio J, et al. Content of trace elements in blood before and after three standard efforts. In: Collery PH, Poirier LA, Littlefield NA, Etienne JC, eds. *Metal Ions in Biology and Medicine.* Paris: John Libbel Eurotext; 1994;557–563.

96. Resina A, Gatteschi L, Castellani W, Gavan P, Parise G, Rubenni MG. Effects of aerobic training and exercise on plasma and erythrocyte magnesium concentration. In: Kies CV, Driskell JA, eds. *Sports Nutrition: Minerals and Electrolytes.* Boca Raton, FL: CRC Press; 1995;189–198.

97. Dressendorfer RH, Wade CE, Keen CL, Scaff JH. Plasma mineral levels in marathon runners during a 20-day road race. *Physician and Sportsmedicine.* 1982; 10:113–118.

98. Cordova A. Changes in plasmatic and erythrocytic magnesium levels after high-intensity exercise in men. *Physiol Behav.* 1992;52:819–821.

99. Rama R, Ibáñez J, Pagés T, Callis A, Palacios L. Plasma and red blood cell magnesium levels and plasma creatinine after a 100 km race. *Rev Esp Fisiol.* 1993;49:43–48.

100. Manore MM, Merkel J, Helleksen M, Skinner JS, Carroll SS. Longitudinal changes in magnesium status in untrained males: effects of two different 12-week exercise training programs and magnesium supplementation. In: Kies CV, Driskell JA, eds. *Sports Nutrition: Minerals and Electrolytes.* Boca Raton, FL: CRC Press; 1995;179–188.

101. Liu L, Borowski G, Rose LI. Hypomagnesemia in a tennis player. *Physician and Sportsmedicine.* 1983; 11:79–80.

102. Williamson SL, Johnson RW, Hudkins PG, Strate SM. Exertional cramps: a prospective study of biochemical & anthropometric variables in bicycle riders. *Cycling Sci.* 1993: Spring, 15–20.

103. Jooste PL, Wolfswinkel JM, Schoeman JJ, Strydom NB. Epileptic-type convulsions and magnesium deficiency. *Aviat Space Environ Med.* 1979;50:734–735.

104. Lukaski HC, Bolonchuk WW, Klevay LM, Milne DB, Sandstead HH. Maximum oxygen consumption as related to magnesium, copper, and zinc nutriture. *Am J Clin Nutr.* 1983;37:407–415.

105. Golf SW, Happel O, Graef V. Plasma aldosterone, cortisol and electrolyte concentrations in physical exercise after magnesium supplementation. *J Clin Chem Clin Biochem.* 1984;22:717–721.

106. Terblanche S, Noakes TD, Dennis SC, Marais DW, Eckert M. Failure of magnesium supplementation to influence marathon running performance or recovery in magnesium-replete subjects. *Int J Sport Nutr.* 1992; 2:154–164.

107. Brilla LA, Haley TF. Effect of magnesium supplementation on strength training in humans. *J Am Coll Nutr.* 1992;11:326–329.

108. Stendig-Lindberg G, Rudy N. Predictors of maximum voluntary contraction force of quadriceps muscles in man: ridge regression analysis. *Magnesium.* 1983; 2:93–104.

109. Arnaud CD, Sanchez SD. Calcium and phosphorus. In: Ziegler EE, Filer LJ Jr, eds. *Present Knowledge in Nutrition*. 7th ed. Washington, DC: International Life Sciences Institute; 1996;245–255.

110. Cade R, Conte M, Zauner C, et al. Effects of phosphate loading on 2,3-diphosphoglycerate and maximal oxygen uptake. *Med Sci Sports Exerc*. 1984;16:263–268.

111. Stewart I, McNaughton L, Davies P, Tristram S. Phosphate loading and the effects of VO_{2max} in trained cyclists. *Res Q Exerc Sport*. 1990;61:80–84.

112. Kreider RB, Miller GW, Williams MH, Somma CT, Nasser TA. Effects of phosphate loading on oxygen uptake, ventilatory anaerobic threshold, and run performance. *Med Sci Sports Exerc*. 1990;22:250–256.

113. Kreider RB, Miller GW, Schenck D, et al. Effects of phosphate loading on metabolic and myocardial responses to maximal and endurance exercise. *Int J Sport Nutr*. 1992;2:20–47.

114. Bredle DL, Stager JM, Breschue WF, Farber MO. Phosphate supplementation, cardiovascular function, and exercise performance in humans. *J Appl Physiol*. 1988;65:1821–1826.

115. Duffy DJ, Conlee RK. Effects of phosphate loading on leg power and high intensity treadmill exercise. *Med Sci Sports Exerc*. 1986;18:674–677.

116. Galloway SDR, Tremblay MS, Sexsmith JR, Roberts CJ. The effects of acute phosphate supplementation in subjects of different aerobic fitness levels. *Eur J Appl Physiol*. 1996;72:224–230.

117. Mannix ET, Stager JM, Harris A, Farber MO. Oxygen delivery and cardiac output during exercise following oral glucose phosphate. *Med Sci Sports Exerc*. 1990;22:341–347.

118. Tremblay MS, Galloway SDR, Sexsmith JR. Ergogenic effects of phosphate loading: physiological fact or methodological fiction? *Can J Appl Physiol*. 1994;19:1–11.

119. Cook JD, Finch CA. Assessing iron status of a population. *Am J Clin Nutr*. 1979;32:2114–2119.

120. Cook JD, Finch CA, Smith NJ. Evaluation of the iron status of a population. *Blood*. 1976;48:449–455.

121. Balaban EP, Cox JV, Snell P, Vaughan RH, Frenkel EP. The frequency of anemia and iron deficiency in the runner. *Med Sci Sports Exerc*. 1989;21:643–648.

122. Colt E, Heyman B. Low ferritin in runners. *J Sports Med Phys Fitness*. 1989;24:13–17.

123. Haymes EM, Spillman DM. Iron status of women distance runners, sprinters, and control women. *Int J Sports Med*. 1989;10:430–433.

124. Risser WL, Lee EJ, Poindexter HBW, et al. Iron deficiency in female athletes: its prevalence and impact on performance. *Med Sci Sports Exerc*. 1988;20:116–121.

125. Clement DB, Lloyd-Smith DR, MacIntyre JG, et al. Iron status in winter Olympic sports. *J Sports Sci*. 1987;5:261–271.

126. Haymes EM, Puhl JL, Temples TE. Training for cross-country skiing and iron status. *Med Sci Sports Exerc*. 1986;18:162–167.

127. Rowland TW, Kelleher JF. Iron deficiency in athletes: insights from high school swimmers. *Am J Dis Child*. 1989;143:197–200.

128. Nickerson HF, Holubets MC, Weller BR, Haas RG, Schwartz S, Ellefson ME. Causes of iron deficiency in adolescent athletes. *J Pediatr*. 1989;114:657–663.

129. Fogelholm M. Indicators of vitamin and mineral status in athlete's blood: a review. *Int J Sport Nutr*. 1995;5:267–284.

130. Robertson JD, Maughan RJ, Milne AC, Davidson RJL. Hematological status of male runners in relation to the extent of physical training. *Int J Sport Nutr*. 1992;2:366–375.

131. Willows ND, Grimston SK, Smith DI, Hanby DA. Iron and hematological status among adolescent athletes tracked through puberty. *Pediat Exer Sci*. 1995;7:253–262.

132. Pate RR, Miller BJ, Davis JM, Slentz CA, Klingshirn LA. Iron status of female runners. *Int J Sport Nutr*. 1993;3:222–231.

133. Dallman PR, Yip R, Johnson C. Prevalence and causes of anemia in the United States, 1976–1980. *Am J Clin Nutr*. 1984;39:437–445.

134. Schmidt W, Maasen N, Trost F, Boning D. Training induced effects on blood volume, erythrocyte turnover haemoglobin oxygen binding properties. *Eur J Appl Physiol*. 1988;57:490–498.

135. Diehl DM, Lohman TG, Smith SC, Kertzer R. Effects of physical training and competition on the iron status of female field hockey players. *Int J Sports Med*. 1986;7:264–277.

136. Nickerson HJ, Holubets M, Tripp AD, Pierce WE. Decreased iron stores in high school female runners. *Am J Dis Child*. 1985;139:1115–1119.

137. Roberts D, Smith D. Serum ferritin values in elite speed and synchronized swimmers and speed skaters. *J Lab Clin Med*. 1990;116:661–665.

138. Blum SM, Sherman AR, Boileau RA. The effects of fitness-type exercise on iron status in adult women. *Am J Clin Nutr*. 1986;43:456–463.

139. Lyle RM, Weaver CM, Sedlock DA, Rajaram S, Martin B, Melby CL. Iron status in exercising women: the effects of oral iron therapy vs increased consumption of muscle foods. *Am J Clin Nutr*. 1992;56:1049–1055.

140. Lampe JW, Slavin JL, Apple FS. Poor iron status of women runners training for a marathon. *Int J Sports Med*. 1986;7:111–114.

141. Lukaski HC, Hoverson BS, Gallagher SK, Bolonchuk WW. Physical training and copper, iron, and zinc status of swimmers. *Am J Clin Nutr*. 1990;51:1093–1099.

142. Taylor C, Rogers G, Goodman C, et al. Hematologic, iron-related and acute-phase protein responses to sustained strenuous exercise. *J Appl Physiol*. 1987; 62:464–469.

143. Green R, Charlton R, Seftel H, et al. Body iron excretion in man. *Am J Med*. 1968;45:336–353.

144. Jacobs RA, Sandstead HH, Munoz JM, Klevay LM, Milne DB. Whole body surface loss of trace metals in normal males. *Am J Clin Nutr*. 1981;34:1379–1383.

145. Haymes EM, Lamanca JJ. Iron loss in runners during exercise: implications and recommendations. *Sports Med*. 1989;7:277–285.

146. Hallberg L, Hogdahl AM, Nilsson L, Rybo G. Menstrual blood loss and iron deficiency. *Acta Med Scand*. 1966;180:639–650.

147. Hallberg L, Rossander-Hulten L. Iron requirements in menstruating women. *Am J Clin Nutr*. 1991;54:1047–1058.

148. Porter AMW. Do some marathon runners bleed into the gut? *Br Med J*. 1983;287:1427.

149. Stewart JG, Ahlquist DA, McGill DB, et al. Gastrointestinal blood loss and anemia in runners. *Ann Intern Med*. 1984;100:843–845.

150. Robertson JD, Maughan RJ, Davidson RJL. Faecal blood loss in response to exercise. *Br Med J*. 1987; 295:303–305.

151. Fisher RL, McMahon LF, Ryan MJ, Larson D, Brand M. Gastrointestinal bleeding in competitive runners. *Dig Dis Sci*. 1986;31:1226–1228.

152. Cooper BT, Douglas SA, Firth LA, Hannagan JA, Chadwick VS. Erosive gastritis and gastrointestinal bleeding in a female runner. *Gastroenterology*. 1987; 92:2019–2023.

153. Paulev PE, Jordal R, Petersen NS. Dermal excretion of iron in intensely training athletes. *Clin Chim Acta*. 1983;127:19–27.

154. Lamanca JJ, Haymes EM, Daly JA, Moffatt RJ, Waller MF. Sweat iron loss of male and female runners during exercise. *Int J Sports Med*. 1988;9:52–55.

155. Waller MF, Haymes EM. The effects of heat and exercise on sweat iron loss. *Med Sci Sports Exerc*. 1996; 28:197–203.

156. Snyder AC, Dvorak LL, Roepke JB. Influence of dietary iron source on measures of iron status among female runners. *Med Sci Sports Exerc*. 1989;21:7–10.

157. Block G, Dresser CM, Hartman AM, Carroll MD. Nutrient sources in the American diet: quantitative data from the NHANES II survey. *Am J Epidemiol*. 1985; 122:13–26.

158. Clement DB, Taunton JE, McKenzie DC, Sawchuk LL, Wiley JP. High- and low-dosage iron supplementation in iron-deficient, endurance-trained females. In: Katch FI, ed. *Sport Health and Nutrition*. Champaign, IL: Human Kinetics; 1986:75–81.

159. Fogelholm M, Jaakkola L, Lampisiarvi T. Effects of iron supplementation in female athletes with low serum ferritin concentrations. *Int J Sports Med*. 1992;13:158–162.

160. Klingshirn LA, Pate RR, Bourque SP, Davis JM, Sargent RG. Effect of iron supplementation on endurance capacity in iron-depleted female runners. *Med Sci Sports Exerc*. 1992;24:819–824.

161. Lamanca JJ, Haymes EM. Effects of iron repletion on VO$_{2max}$, endurance, and blood lactate. *Med Sci Sports Exerc*. 1993;25:1386–1392.

162. Newhouse IJ, Clement DB, Taunton JE, McKenzie DC. The effects of prelatent/latent iron deficiency on work capacity. *Med Sci Sports Exerc*. 1989;21:263–268.

163. Rowland TW, Deisroth MB, Green GM, Kelleher JF. The effect of iron therapy on the exercise capacity of nonanemic iron-deficient adolescent runners. *Am J Dis Child*. 1988;142:165–169.

164. Yoshida T, Udo M, Chida M, Ichioka M, Makiguchi K. Dietary iron supplement during severe physical training in competitive distance runners. *Sports Training Med Rehab*. 1990;1:279–285.

165. Davies KJA, Donovan CM, Refino CJ, Brooks GA, Packer L, Dallman PR. Distinguishing effects of anemia and muscle iron deficiency on exercise bioenergetics in the rat. *Am J Physiol*. 1984;246:E535–E543.

166. Finch CA, Gollnick PD, Hlastala MP, Miller LR, Dillmann E, Mackler B. Lactic acidosis as a result of iron deficiency. *J Clin Invest*. 1979;64:129–137.

167. Davies KJA, Maguire JJ, Brooks GA, Dallman PR, Packer L. Muscle mitochondrial bioenergetics, oxygen supply, and work capacity during dietary iron deficiency and repletion. *Am J Physiol*. 1992;242:E418–E427.

168. Celsing F, Blomstrand E, Werner B, Pihlstedt P, Ekblom B. Effects of iron deficiency on endurance and muscle enzyme activity in man. *Med Sci Sports Exerc*. 1986;18:156–161.

169. Aruoma OL, Bomford A, Oiksib RJ, Halliwell B. Nontransferrin-bound iron in plasma from hemochromatosis patients: effect of phlebotomy therapy. *Blood*. 1988;72:1416–1419.

170. Salonen JT, Nyyssonen K, Korpela H, Tuomlehto J, Seppanen R, Salonen R. High stored iron levels are associated with excess risk of myocardial infarction in eastern Finnish men. *Circulation*. 1992;86:803–811.

171. Stevens RG, Jones DY, Micozzi MS, Taylor PR. Body iron stores and the risk of cancer. *N Engl J Med*. 1988;319:1047–1052.

172. Dressendorfer RH, Sockolov R. Hypozincemia in athletes. *Physician Sportsmedicine*. 1980;8:97–100.

173. Haralambie G. Serum zinc in athletes in training. *Int J Sports Med*. 1981;2:136–138.

174. Fogelholm M, Rehunen S, Gref CG, et al. Dietary intake and thiamin, iron, and zinc status in elite Nordic skiers during different training periods. *Int J Sport Nutr*. 1992;2:351–365.

175. Singh A, Smoak BL, Patterson KY, LeMay LG, Veillon C, Deuster PA. Biochemical indices of selected trace minerals in men: effect of stress. *Am J Clin Nutr*. 1991;53:126–131.

176. Miyamura JB, McNutt SW, Lichton IJ, Wenkam NS. Altered zinc status of soldiers under field conditions. *J Am Diet Assoc*. 1987;87:595–597.

177. Couzy F, Lafargue P, Guezennec CT. Zinc metabolism in the athlete: influence of training, nutrition, and other factors. *Int J Sports Med*. 1990;11:263–266.

178. Anderson RA, Polansky MM, Bryden NA. Strenuous running: acute effects on chromium, copper, zinc, and selected clinical variables in urine and serum of male runners. *Biol Trace Elem Res*. 1984;6:327–336.

179. Van Rij AM, Hall MT, Dohm GL, Bray J, Pories WJ. Changes in zinc metabolism following exercise in human subjects. *Biol Trace Elem Res*. 1986;10:99–106.

180. Deuster PA, Day BA, Singh A, Douglass L, Moser-Veillon PB. Zinc status of highly trained women runners and untrained women. *Am J Clin Nutr*. 1989;49:1295–1301.

181. Tipton K, Green NR, Haymes EM, Waller MF. Zinc loss in sweat of athletes exercising in hot and neutral temperatures. *Int J Sport Nutr*. 1993;3:261–271.

182. Singh A, Failla ML, Deuster PA. Exercise-induced changes in immune function: effects of zinc supplementation. *J Appl Physiol*. 1994;76:2298–2303.

183. Oh SH, Deagen JT, Whanger PD, Weswig PH. Biological function of metallothionein: V. Its induction in rats by various stressors. *Am J Physiol*. 1978;234:1978;234:E282–E285.

184. Ohno H, Sato Y, Ishikawa M, et al. Training effects on blood zinc levels in humans. *J Sports Med Phys Fitness*. 1990;30:247–253.

185. Fogelholm M. Micronutrient status in females during a 24-week fitness-type exercise program. *Ann Nutr Metab*. 1992;36:209–218.

186. Ohno H, Yamashita K, Doi R, Yamamura K, Kondo T, Taniguchi N. Exercise-induced changes in blood zinc and related proteins in humans. *J Appl Physiol*. 1985;58:1453–1458.

187. Nosaka K, Clarkson PM. Changes in plasma zinc following high force eccentric exercise. *Int J Sport Nutr*. 1992;2:175–184.

188. Pennington JAT, Young BE, Wilson DB. Nutritional elements in U.S. diets: results from the total diet study, 1982 to 1986. *J Am Diet Assoc*. 1989;89:659–664.

189. Patterson KY, Holbrook JT, Bodner JE, Kelsay JL, Smith JC, Veilon C. Zinc, copper, and manganese intake and balance for adults consuming self-selected diets. *Am J Clin Nutr*. 1984;40:1397–1403.

190. Nieman DC, Butler JV, Pollet LM, Dietrich SJ, Lutz RD. Nutrient intake of marathon runners. *J Am Diet Assoc*. 1989;89:1273–1278.

191. Krotkiewski M, Gudmundsson M, Backstrom P, Mandroakas K. Zinc and muscle strength and endurance. *Acta Physiol Scand*. 1982;116:309–311.

192. Lukaski HC, Bolonchuk WW, Klevay LM, Milne DB, Sandstead HH. Changes in plasma zinc content after exercise in men fed a low-zinc diet. *Am J Physiol*. 1984;247:E88–E93.

193. Chandra RK. Excessive intake of zinc impairs immune responses. *JAMA*. 1984;252:1443–1446.

194. Hooper PL, Visconti L, Garry PJ, Johnson GE. Zinc lowers high-density lipoprotein-cholesterol levels. *JAMA*. 1980;244:1960–1961.

195. Goodwin JA, Hunt WC, Hooper P, Garry PJ. Relationship between zinc intake, physical activity, and blood levels of high-density lipoprotein cholesterol in a healthy elderly population. *Metabolism*. 1985;34:519–523.

196. Crouse SF, Hooper PL, Atterbom HA, Papenfuss RL. Zinc ingestion and lipoprotein values in sedentary and endurance-trained men. *JAMA*. 1984;252:785–787.

197. O'Dell BL. Copper. In: *Present Knowledge in Nutrition*. 5th ed. Washington, DC: The Nutrition Foundation; 1984:506–518.

198. Haralambie G. Changes in electrolytes and trace elements during long-lasting exercise. In: Howald H, Poortmans J, eds. *Metabolic Adaptations to Prolonged Physical Exercise*. Basel: Birkhauser Verlag; 1975:340–351.

199. Resina A, Fedi S, Gatteschi L, et al. Comparison of some serum copper parameters in trained runners and control subjects. *Int J Sports Med*. 1990;11:58–60.

200. Resina A, Gatteschi L, Rubenni MG, Giamberardino MA, Imreh F. Comparison of some serum copper parameters in trained professional soccer players and control subjects. *J Sports Med Phys Fitness*. 1991;31:413–416.

201. Bordin D, Sartorelli L, Bonanni G, Mastrogiacomo I, Scalco E. High intensity physical exercise induced effects on plasma levels of copper and zinc. *Biol Trace Elem Res*. 1993;36:129–134.

202. Wang W-C, Hainonen D, Mukela P, Nauto V. Serum selenium, zinc and copper in Swedish and Finnish

orienteers: a comparative study. *Analyst*. 1995; 120:837–840.

203. Dowdy RP, Burt J. Effect of intensive long-term training on copper and iron nutriture in man. *Fed Proc*. 1980;39:786.

204. Ohno H, Yahata T, Hirata F, et al. Changes in dopamine-beta-hydroxylase and copper and catecholamine concentrations in human plasma with physical exercise. *J Sports Med Phys Fitness*. 1984;24:315–320.

205. Anderson RA, Bryden NA, Polansky MM. Acute exercise effects on urinary losses and serum concentrations of copper and zinc of moderately trained and untrained men consuming a controlled diet. *Analyst*. 1995; 120:867–870.

206. Aruoma OI, Reilly T, MacLaren D, Halliwell B. Iron, copper and zinc concentrations in human sweat and plasma: the effect of exercise. *Clin Chim Acta*. 1988; 177:81–88.

207. Levander OA, Burk RF. Selenium. In: Ziegler EE, Filer LJ Jr, eds. *Present Knowledge in Nutrition*. 7th ed. Washington, DC: International Life Sciences Institute; 1996:320–328.

208. Jenkins RR. Exercise, oxidative stress, and antioxidants: A review. *Int J Sport Nutr*. 1993;3:356–375.

209. Halliwell B. Antioxidants. In: Ziegler EE, Filer LJ Jr, eds. *Present Knowledge in Nutrition*. 7th ed. Washington, DC: International Life Sciences Institute; 1996: 596–603.

210. Clarkson PM. Antioxidants and physical performance. *Crit Rev Food Sci Nutr*. 1995;35:131–141.

211. Snook JT, Cummin D, Good PR, Grayzar J. Mineral and energy status of groups of male and female athletes participating in events believed to result in adverse nutritional status. In: Kies CV, Driskell JA, eds. *Sports Nutrition: Minerals and Electrolytes*, Boca Raton, FL: CRC Press; 1995.

212. Dragan I, Dinu V, Mohora M, Cristea E, Ploesteanu E, Stroescu V. Studies regarding the antioxidant effects of selenium on top swimmers. *Rev roum Physiol*. 1990; 27:15–20.

213. Dragan I, Dinu V, Cristea E, Mohora M, Ploesteanu E, Stroescu V. Studies regarding the effects of an antioxidant compound in top athletes. *Rev roum Physiol*. 1991;28:105–108.

214. Tessier F, Margaritis I, Richard M, Moynot C, Marconnet P. Selenium and training effects of the glutathione system and aerobic performance. *Med Sci Sports Exerc*. 1995;27:390–396.

215. Tessier F, Hida H, Favier A, Marconnet P. Muscle GSH-Px activity after prolonged exercise training and selenium supplementation. *Biol Trace Element Res*. 1995;47:279–285.

216. Stoecker BJ. Chromium. In: Ziegler EE, Filer LJ Jr, eds. *Present Knowledge in Nutrition*. 7th ed. Washington, DC: International Life Sciences Institute; 1996: 344–353.

217. Trent LK, Thieding-Cancel D. Effects of chromium picolinate on body composition. *J Sports Med Phys Fitness*. 1995;35:273–280.

218. Anderson RA, Bryden NA, Polansky MM, Thorp JW. Effects of carbohydrate loading and underwater exercise on circulating cortisol, insulin and urinary losses of chromium and zinc. *Eur J Appl Physiol*. 1991; 63:146–150.

219. Clarkson PM. Nutritional ergogenic aids: chromium, exercise, and muscle mass. *Int J Sport Nutr*. 1991; 3:289–293.

220. Clarkson PM, Haymes EM. Trace mineral requirements for athletes. *Int J Sport Nutr*. 1994;4:104–119.

221. Lefavi RG, Anderson RA, Keith RE, Wilson GD, McMillan JL, Stone MH. Efficacy of chromium supplementation in athletes: emphasis on anabolism. *Int J Sport Nutr*. 1992;2:111–122.

222. Anderson RA, Polansky MM, Bryden NA, Roginski EE, Patterson KY, Reamer DC. Effect of exercise (running) on serum glucose, insulin, glucagon, and chromium excretion. *Diabetes*. 1982;31:212–216.

223. Gatteschi L, Castellani W, Galvan P, Parise G, Resina A, Rubenni MG. Effects of aerobic exercise on plasma chromium concentrations. In: Kies CV, Driskell JA, eds. *Sports Nutrition: Minerals and Electrolytes*. Boca Raton, FL: CRC Press; 1995:199–204.

224. Anderson RA, Bryden NA, Polansky MM, Reiser S. Urinary chromium excretion and insulinogenic properties of carbohydrates. *Am J Clin Nutr*. 1990;51:864–868.

225. Anderson RA, Bryden NA, Polansky MM, Deuster PA. Exercise effects on chromium excretion of trained and untrained men consuming a constant diet. *J Appl Physiol*. 1988;64:249–252.

226. Evans GW. The effect of chromium picolinate on insulin controlled parameters in humans. *Int J Biosocial Med Res*. 1989;11:163–180.

227. Hasten DL, Rome EP, Franks BD, Hegsted M. Effects of chromium picolinate on beginning weight training students. *Int J Sport Nutr*. 1992;2:343–350.

228. Clancy S, Clarkson PM, DeCheke ME, et al. Effects of chromium picolinate supplementation on body composition, strength, and urinary chromium loss in football players. *Int J Sport Nutr*. 1994;4:142–153.

229. Hallmark MA, Reynolds TH, DeSouza CA, Dotson CO, Anderson RA, Roger MA. Effects of chromium and resistive training on muscle strength and body composition. *Med Sci Sports Exerc*. 1996;28:139–144.

230. Stearns DM, Wise JP Sr, Patierno SR, Wetterhahn KE. Chromium (III) picolinate produces chromosome damage in Chinese hamster ovary cells. *FASEB J.* 1995; 9:1643–1649.

231. McCarty MF. Chromium (III) picolinate (letter). *FASEB J.* 1996;10:365–367.

232. Stearns DM, Belbruno JJ, Wetterhahn KE. A prediction of chromium (III) accumulation in humans from chromium dietary supplements. *FASEB J.* 1995; 9:1650–1657.

CHAPTER 6

Antioxidant Supplementation for Persons Who Are Physically Active

Mitchell Kanter

A free radical is chemically defined as a molecule capable of independent existence that contains one or more unpaired electrons in an orbital.[1] In nature, atoms and molecules tend to be most stable when they contain pairs of electrons in an orbital. Therefore, free radicals tend to be highly reactive species that can interact with numerous biologic molecules and set in motion a series of damaging reactions.[2]

During the past 25 years, the study of free radicals and their potential role in the etiology of various disease conditions has increased dramatically. Indeed, numerous epidemiologic and experimental studies conducted in recent years strongly implicate free radicals in the development of diverse disease conditions such as cancer, cardiovascular disease, autoimmune diseases,[3] and thermal injury,[4] as well as the aging process[5,6] (see Table 6–1).

A link between physical exercise and free radicals has been established as well. However, it is difficult to draw definitive conclusions about the link between exercise and free radicals, largely because of differences in experimental protocols, the use of various subpopulation groups, and the equivocal nature of the markers used to measure free radicals in living systems. Although it can be stated with some level of certainty that oxidant stress occurs during exercise, the physiologic implications of this effect remain to be elucidated.

Nevertheless, the suggestion that free radicals may, in essence, represent the "dark side" of physical activity has led to the extensive study of nutritional antioxidants as a means of diminishing the potential harmful effects of reactive oxygen species. To date, vitamins E and C have been the most well-studied antioxidants under exercising conditions. Results of these studies have been equivocal as well. Under particular environmental conditions,[7] and with certain population groups,[8] vitamin supplementation has proven to be efficacious, but numerous other studies have produced mixed results.[9–14]

A burgeoning area of research has been the study of various "phytonutrients" that exist in common foods and ingredients. Many of these compounds are reported to have antioxidant properties in in vitro studies. Nevertheless, their efficacy in subjects who are physically active remains to be determined.

GENERAL RESEARCH FINDINGS

There are various pathways for the production of free radicals in living systems; one pathway involves the enzymatic reduction of oxygen through the cytochrome chain. Although this pathway represents the body's principal means of energy generation, the reduction of molecular oxygen also leads to the generation of free radical species.

As a result of studies conducted by Dillard et al[15,16] and Tappel[17] in the 1970s, and Davies et al[18] and Jenkins et al[19] in the early 1980s, a link

Table 6–1 Clinical Conditions Purportedly Involving Free Radical Generation

	Condition
Cardiovascular	Adriamycin cardiotoxicity Atherosclerosis Keshan disease (selenium deficiency)
Eye	Cataracts Degenerative retinal damage
Gastrointestinal tract	Oral iron poisoning Pancreatitis
Inflammatory-immune injury	Autoimmune diseases Rheumatoid arthritis
Lung	Cigarette smoke effects Emphysema Pollutant damage
Neuromuscular diseases	Multiple sclerosis Muscular dystrophy Parkinson's disease
Red blood cell	Lead poisoning Malaria Sickle cell anemia
Skin	Solar radiation Thermal injury
Additional	Aging Alcohol-induced iron overload Cancer Drug-induced reactions Ischemia-reperfusion injury Radiation injury

Source: Adapted with permission from H.B. Halliwell, Oxident and Human Disease: Some New Concepts, *FASEB Journal*, Vol. 1, pp. 358–364, © 1987, Federation of American Societies for Experimental Biology.

among physical exercise, increased oxygen consumption, and free radical production through the cytochrome chain has been established. It has been estimated that for every 25 oxygen molecules reduced through the cytochrome chain during normal respiration, one free radical is produced.[20] Coupled with the fact that the rate of whole body oxygen consumption during exercise may increase 10- to 15-fold, and that oxygen flux in an active muscle may increase 100-fold,[21] it is easy to understand how an increased metabolism can greatly increase free radical production. This relationship between an apparently healthful act (exercise) and a series of reactions that can, among other things, damage various organ systems has been troublesome to many researchers. The so-called "oxygen paradox" evoked by exercise prompted Jenkins to state that, "elemental and gaseous oxygen presents a conundrum in that it is simultaneously essential for and potentially destructive to human life."[22]

It should be noted, however, that an increase in exercise-induced oxygen consumption is not the only mechanism that has been linked to the production of free radicals in persons who are physically active. For example, transient tissue hypoxia, which may occur with heavy weight lifting or high-intensity anaerobic work, can lead to an increase in hydrogen ions, which can, in turn, react with superoxide anions to produce additional reactive oxygen species.[22] Tissue hypoxia can also lead to the freeing of transitional metals such as iron and copper from their normal transporters. These free metals can further catalyze free radical reactions.

It has also been suggested that reperfusion of hypoxic muscle after a period of particularly stressful activity can result in postischemic injury, including edema formation, microvascular dysfunction, and muscle necrosis.[23] The widely held hypothesis about ischemia-reperfusion injury suggests that xanthine is formed after adenosine triphosphate (ATP) and other high-energy phosphates are depleted through anaerobic metabolism. Simultaneously, calcium influx and protease activation in damaged tissues stimulate the conversion of xanthine dehydrogenase to xanthine oxidase. With reperfusion and the reintroduction of molecular oxygen into the microenvironment, xanthine oxidase catalyzes xanthine to uric acid.[24] Toxic reactive oxygen metabolites are produced as metabolic by-products.

Tissue trauma and inflammation, which result in the release of phagocytic cells such as neutrophils, have also been implicated in free radical production through activity of enzymes such as NADPH oxidase.[25]

Other mechanisms purported to induce oxidant stress with exercise include substrate depletion (purportedly through a diminution in pentose shunt-generated NADPH activity and, ultimately, a decline in tissue glutathione reductase activity[26]) and mechanical trauma (through joint compression of synovial fluid).[27] Further, a study by Salo et al[4] suggested that exercise-in-

duced hyperthermia could trigger oxidative stress by promoting mitochondrial uncoupling, loss of respiratory control, and, ultimately, free radical production.

Despite the large number of potential mechanisms that apparently promote free radical generation under exercising conditions, it should be pointed out that the true biologic implications of these effects have yet to be determined. While discussing the role of oxidants in human diseases, Halliwell questioned whether free radicals are a major cause of tissue injury or are merely produced during injury. He attributed the relative lack of understanding of this issue to inadequate experimental techniques, as well as an overemphasis on lipid peroxidation as a mechanism of oxidant injury.[3] Although Halliwell was discussing the relationship between oxidant stress and disease, a review of the exercise literature would suggest that the points he raised are pertinent to physical activity as well.

MEASUREMENT OF FREE RADICAL PRODUCTION IN EXERCISE STUDIES

Few studies have actually measured exercise-induced free radical production. Davies et al[18] were one of the only groups to directly measure free radicals in animal tissue through electron paramagnetic resonance (EPR). Although their study was published approximately 15 years ago, their results have never been replicated, and their ability to have accurately quantified free radical generation under biologic conditions has been questioned.

Most of the studies that have looked at exercise-induced oxidant stress have actually measured indirect markers of lipid peroxidation, and not free radical generation. The majority of these markers, including tissue malondialdehyde production [through gas chromatography or high-performance liquid chromatography], conjugated diene formation, chemiluminescence, and expired breath pentane and ethane, represent minor reaction pathways in highly complex systems.[1] Most have been criticized for their lack of specificity, sensitivity, and reproducibility.[28,29] Nevertheless, much of our understanding and beliefs about exercise-induced free radicals are based on the results of studies that have used combinations of these methodologies. Coupled with the fact that these studies have involved various modes of exercise and numerous population groups, it is understandable why our current knowledge of the relationship between exercise and free radicals is tenuous. New, promising methods such as the use of spin traps, monoclonal antibodies, and flow cytometry should shed greater light in the future on the role of free radicals in exercise-induced tissue damage. A few recent studies have looked at the effects of exercise on the susceptibility of the low-density lipoprotein (LDL) subfraction to oxidation; results of these studies suggest that strenuous exercise promotes oxidative changes to LDL.[30] This methodology represents a novel approach to studying exercise-induced oxidative stress, and preliminary results imply that exercise does, in fact, promote free radical generation.

ENDOGENOUS ANTIOXIDANT PROTECTION

Despite the uncertainty surrounding our understanding of the relationship between exercise and free radicals, the relatively consistent finding of an increase in antioxidant enzyme activity in various tissues of subjects who are trained is highly suggestive of a protective adaptation to the habitual stress of exercise.[19,31-37] It also suggests that a bout of exercise may outstrip the inherent capacity of the protective endogenous antioxidant enzyme system[35,38] (particularly in a person who does not habitually exercise), necessitating greater protection. The findings of various research studies suggest that this added protection could come in the form of an exogenous supplement.[7,39-43]

ANTIOXIDANT SUPPLEMENTATION

By far, vitamins E and C have been the most well-researched nutritional antioxidants in subjects who exercise. Vitamin E is considered to be important because of its association with cell membranes.[44] Of the various forms of vitamin E that exist in nature, alpha tocopherol has the highest biologic activity and the greatest free radical scavenging ability.[45] Vitamin E toxicity is not widely reported, and intakes as high as 200 times the recommended dietary allowance have been ingested without apparent complications.[46] This information has prompted some researchers to suggest that persons who are physically active should consider supplementing at levels in excess of 10 times the current recommended dietary intake (RDI).[47] Vitamin C also serves as an important antioxidant and free radical scavenger; it is extremely labile, and it is highly susceptible to a number of environmental factors including temperature, smog, and cigarette smoke.[48] The labile nature of vitamin C has led some researchers to suggest that persons who are physically active likely require greater than RDI levels.

There is little doubt that vitamin deficiencies in general can impair one's ability to do physical work. Animal studies by Gohil et al[43] and Davies et al[18] indicated that vitamin E deficiency impaired performance, and Salminen and Vihko[49] demonstrated greater susceptibility to lipid peroxidation in rats fed a vitamin E-deficient diet. However, vitamin deficiencies (particularly deficiencies of vitamins E and C) in healthy human subjects are rare, and data from subjects who are well-fed who consume vitamin supplements have produced contradictory results.

Studies by Sumida et al,[42] Cannon et al,[50] and Rokitzi et al[40] reported declines in post-exercise serum enzymes indicative of muscle tissue damage in subjects who consumed 300 to 800 IU vitamin E for 4 to 8 weeks (Rokitzi's subjects consumed 200 mg vitamin C per day as well). Hartmann et al[39] demonstrated that short-term vitamin E supplementation (800 mg administered 12 and 2 hours before exercise and 22 hours after exercise) reduced DNA damage in peripheral white blood cells after exhaustive exercise, and Kanter et al[51] recently reported a 35% increase in T-lag time (indicative of a diminished LDL oxidation rate) in subjects who consumed 1000 IU vitamin E daily for 1 week before exercise.

Various studies have demonstrated beneficial physiologic effects of vitamin C supplementation in persons who are physically active as well. Jakeman and Maxwell[52] reported more rapid recovery of maximal voluntary contraction in subjects who consumed 400 mg vitamin C per day for 21 days; Kaminski and Boals[53] reported less calf soreness in subjects who consumed 3 g vitamin C for 3 days before and 4 days after strenuous calf exercise; and Peters et al[54] noted fewer cases of self-reported upper respiratory tract infection in runners who consumed 600 mg vitamin C per day for 3 weeks before a 42-km road race.

All of the aforementioned studies suggest tangible benefits of vitamins E and C supplementation for combating detrimental physiologic processes that may be initiated by physical activity. Coupled with the results of various studies[16,17,41,42,55,56] that have demonstrated declines in lipid peroxidation markers after exercise in subjects who consumed supplements before exercise, it would appear that vitamin supplementation for persons who are physically active is warranted.

However, it should be noted that contradictory data do exist. Studies by Warren et al, Robertson et al, and Helgheim et al[57–59] have reported no effect of vitamin E supplementation on changes in serum enzyme levels after exercise, and Nieman et al[60] found no beneficial effects of vitamin C supplementation on markers of immune function after a 2.5-hour run. Results of studies that used antioxidant mixtures have produced contradictory findings as well.[41,61,62]

Despite conflicting results in the literature, one could argue that persons who are physically active might benefit from supplementation for a number of reasons. Recent data indicate that the "typical" North American diet provides about two thirds of the recommended daily value of vitamin E.[63] Further, data from the ongoing National Health and Nutrition Examination Survey (NHANES) longitudinal study in the United States suggest that 90% of the study participants failed to ingest the recommended daily intake of five servings of fruits and vegetables per day.[64] Of course, these dietary staples are excellent sources of numerous vitamins and minerals; failure to ingest sufficient quantities of fruits and vegetables would suggest suboptimal intake of various antioxidant nutrients as well.

POTENTIAL OF NONTRADITIONAL NUTRIENTS

This chapter has focused primarily on the potential of more traditional nutrients (particularly vitamins E and C) for persons who are physically active. It should be noted, however, that a burgeoning area of research involves the study of less well-researched nutrients that presently exist in many of the common foods that we eat.[45,65] These phytonutrients have been studied more in relation to various disease conditions and generally in in vitro systems or in animal models. Nevertheless, some of these compounds do warrant mention in an chapter dealing with the antioxidant needs of persons who are physically active; their efficacy may or may not be demonstrated in future studies.

Examples of these nontraditional compounds include various phenolics and isoflavones, such as genestein in soy, caffeic and ferulic acid in oats, and lycopene in tomatoes. Preliminary research suggests, for example, that caffeic and ferulic acid can inhibit rat liver xanthine oxidase activity,[66] and that genestein from soy can inhibit in vitro lipoprotein oxidation in serum.[67] Further, green tea catechins have exhibited antimutagenic effects in cultured Chinese hamster cells.[68] Certainly, most of this research is in its preliminary stages. Much more research will need to be done to further establish the properties, efficacy, and safety of these compounds before they are used as food additives and supplements. Nevertheless, preliminary data have demonstrated that these compounds possess antioxidant potential. They also underscore the importance of eating whole foods, as opposed to relying heavily on supplements as a means of boosting antioxidant intake. As stated previously, the majority of these compounds exist in common foods. Failure to eat a diet that contains a variety of foods diminishes one's ability to consume many of these natural antioxidant compounds.

CONCLUSION

Although conflicting data exist, the preponderance of available information suggests that physical exercise promotes an increase in free radical generation. However, few studies have actually measured exercise-induced free radicals directly, primarily because of a lack of sophisticated methodologies to measure this phenomenon. Instead, researchers have relied heavily on the measurement of lipid peroxidation as the principal indicator of exercise-induced free radicals. It should be noted that free radicals can also alter inactive enzyme complexes, damage DNA and RNA, and promote mutations and cancer, among other things. However, few studies to date dealing with exercise and oxidant stress have measured these outcomes. It should also be noted that free radical species are continuously produced in the human body, and that some have beneficial effects,[69] notably as a part of the body's natural immune system. It is not presently known if long-term ingestion of antioxidant compounds will impact on these positive aspects of free radical generation.

The preponderance of available evidence suggests that antioxidant supplementation, particularly with the vitamins C and E, has favorable effects on markers of lipid peroxidation after exercise. Although the physiologic implications of these effects remain to be elucidated, the prudent use of an antioxidant supplement can provide insurance against a suboptimal diet and/or the increased demands of physical activity. Future research may uncover additional nutritional antioxidants that can benefit the person who is physically active.

Numerous additional questions about the antioxidant needs for physical activity remain to be answered. Little is known about the needs of women who are physically active, particularly those who habitually consume a calorie-restricted diet, or the effects of monthly menstrual blood loss (coupled with exercise) on antioxidant requirements. The needs of the "weekend warrior"—a person who participates in strenuous activity sporadically—versus those of someone who exercises habitually have not been addressed adequately, nor have the needs of the aging athlete. A study by Meydani et al[70] suggested that persons who are elderly and physically active can benefit from antioxidant supplementation more than their younger counterparts, but follow-up studies have not been reported to date.

Dietary issues need to be addressed as well. How much supplementation is too much, and can chronically increased antioxidant intake have an adverse impact on the positive effects of free radicals in living systems? Does a high carbohydrate diet increase antioxidant needs, particularly of the fat-soluble vitamin E? Does a high polyunsaturated fat intake or increased iron intake affect needs? Obviously, there are a number of issues about the antioxidant needs of a person who is physically active that need to be elucidated. Future research using newer, more sophisticated methodologies should provide answers to many of these questions.

REFERENCES

1. Halliwell B, Chirico S. Lipid peroxidation: its mechanism, measurement and significance. *Am J Clin Nutr.* 1993;57(suppl):715S-725S.
2. Kanter M. Free radical and exercise: effects of nutritional antioxidant supplementation. In: Holloszy J, ed. *Exercise and Sports Science Reviews.* Baltimore: Williams & Wilkins; 1995;23:375–397.
3. Halliwell B. Oxidants and human disease: some new concepts. *FASEB J.* 1987;1: 358–364.
4. Salo DC, Donovan CM, Davies KJA. HSP70 and other possible heat shock or oxidative stress proteins are induced in skeletal muscle, heart and liver during exercise. *Free Radic Biol Med.* 1991;11:239–246.

5. Harman D. The aging process. *Proc Nat Acad Sci USA.* 1981;78:7124–7128.

6. Pearl, R. *The Rate of Living.* New York: Kopf; 1928.

7. Simon-Schnass I, Pabst H. Influence of vitamin E on physical performance. *Int J Vitam Nutr Res.* 1988; 58:49–54.

8. Meydani M. Protective role of dietary vitamin E on oxidative stress in aging. *Age.* 1992;15:89–93.

9. Keith RE. (1989). Vitamins in sport and exercise. In: Hickson JE, Wolinsky I, eds. *Nutrition in Exercise and Sport.* Boca Raton, FL: CRC Press.

10. Bramich K, McNaughton L. The effects of two levels of ascorbic acid on muscular endurance, muscular strength, and on VO_{2max}. *Int Clin Nutr Rev.* 1987;7: 5–8.

11. Keren G, Epstein Y. The effect of high dosage vitamin C intake on aerobic and anaerobic capacity. *J of Sports Med.* 1980;20:145–148.

12. Talbot D, Jamieson J. An examination of the effect of vitamin E on the performance of highly trained swimmers. *Can J of Appl Sports Sci.* 1977;2:67–71.

13. Sharman IM, Down MG, Norgan NG. The effects of vitamin E on physiological function and athletic performance of trained swimmers. *J of Sports Med.* 1976;16:215–225.

14. Shephard RJ, Campbell R, Pimm P, Stuart D, Weight GR. Vitamin E, exercise, and the recovery from physical activity. *Eur J Appl Physiol.* 1974;33:119–124.

15. Dillard CJ, Dumelin EE, Tappel AL. Effect of dietary vitamin E on expiration of pentane and ethane by the rat. *Lipids.* 1976;12(1):109–114.

16. Dillard CJ, Litov RE, Savin RE, Dumelin EE, Tappel AL. Effects of exercise, vitamin E, and ozone on pulmonary function and lipid peroxidation. *J of Appl Physiol.* 1978;45(6):927–932.

17. Tappel A. Lipid peroxidation damage to cell components. *Fed Procs.* 1973;32:1870–1876.

18. Davies KJA, Quintanilha AT, Brooks GA, Packer L. Free radicals and tissue damage produced by exercise. *Biochem Biophys Res Commun.* 1982;107(4):1198–1205.

19. Jenkins RR, Friedland R, Howald H. The adaptation of the hydroperoxide enzyme system to increased oxygen use. *Med Sci Sports Exerc.* 1982;14(2):148.

20. McCord JM. Superoxide, superoxide dismutase and oxygen toxicity. *Rev of Biochem Toxi.* 1979;109–121.

21. Sen CK. Oxidants and antioxidants in exercise. *J Appl Physiol.* 1995;79:675–682.

22. Jenkins RR. Exercise, oxidative stress, and antioxidants: a review. *Int J Sports Nutr.* 1993;3:356–375.

23. Rubin BB, Romaschin A, Walker PM, Gute DC, Korthuis RJ. Mechanisms of postischemic injury in skeletal muscle: intervention strategies. *J Appl Physiol.* 1996;80(2):369–387.

24. Hamvas A, Palazzo R, Kaiser L, et al. Inflammation and oxygen free radical formation during pulmonary ischemia-reperfusion injury. *J Appl Physiol.* 1992; 72(2):621–628.

25. Ward PA, Till GO, Johnson KJ. Oxygen-derived free radicals and inflammation. In: Ledbetter W, Buckwalter J, Gordon W, eds. *Sports-Induced Inflammation*, Park Ridge, IL: American Academy of Orthopedic Surgeons; 1990:315–324.

26. Dernbach AR, Sherman WM, Simonsen JC, Flowers KM, Lamb DR. No evidence of oxidant stress during high-intensity rowing training. *J Appl Physiol.* 1993; 74(5): 2140–2145.

27. Symons MCR. Formation of radicals by mechanical processes. *Free Rad Res Commun.* 1988;5:131–139.

28. Wong SHY, Knight JA, Hopfer SM, Zaharia O, Leach CN, Sunderman FW. Lipoperoxides in plasma as measured by liquid-chromatographic separation of malondialdehyde-thiobarbituric acid adduct. *Clin Chem.* 1987;33(2):214–220.

29. Halliwell B, Gutteridge JMC. *Free Radicals in Biology and Medicine.* Oxford: Clarendon Press; 1985:162–164.

30. Sanchez-Quesada JL, Homs-Serradesanferm R, Serrat-Serrat J, Serra-Grima JR, Gonzalez-Sastre F, Ordonez-Llanos J. Increase of LDL susceptibility to oxidation occurring after intense, long duration aerobic exercise. *Atherosclerosis.* 1995;118(2):297–305.

31. Hamaren J, Powers S, Lawler J, Criswell D, Lowenthal D, Pollack M. Exercise training-induced alterations in skeletal muscle oxidative and antioxidant enzyme activity. *Int J Sports Med.* 1993;13:412–416.

32. Girten B, Oloff C, Plato P, Eveland E, Merola AJ, Kazarian L. Skeletal muscle antioxidant enzyme levels in rats after simulated weightlessness, exercise and dobutamine. *The Physiologist.* 1989;32(1): S59–S60.

33. Alessio HM, Goldfarb AH. Lipid peroxidation and scavenger enzymes during exercise: adaptive response to training. *J Appl Physiol.* 1988a;64(4):1333–1336.

34. Ji LL, Stratman FW, Lardy HA. Antioxidant enzyme systems in rat liver and skeletal muscle: Influences of selenium deficiency, chronic training, and acute exercise. *Arch Biochem Biophys.* 1988;263:150–160.

35. Ohno H, Sato Y, Yamashita K, et al. The effect of brief physical exercise on free radical scavenging enzyme systems in human red blood cells. *Can J Physiol Pharmacol.* 1986;64:1263–1265.

36. Higuchi M, Cartier LJ, Chen M, Holloszy JO. Superoxide dismutase and catalase in skeletal muscle: adaptive response to exercise. *J Gerontol.* 1985;40(3):281–286.

37. Kanter MM, Hamlin RL, Unverferth DV, Davis HW, Merola AJ. Effect of exercise training on antioxidant

enzymes and cardiotoxicity of doxorubicin. *J Appl Physiol.* 1985;59:1298–1303.

38. Pincemail J, Camus G, Roesgen A, et al. Exercise induces pentane production and neutrophil activation in humans: effect of propranolol. *Eur J Appl Physiol.* 1990;61:319–322.

39. Hartmann A, Nies AM, Grunert-Fuchs M, Poch B, Speit G. Vitamin E prevents exercise-induced DAN damage. *Mutat Res.* 1995;346:195–202.

40. Rokitzi L, Logemann E, Sagredos AN, Murphy M, Wetzel-Roth W, Keul J. Lipid peroxidation and antioxidative vitamins under extreme endurance stress. *Acta Physiol Scand.* 1994;154:149–154.

41. Kanter MM, Nolte LA, Holloszy JO. Effects of an antioxidant vitamin mixture on lipid peroxidation at rest and postexercise. *J Appl Physiol.* 1993;74:965–969.

42. Sumida S, Tanaka K, Kitao H, Nakadomo F. Exercise-induced lipid peroxidation and leakage of enzymes before and after vitamin E supplementation. *Int J Biochem.* 1989;21:835–838.

43. Gohil K, Packer L, De Lumen B, Brooks GA, Terblanche SE. Vitamin E deficiency and vitamin C supplements: exercise and mitochondrial oxidation. *J Appl Physiol.* 1986;60:1986–1991.

44. Bjorneboe A, Bjorneboe GA, Drevon CA. Absorption, transport and distribution of vitamin E. *J Nutr.* 1990;120:233–242.

45. Niki E, Kawakami A, Saito M, Yamamoto Y, Tsuchiya T, Kamiya Y. Effect of phytyl side chain of vitamin E on its antioxidant activity. *J Biol Chem.* 1985;260:2191–2196.

46. Bendich A, Machlin LJ. Safety of oral intake of vitamin E. *Am J Clin Nutr.* 1988;48:1088–1089.

47. Horwitt MK, Harvey CC, Dahm DJ, Searcy MT. Relationship between tocopherol and serum lipid levels for determination of nutritional adequacy. *Ann NY Acad Sci.* 1972;203:233–236.

48. Zapsilas C, Anderle Beck R. *Food Chemistry and Nutritional Biochemistry.* New York: John Wiley and Sons; 1985:273–275.

49. Salminen A, Vihko V. Lipid peroxidation in exercise myopathy. *Exp Mol Pathol.* 1983;38:380–388.

50. Cannon JG, Orencole SF, Fielding RA, et al. Acute phase response to exercise: interaction of age and vitamin E on neutrophils and muscle enzyme release. *Am J Physiol.* 1990;259:R1214–R1219.

51. Kanter MM, Bartoli WP, Eddy DE, Horn MK. Effects of short term vitamin E supplementation on lipid peroxidation, inflammation, and tissue damage during and following exercise. *Med Sci Sports Exerc.* 1997;29(5):S40.

52. Jakeman P, Maxwell S. Effect of antioxidant vitamin supplementation on muscle function after eccentric exercise. *Eur J Appl Physiol.* 1993;67:426–430.

53. Kaminski M, Boals R. An effect of ascorbic acid on delayed-onset muscle soreness. *Pain.* 1992;50:317–321.

54. Peters EM, Goetzsche JM, Grobbelaar B, Noakes TD. Vitamin C supplementation reduces the incidence of postrace symptoms of upper-respiratory-tract infection in ultramarathon runners. *Am J Clin Nutr.* 1993;57:170–174.

55. Kumar CT, Reddy VK, Prasad M, Thyagaraju K, Reddanna P. Dietary supplementation of vitamin E protects heart tissue from exercise-induced oxidant stress. *Mol Cell Biochem.* 1992;111:109–115.

56. Packer L. Vitamin E, physical exercise, and tissue damage in animals. *Medical Biology Helsinki.* 1984;62:105–109.

57. Warren JA, Jenkins RR, Packer L, Witt EH, Armstrong RB. Elevated muscle vitamin E does not attenuate eccentric exercise-induced muscle injury. *J Appl Physiol.* 1992;72(6):2168–2175.

58. Robertson JD, Maughan RJ, Duthie GG, Morrice PC. Increased blood antioxidant systems of runners in response to training load. *Clin Sci.* 1991;80:611–618.

59. Helgheim I, Hetland O, Nilsson S, Ingjer F, Stromme SB. The effects of vitamin E on serum enzyme levels following heavy exercise. *Eur J Appl Physiol.* 1979;40:283–289.

60. Nieman DC, Nehlsen-Cannarella SL, Henson DA, et al. Carbohydrate, ascorbic acid, and the immune response to running. *Int J Sports Med.* (In press).

61. Kanter MM, Eddy DE. Effect of antioxidant supplementation on serum markers of lipid peroxidation and skeletal muscle damage following eccentric exercise. *Med Sci Sports Exer.* 1992;24(5):S17.

62. Viguie CA, Packer L, Brooks GA. Antioxidant supplementation affects indices of muscle trauma and oxidant stress in human blood during exercise. *Med Sci Sports Exerc.* 1989;21:S16.

63. Goldfarb AH, Sen CK. Antioxidant supplementation and the control of oxygen toxicity during exercise, In: Sen CK, Packer L, Hanninen O, eds. *Exercise and Oxygen Toxicity.* Amsterdam: Elsevier; 1994:163–189.

64. Patterson BH, Block G, Rosenberger WF, Pee D, Kahle LL. Fruit and vegetables in the American diet: data from the NHANES II survey. *Am J Public Health.* 1990;80:1443–1449.

65. Namiki M. Antioxidants/antimutagens in food. *Critical Reviews in Food Science and Nutrition.* 1990;29(4):273–300.

66. Talla SRR, Halter RC, Dwivedi C. Xanthine oxidase inhibitory activity of caffeic, chlorogenic and ferulic acids. *Biochem Arch.* 1996;12(4):245–247.

67. Hodgson JM, Croft KD, Puddey IB, Mori TA, Beilin LJ. Soybean isoflavonoids and their metabolic products inhibit in vitro lipoprotein oxidation in serum. *J Nutr Biochem.* 1996;7(12):664–669.

68. Kuroda Y. Bio-antimutagenic activity of green tea catechins in cultured Chinese hamster V79 cells. *Mutation Res Environ Mut Rel Subj.* 1996;361(2):179–186.

69. Arouma OI. Free radicals and antioxidant strategies in sports. *J Nutr Biochem.* 1994;5:370–381.

70. Meydani M, Evans WJ, Handelman G, et al. Protective effect of vitamin E on exercise-induced oxidative damage in young and older adults. *Am J Physiol.* 1993;264:R992–R996.

CHAPTER 7

Nutritional Ergogenic Aids

Edmund R. Burke

Studies of the dietary practices of athletes report that nutritional supplements are commonly used during both training and competition.[1,2] In addition, there is significant evidence to suggest that athletes use a number of supplements concurrently and in higher doses.[3]

Athletes have increased their use of nutritional ergogenic aids because they are bombarded with advertisements, both electronically and in print, about the effect of nutrition and supplementation upon performance. Many believe nutritional ergogenic aids improve performance and aid in recovery. As in the past, and probably in the future, many of the claims advertised and written about supplements are not supported by published studies. In some instances, no scientific research is found to substantiate the claims or information is from non–peer-reviewed journals; and in other cases, research findings are extrapolated to inappropriate applications.[4]

This increased exposure in advertising has occurred primarily because of the passage of the Dietary Supplement Health and Education Act (DSHEA) in 1994,[5] creating a new category called "dietary supplements," which includes vitamins, minerals, amino acids, herbs and other botanical preparations that do not fall under Food and Drug Administration (FDA) approval. This has also led to an increase in the number of nutritional ergogenic aids on the market. Nutritional supplements are now classified as foods, and not "food additives" and drugs. An interesting and somewhat controversial section of the act allows manufacturers to publish limited information about the benefits of dietary supplements in the form of statements of support as well as so-called "structure and function claims."

This chapter will provide an overview of several (not all-inconclusive) nutritional ergogenic aids that have received attention in the popular press and scientific literature in recent years. Some have been shown to enhance exercise performance, while some have no effect on performance and others need additional studies to substantiate their effectiveness. Also, the possible mechanisms of these nutritional ergogenic aids and their effectiveness and safety will be discussed.

BETA-HYDROXY BETA-METHYLBUTYRATE

Beta-hydroxy beta-methylbutyrate (HMB) is an important compound made in the body and a metabolite of the essential amino acid leucine. In addition to the amount synthesized in the body, the body can make HMB from foods containing the branched-chain amino acid (BCAA) leucine.

Several studies done with both animals and humans have found that subjects supplemented with HMB have a decreased stress-induced muscle protein breakdown.[6,7] Studies with humans have found that HMB may enhance increases in both muscle size and strength when combined with resistance training.

In this two-part study conducted by Nissen et al[7] (funded by Environmental and Applied Science, which holds the patent for HMB), 41 male volunteers ages 19 to 29 years who weighed an average of 180 lb were randomized among the following three levels of HMB supplementation: 0, 1.5, or 3 g of HMB per day and two different levels of protein (117 or 175 g per day). The subjects controlled their food intake by selecting meals from a list of prepared entrees; the same meals were used during the baseline-data collecting week, and then repeated during each week of the study. The participants also lifted weights for 1.5 hours, 3 days a week for 3 weeks.

The results of this first study indicated that HMB improved strength and lean body mass. Subjects gained lean body mass in the following dose-responsive manner: 0.88 lb for the group receiving no HMB, 1.76 lb for the group ingesting 1.5 g of HMB, and 2.64 lb for the group receiving 3 g of HMB per day.

Researchers also found that subjects receiving HMB supplementation lifted more weight than subjects who did not receive supplements during all 3 weeks. Those subjects receiving HMB were able to do more abdominal exercises (subjects who did not receive supplements increased performance by 14%, and subjects who received supplements increased performance by 50%). Additionally, total strength (combining increases for upper- and lower-body exercises) increased 8% in subjects who did not receive supplements, 13% in subjects who received 1.5 g of HMB, and 18.4% in the subjects who received 3 g HMB.

In the second part of the study, 32 male volunteers (ages 19 to 22 years) participated. These men were divided into two groups—those receiving no HMB or those receiving 3 g of HMB per day—and they lifted weights for 2 to 3 hours per day, 6 days a week for 7 weeks. The early measurements in the study indicated that the subjects who received HMB developed significantly more fat-free mass [measured by total body electrical conductivity (TOBEC)] than those who lifted weights but did not take HMB.

Bench-press strength was almost three times greater in the group receiving HMB, and strength increases for the squat, although not statistically significant, were also greater. In both parts of the study, it is important to note that the control groups started out much stronger than the HMB-supplemented groups. It is not surprising, then, that the control group members, who were more highly trained, had lesser strength gains from the same exercise protocol than did the lesser-trained experimental HMB groups.

The exact mechanism of the effect of HMB on muscle metabolism is not known, but at least two hypotheses have been proposed.

HMB may be an essential component of the cell membrane: Scientists propose that under stressful situations, the body may not make enough HMB to satisfy the increased needs of tissues. It could also be that stress may alter enzymes or concentration of certain biochemicals that decrease normal HMB production. Either scenario would require dietary supplementation of HMB for muscle or the immune system to maximally function.

A second hypothesis is that HMB regulates enzymes responsible for muscle tissue breakdown. This theory is supported by the evidence found in several studies where biochemical indicators of muscle damage were decreased [creatine phosphokinase (CPK) and 3-methylhistidine]. Additionally, a recent study using isolated chick and rat muscle indicated that HMB can directly decrease muscle protein breakdown.[8]

The large database of animal data along with results of some human studies all indicate that HMB holds great promise as a tool to maximize muscle function and muscle mass as well as maximizing health in both animals and humans. HMB appears to have applications for persons suffering from muscle-wasting diseases and may be able to slow the loss of lean tissue, which usually occurs with the aging process. Current research is underway that ranges from basic studies designed to elucidate the biochemical action of HMB to studies assessing the impact of HMB on wasting diseases and maintaining lean mass in women who are losing weight.[9]

Several studies have been completed, and they all show that HMB is safe and effective for men and women over the short term. Human studies have been conducted with up to 4 g/day of HMB being administered for up to 4 weeks. The authors report no toxicity at these levels.[6] No long-term research has been conducted.

BORON

Boron is a trace element that influences calcium and magnesium metabolism. Claims have been made by companies that boron increases testosterone levels and thereby increases growth and strength. These claims are largely based on a study of boron and the prevention of osteoporosis by Nielsen.[10] He noted that boron supplementation in postmenopausal women for 48 days (after they had been deprived of boron for 4 months) doubled their serum testosterone levels. However, continued supplementation did not increase testosterone levels any further, and boron supplementation in males did not increase serum testosterone levels at all. In another study, bodybuilders were given boron supplementation. Although serum boron levels increased, there were no significant increases in serum testosterone, lean body mass, or strength.[11]

BRANCHED-CHAIN AMINO ACIDS

Mixtures of amino acids have become popular during the last few years because of the availability of large amounts of food-grade L-amino acids. Most free-form amino acids are produced by microbial fermentation in Japan, accounting for the great expense of free-form amino acids as a sole dietary nitrogen source.[12] Proponents of free-form amino acid mixtures claim that absorption is complete with no fecal residue occurring, the absorption of nitrogen is more rapid from these mixtures than from food proteins, amino acid compositions can be manipulated to optimize energy or protein synthesis for athletes, and various physiologic parameters can be influenced, such as hormone release. More research about free-form amino acid mixtures is needed to help support the claims of many manufacturers.

Although far from conclusive, there are some data that suggest that individual amino acid supplementation may be beneficial for some types of exercise performance, particularly very high-intensity, endurance exercise of over several hours and when training volume is increased. Examples include BCAAs (leucine, isoleucine, and valine), tryptophan, glutamate, aspartates, and potential growth-hormone-stimulating amino acids.[13] Although there has been some talk about this, few studies concurrently support the concept of increasing the ingestion of these types of amino acids.

A more recent area of research focuses on amino acids and their contribution to the reduction of fatigue of the central nervous system (CNS) (central fatigue) during long-term exercise. The mechanisms of central fatigue are largely unexplored, but the central fatigue hypothesis suggests that increased brain serotonin (5-HT) can cause a deterioration in sport and exercise performance. In general, the central fatigue hypothesis suggests that increased concentrations of brain 5-HT can impair CNS function, leading to premature fatigue.[14]

There is now evidence that exercise-induced increases in the plasma-free tryptophan f-TRP/BCCA ratio are associated with increased brain 5-HT and the onset of fatigue during prolonged exercise. When drugs are administered to alter brain 5-HT, they result in the predicted effects on exercise performance. The influence of amino acids or other nutritional manipulations of f-TRP/BCCA on exercise is less established.[15]

Davis and Bailey[16] propose that changing the f-TRP/BCAA ratio can reduce central fatigue. There are two ways to change this ratio. The first is to reduce the amount of f-TRP. TRP is normally bound to albumin and not found in high levels in the free state. However, with prolonged exercise, there is an increase in plasma fatty acids that also bind to albumin, thus increasing the amount of f-TRP, resulting in an increased shift. Consuming carbohydrate-rich products during prolonged exercise will reduce the amount of free fatty acids (FFAs) released, thus decreasing the amount of f-TRP. The second way to change this ratio is to increase the amount of BCAAs in the blood so that they compete with the tryptophan for transport across the blood-brain barrier. In theory, the greater the circulating levels of BCAAs, the smaller the amount of tryptophan to cross the blood-brain barrier; however, large amounts of BCAA ingestion can lead to gastrointestinal (GI) upset and diarrhea.

It will take years of controlled research investigating the hypotheses presented before definitive conclusions can be drawn about the proposed ergogenic value of amino acid supplementation for strength and endurance athletes[17] and as a mediator of central fatigue during prolonged exercise.

CAFFEINE

The effects of caffeine on exercise and athletic performance have been extensively studied during the last few years. Better controlled studies and more sophisticated instrumentation for laboratory tests have revealed more accurate information. Significant changes in performance in caffeine-treated groups were noted in exercise times of greater than 30 minutes.

Early studies investigating caffeine ingestion found significantly higher plasma FFA concentration in persons ingesting various levels of caffeine before exercise when compared to control groups in five studies using subjects who train.[18-22] Two of these studies indicated increased times to exhaustion or total work, two reported nonsignificant changes, and one did not report any changes. Knapik et al[21] indicated increases in lactate, FFAs, glycerol, and glucose. One study[23] reported an increase in lactate, but another study[24] indicated nonsignificant changes in the lactate concentration as well as heart rate, VO_{2max}, respiratory quotient, and FFAs. Another

study of marathon runners did not report performance change, but did indicate an increase in lactate but nonsignificant changes in heart rate, VO_{2max}, FFAs, glucose, or triglycerides.[25]

Although the effects of caffeine have been investigated extensively, not much has been done about how it might alter a person's work output while the perception of effort remains constant. A recent study[26] addressed this subject. Researchers recruited 10 recreational and competitive runners and competitive triathletes to complete six exercise trials on an exercise bike that allowed for altering the resistance while keeping the effort constant.

One hour before testing, half the subjects were given 6 mg of caffeine per kilogram of bodyweight, whereas the placebo group received glucose. Next, the subjects were asked to cycle at different rates of perceived exertion. Each subject cycled for 10 minutes lightly, 10 minutes somewhat heavily, and 10 minutes heavily. A computer that interfaced with the cycle recorded work outputs of the subjects based on the force applied to the pedals. The results of this study indicate that although the perception of effort was constant, the experimental group's work output was significantly greater than that of the control group.

However, there is a lack of well-controlled field studies to determine the applicability of laboratory results to the athletic world. Caffeine does not appear to enhance performance during incremental exercise tests lasting 8 to 20 minutes and during sprinting lasting less than 90 seconds, although research examining sprinting is rare. In addition, the mechanisms responsible for any improvement in endurance and short-term exercise have not been clearly established.[27]

Because tolerance to caffeine is developed by users, subjects are required to refrain from caffeine for a couple of days before the study. Fisher et al[24] reported significant changes in metabolism and performance of subjects only after the withdrawal period of caffeine.

The general consensus of research indicates that the ingestion of caffeine increases FFAs and glycerol more than just exercise alone. The time to exhaustion appeared to increase in several studies as well.[28] Athletes need to be aware that more than five cups of coffee may produce urinary caffeine levels unacceptable for competition. Other side effects include diuresis, which may lead to dehydration, and stomach upset from increased gastric secretion.

Caffeine occurs naturally or is added to many commonly consumed items, including coffee, tea, chocolate, soft drinks, and pain relievers. The International Olympic Committee has set a tolerance limit for caffeine in the urine at 12 μg/mL; therefore, ingesting caffeine with the intention of improving performance is not prohibited. Consuming 3 to 6 mg of caffeine per kg (2 cups for 150-pound person) one hour before exercise improves endurance performance without raising caffeine levels above the International Olympic Committee doping threshold (urine caffeine = 6 to 8 cups; 12 μg/ml). Because it is considered doping, the use of caffeine becomes a question of sports ethics.

CHOLINE

Choline is an amine and is part of phospholipids found in plant and animal foods. There is no dietary requirement for this substance. Choline can be made by the body from methionine, an essential amino acid. Choline is a precursor of acetylcholine (neurotransmitter) and phosphatidylcholine (lecithin), a component of lipoproteins. Based on these functions, choline supplementation has been hypothesized to affect nerve transmission, increase strength, or facilitate loss of body fat.

A few studies have demonstrated a significant reduction in plasma choline levels after exercise.[29] The reduction in plasma choline levels associated with strenuous exercise (for example, long-distance running or extended swimming) may reduce acetylcholine contents, and thus its release, and could thereby affect nerve impulses, which would impair endurance and performance. It has been hypothesized that the replacement of choline lost during exercise or prevention of that loss could influence neuronal

release of acetylcholine and, subsequently, affect measures of athletic performance and fatigue.

The running and swimming exercise paradigms used in a series of experiments with trained athletes produced similar depletions in plasma choline levels after that particular exercise.[30,31] Running 20 miles or swimming for 2 hours led to a significant decrease in plasma choline levels (40% to 50%). However, Spector et al[32] failed to show a decrease in plasma choline levels after either brief (approximately 2 minutes' duration), but highly intensive exercise or longer (approximately 73 minutes' duration) submaximal exercise on a stationary bicycle. Apparently, the duration and type of exercise are important determinants of whether plasma choline levels will decrease after exercise.

In the previous study by Spector, providing 2 g of free choline before exercise prevented a decrease in choline levels (25% to 40% percent) and increased choline levels above baseline values for up to 2 hours after exercise. Randomized placebo-controlled cross-over studies found improvements in running times and a timed swim test, and suggested that performance in these activities is sensitive to changes in choline levels.[30] In one study, long-distance runners improved running times by an average of 5 minutes over a 20-mile course when compared with those taking a placebo.[33] In a second study, a higher percentage of swimmers who took choline before their swim experienced an improved performance on a timed swim test than when they consumed a placebo. The implication that a decline in plasma choline can lead to impaired acetylcholine release and ultimately to a decrement in physical performance is largely theoretical and warrants more research.[34] There is no research to support that choline increases strength or facilitates the loss of body fat.[35]

CHROMIUM PICOLINATE

Chromium is the active component of the glucose tolerance factor—an essential co-factor that potentiates the actions of insulin in carbohydrate, lipid, and protein metabolism. Chromium augments the effects of insulin at target tissues and promotes glucose transport. Since insulin also regulates protein synthesis, chromium enhances protein synthesis by promoting amino acid uptake. Although chromium helps to potentiate the function of insulin, it is a nutrient, not a drug. Picolinic acid is a natural derivative of the amino acid tryptophan and is believed to facilitate chromium absorption.[36] The "enhanced bioavailability" of chromium picolinate forms the basis for misleading claims that it increases muscle mass, decreases body fat, and increases energy.[37]

The promotion of chromium picolinate is due to a well-orchestrated marketing campaign initiated by both Nutrition 21 (a supplement company in San Diego) and their consultant chemist Gary Evans.[38] Nutrition 21 holds the exclusive U.S. license on the patent rights to the synthetic process for chromium picolinate. The supplement is sold through distributors to the public. Unfortunately, patenting laws do not require that claims for health products be valid.[36]

Marketing claims for chromium picolinate are based on two poorly controlled, unpublished research studies cited in a review article by Evans.[38] During 6 weeks of weight lifting, subjects received 200 µg of chromium picolinate daily. Results showed small increases in lean body mass (1.6 to 2.6 kg) and a decrease in percent body fat (3.6%) that Evans attributed to chromium picolinate supplementation. However, these small changes could have been due to errors in estimating body composition via skinfolds. In addition, the chromium status of the subjects before or during the studies was not evaluated.

Clancy and researchers examined the effects of chromium picolinate supplementation on football players during spring training.[39] Training included weight lifting 4 days per week and running 2 days per week. Subjects were given either 200 µg of chromium picolinate or a placebo for 9 weeks. The subjects on supplemental chromium had urinary chromium losses (attributed to the supplement) that were five times

greater than those of the placebo group. No significant changes in strength or body composition were observed between the chromium-supplemented and control groups.

Hallmark et al[40] evaluated the effects of chromium picolinate supplementation and weight training for 12 weeks on muscle strength, body composition, and chromium excretion. Subjects weight lifted 3 days per week and received either 200 µg of chromium picolinate or a placebo. Weight training significantly increased the muscular strength of both groups. The subjects on supplemental chromium had urinary chromium losses (attributed to the supplement) that were nine times greater than those of the placebo group. However, there were no significant changes in strength or body composition between the chromium-supplemented and control groups.

In November 1996, the Federal Trade Commission (FTC) ordered Nutrition 21 and two other companies to stop making unsubstantiated weight loss and health claims (eg, reduced body fat, increased muscle mass, and increased energy) for chromium picolinate.[41] Although the product is still widely available, under the FTC settlement, the companies are prohibited from making any of the challenged claims in the future unless they can be verified by reliable research. In addition, animal studies have reported that chromium picolinate causes damage to DNA due to enhanced bioavailability.

COLLOIDAL MINERALS

In recent years, many colloidal mineral solutions have appeared on the market, sold as mineral and trace element supplements. Colloidal mineral manufacturers have aggressively marketed the athletes about the importance of mineral and trace elements to help improve their health and athletic performance. Although minerals and trace elements are important for health, these manufacturers have made exaggerated and unfounded claims that lack scientific support and experimental evidence. Recently, Schauss[42] reported that an extensive search of more than

2000 medical and scientific journals did not reveal a single reference on colloidal mineral intake in humans before 1996.

Basically, colloidal minerals are a mixture of clay and water. When water, the dispersing agent, is mixed with clay, the dispersed colloid, a colloidal mineral, is created. When an element is soluble, it is usually more absorbable than when it is insoluble. Calling a product colloidal makes a product insoluble by definition. If it was a soluble solution, it could not be colloidal. So, how can these minerals and trace elements be more absorbable? This is a question that many of these manufacturers have to answer or stop making such claims.[43]

The minerals contained in these products evolved through a lengthy process of minerals settling within the clay that was formed during the Ice Age. The minerals in clay come from secondary minerals that have been recrystallized in solution through geothermal forces from minerals primarily found in granitic rocks. The clay forms through a lengthy process involving glaciation and weathering. In essence, clay is a glacial byproduct found throughout North America and northern Europe and Asia. Depending on the host rock source of the minerals, specific types of clay accumulate in the valleys where most of the clay settled. The most common examples are montmorillonite, benonite, kaolinite, and vermiculite. These minerals contain large amounts of aluminum.

Clay minerals are essentially hydrous aluminum silicates. In some of these minerals, magnesium or iron substitute in part for the aluminum, and alkalies or alkaline earth may be present as essential constituents.[44] Herein lies the concern. Some colloidal mineral products claim that they contain between 1800 and 4400 parts per million (ppm) of aluminum. By composition, foodstuffs contain no more than 10 ppm as bound complexes that are often difficult to absorb. Because of the lack of any long-term research on the effect of consuming colloidal minerals, it is unknown whether they can contribute to the increased incidence of neurodegenerative diseases, such as Alzheimer's disease. Aluminum has been implicated in the possible cause of Alzheimer's disease when aluminum deposits in microscopic clusters of aluminum-containing neurofibrillary tangles and granulovacuolar degeneration of the neurons. More research needs to be conducted to see what role aluminum plays in this disease.

Fortunately, until research is completed on the benefits and safety of colloidal minerals, many other products are available in the marketplace that offer athletes safe and reasonable levels of mineral supplementation. Until such research is conducted, colloidal minerals should be avoided. Methods exist in the research community that would allow for proper testing of these products. Long-term studies of the safety of colloidal minerals are certainly needed in light of the claims being made for these products.

CONJUGATED LINOLEIC ACID

A recently proposed new ergogenic aid is a fatty acid called conjugated linoleic acid (CLA). The proposed ergogenic effect of CLA is the possibility of it reducing catabolism because of its antioxidant properties; although animal studies can support this hypothesis,[45] human studies have not been published.

Pariza, head of the Food Research Institute at the University of Wisconsin, has studied CLA for 16 years and has discovered immune stimulation from CLA in mice, rats, and chicks. More relevant to athletes, Park, a graduate student in food microbiology and toxicology at the university, found that sedentary adult mice, rats, and chicks that received CLA supplements produced more lean muscle and less body fat. Results also revealed below-normal abdominal fat in mice that were fed CLA. Further analysis showed that CLA reduced body fat in the mice by 50% or more.[46] The data indicate that CLA is a regulator of body-fat accumulation and retention. The authors suggest that when animals ingest CLA at approximately 0.1% of the diet (dry weight), it will incorporate into the phospholipid membranes of the cells and, in so doing, increase the process that enables nutrients to enter active cells rather than fat cells.

Some researchers have hypothesized that CLA, when absorbed into cell membranes (including those of muscles), could change responsiveness to certain hormone stimulatory and/or inhibitory factors that are known to play a part in the way a cell grows and develops, although no tests have been published. Or, the effects could be related to a counteractive influence on the adverse effects of certain catabolic hormones.[47]

Many of the animal studies have reported improved feed efficiency. Fats like CLA have been known to show unique sparing effects. In other animal experiments, "structured lipids"—artificially made fats—with which CLA shares many traits, have resulted in higher albumin concentration and nitrogen retention (both associated with increased muscle growth).[48] One experiment showed that certain fats related to CLA showed a significant increase in skeletal muscle protein synthesis rates.[49] CLA, it seems, may possess unique protein-sparing abilities.

Although no human studies have been published in peer review journals, manufacturers of CLA suggest that CLA seems to do its work best in daily doses of 2 to 5 g. This is anecdotal evidence—science hasn't definitively weighed in on the subject as far as humans are concerned. More research needs to be done. Currently, no side effects have ever been reported with its use in humans or animals in the dosages described in the previous studies.

CREATINE MONOHYDRATE

The use of creatine (Cr) in its supplemental form, Cr monohydrate, has become widespread. Cr is derived from the amino acids arginine, glycine, and methionine. It is normally found in meat or fish in quantities of approximately 5 g Cr per kilogram of meat.

The discovery that the Cr and phosphocreatine (PCr) content in human muscle can be increased by oral ingestion of supplemental Cr has led to numerous studies examining its benefits on exercise performance. Judging from the current research results, Cr monohydrate supplementation in healthy persons has an impact on performance during high-intensity, intermittent exercise and increases the rate of PCr resynthesis during the recovery phase of intermittent high-intensity exercise. Improvements in performance are particularly evident in persons who already have low levels of muscle Cr and PCr (less than 120 mmol·kg^{-1}) and who may be vegetarians. In these subjects, Cr monohydrate supplementation has been proven to increase both Cr and PCr muscle concentration by as much as 30%.[50]

Subjects who received Cr monohydrate supplements demonstrated a reduction in the accumulation of plasma lactate, ammonia, and hypoxanthine, indicating an alteration in energy metabolism and an attenuation of adenosine triphosphate (ATP) degradation.[51] Thus, higher supplemental levels of Cr seem to enhance the muscle's ability to sustain the high ATP turnover rates encountered during strenuous exercise. Another reported potential benefit is an increase in body mass that results from the ingestion of Cr monohydrate; however, the composition of the weight gain remains a point of discussion.[52]

Increased Cr and PCr levels attenuate ATP degradation during high-intensity muscular activity.[53] This is likely a result of an increased rate of ATP resynthesis from adenosine diphosphate (ADP). The increased availability of PCr as an energy source may decrease the usual dependence on anaerobic glycolysis for resynthesis of ATP. Thus, the accumulation of lactate and [H+] associated with maximal rates of glycolysis is delayed, allowing the muscle to generate a high force for an extended time. Increases in performance during intermittent exercise are most likely explained by a greater availability of PCr in the activated muscles, particularly the type II muscle fibers, as a result of a higher rate of resynthesis during recovery periods. Higher Cr and PCr concentrations before exercise, as well as a smaller decrease in muscle pH, may also increase the amount of PCr available during the next exercise bout after a rest period.

Although the length of the Cr ingestion period in most Cr supplementation studies was relatively short (5 to 6 days), the weight gain in subjects after supplementation was significant compared to subjects who received a placebo.[54] The most logical explanation is an increase in total body water; however, an increase in lean tissue cannot be ruled out. There is evidence that Cr is a positive effector in regulating the biosynthesis of actin, myosin, and Cr kinase by developing muscle cells.

What about this so-called loading phase that everyone seems to follow before receiving a maintenance dose? Is it really needed? A recent study at Karolinska Institute in Sweden compared the effects of two different supplementation schemes. One involved taking 20 g of Cr a day for 6 days followed by 2 g per day for an additional month; another group took 3 g of Cr daily for 1 month. Interestingly, both schemes worked equally well (approximately a 20% increase in muscle Cr). Thus, 3 g (as contained in about 1 to 2 tsp) of Cr a day is an effective way to supplement. The loading phase may be unnecessary.[55] In addition, this research suggested that taking Cr with a carbohydrate drink will help maximize muscle loading.

However, not all research results about Cr are positive. Burke et al conducted a study to determine the effect of Cr supplementation on performance of a single-effort sprint by elite swimmers.[56] Thirty-two elite swimmers (18 males and 14 females; age = 17 to 25 years) were tested on two occasions, 1 week apart. Tests done were 25-m, 50-m, and 100-m maximal effort sprints, each with approximately 10 minutes of active recovery. A 10-second maximal leg ergometry test was also undertaken. Swimmers were divided into two groups matched for sex, stroke and event, and sprint time over 50 m, and groups were randomly assigned to 5 days of Cr supplementation (20 g/day) or placebo before the second trial. Results revealed no significant differences between the group means for sprint times or between 10-second maximal leg ergometry power and work. This study did not support the hypothesis

that Cr supplementation enhances single-effort sprint ability of elite swimmers.[56]

Lastly, research needs to focus on the physiologic consequences of long-term Cr supplementation and determination of adequate dosages to maximize and maintain increased muscle levels of Cr. There have been anecdotal reports of muscle cramping by athletes supplementing with Cr. At this time, taking doses greater than 5 g/d for long periods does not seem warranted, especially when no one knows what health concerns could arise from long-term high doses of Cr.

DEHYDROEPIANDROSTERONE

Dehydroepiandrosterone (DHEA) was first isolated from urine in 1934, and in 1944, DHEA's precursor dehydroepiandrosterone-3-sulfate (DHEAS) was isolated from urine. DHEA is a metabolic precursor for at least two hormones—testosterone and estradiol. Although DHEAS is the most abundant circulating adrenal hormone in humans, its physiologic role and that of DHEA are poorly understood.

DHEA has been labeled by the popular press as the "youth hormone" because its levels peak during early adulthood. Several studies have suggested positive correlations between increased plasma levels of DHEA and improved vigor, health, and well-being in persons in their 40s. One randomized, placebo-controlled, crossover study examined the effect of oral DHEA 50 mg administered daily for 6 months in 13 men and 17 women age 40 to 70 years.[57] Within 2 weeks of replacement therapy, the subjects' DHEA and DHEAS levels reached those associated with young adults in their twenties. The results showed an increase in the bioavailability of serum insulin-like growth factor I (IGF-I), as reflected by an increase in IGF-I and a decrease in IGF-binding protein-I. This change was accompanied by a perceived increase in physical and psychological well-being among men (67%) and women (84%), with no change in libido.

Is DHEA anabolic? By modifying cortisol output, DHEA may indeed exert anabolic effects. Scientists originally thought that it might competitively bind to cortisol-cell receptors in a manner analogous to anabolic steroids. But studies failed to prove this hypothesis.[58] Other studies involving DHEA and liver-cortisol receptors show that the former directly decreases the latter in that organ by 50%.[59] If this were to occur in muscle tissue as well, the anabolic effect would be comparable to that of anabolic steroids. However, no proof of this currently exists. Yet, DHEA is a precursor to testosterone and estrogen.

Another possible anticatabolic effect of DHEA would come as a result of its conversion into other hormones associated with cortisol inhibition, including testosterone and estrogen. So, the next question, and perhaps the most confusing to athletes, is, "Does DHEA convert into testosterone in the body?"

DHEA can take several different hormonal pathways. The one that it follows depends on several factors, including existing levels of other hormones, such as testosterone and estrogen, for which DHEA serves as a precursor. It can also take a few metabolic "back roads" if it interacts with certain enzymes along the sex-steroid passageway. Thus, it can turn into a less desirable byproduct of testosterone called dehydrotestosterone (DHT), which is associated with male pattern baldness, prostate enlargement, and acne.

Another interesting aspect of DHEA is its relationship to insulin levels. Several studies of humans have found that insulin infusion acutely decreases serum DHEA and DHEAS and that increased serum DHEA and DHEAS levels are associated with improvement in insulin resistance or hyperinsulinemia over a broad range of ages.[60] Because it is well-established that weight loss is associated with improved insulin sensitivity, some researchers have postulated that DHEA and DHEAS may be helpful in weight loss and "muscle toning." However, studies of humans have failed to demonstrate a beneficial effect of DHEA on body composition or energy expenditure at either pharmacologic or physiologic replacement dosages for 1 to 3 months.[61] Therefore, a significant role for DHEA in weight management is highly unlikely.

Until recently, DHEA was a prescription drug. Because of the 1994 Dietary Supplement Act, it is now sold over the counter. It is important to keep in mind that the beneficial effects of DHEA administration in humans have not been clearly established. Furthermore, the effects of chronic DHEA administration are not known. Long-term safety has not been established, and as with other hormones, adverse effects may not appear for years. DHEA is not recommended for athletic use until its benefits and risks are better understood.[62]

As noted, there are some possible side effects to taking this supplement. Both males and females have reported acne flare-ups, unwanted hair growth, irritability, and rapid heartbeat when taking doses of more than 100 mg/day. It should also be noted that DHEA has been added to the banned list by both the U.S. Olympic Committee (USOC) and the National Football League (NFL). Other sports are currently reviewing this product and are expected to follow the same action as the USOC and the NFL.

A "safe" alternative to DHEA is also being promoted—Mexican yams. Although Mexican yams contain a DHEA precursor (plant sterol) for the semisynthetic production of DHEA in the laboratory, the idea that the body can convert this plant sterol to testosterone is a complete scam.

DIHYDROXYACETONE AND PYRUVATE

Consuming foods rich in complex carbohydrates, such as breads, pasta, and rice, is the preferred way to supercompensate the body's glycogen stores; however, in the early 1980s, glucose polymer drinks became commercially available to facilitate the supercompensation process without added bulk in the intestinal tract. More recently, the combination of dihydroxyacetone and pyruvate (DHAP), two 3-carbon intermediates from the glycolytic process, has been shown to increase muscle glycogen stores more effectively than a glucose polymer.[63]

In two double-blind repeated measure studies, Stanko and his colleagues,[64,65] using subjects who do not train, reported that 75 g DHA and 25 g of pyruvate significantly improved arm and leg ergometer performance compared to a carbohydrate placebo. The authors thought that the effect could be attributed to either enhanced muscle glycogen storage or increased blood glucose extraction by the exercising muscle.

The authors found that supplementation with DHAP for 7 days significantly increased muscular endurance in both the arms and legs by 20% as measured by muscle biopsy results.[64,65] More specifically, the pyruvate mixture increased the time it took to exhaust arm muscles by 23 minutes and leg muscles by 13 minutes.

Stanko's results are supported by a third study by Robertson et al,[66] who found that when subjects ingested the DHAP mixture in a double-blind design, with each subject assigned to one of two dietary combinations, more than a 20% decrease in perceived level of exertion occurred, meaning the subjects thought that the task was easier to do. Both diets had a composition of 15% protein, 30% fat, and 55% carbohydrate, with the treatment diet substituting 75 g of DHAP for some of the carbohydrate.

According to the previously mentioned studies, DHAP improves exercise performance primarily by enhancing the transport of glucose into the muscle cell. This process is known as "glucose extraction" and refers to the amount of glucose extracted by the muscles from circulating blood. In fact, the pyruvate mixture increased glucose extraction after 1 hour of exercise almost 300% in the study that measured arm endurance,[64] 150% in the study that measured perceived exertion,[66] and more than 60% in the study measuring leg endurance.[65] Glucose extraction was also increased at rest with the pyruvate mixture, which may not sound important but led to a 50% increase in muscle glycogen.[65]

No major metabolic side effects were seen in subjects fed only pyruvate or DHAP in the previous studies; however, diarrhea and intestinal gas were seen in a few of the subjects.

Although results of these three well-controlled studies show an ergogenic effect with DHAP with subjects who do not train, data need to be forthcoming with subjects who train intensely. More research is needed to determine how and why pyruvate may enhance athletic performance. Before preliminary research is used to promote pyruvate to athletes, it should be noted that commercial pyruvate preparations contain only 500 mg to 1 g pyruvate and may not contain DHA.

EPHEDRA/MA HUANG

Ephedra, or as the Chinese call it, Ma Huang, has been used in Chinese medicine for more than 5000 years. It has been used in Traditional Chinese Medicine as a bronchodilator and a stimulant to the CNS.

The use of Ephedra in modern medicine began in 1923 with the discovery of the alkaloid compound ephedrine. Synthetic manufacture of ephedrine began shortly thereafter in 1927.[67]

It is used as an ingredient in many over-the-counter (OTC) drugs because of its effectiveness as a bronchodilator and decongestant. Ephedra (ephedrine) acts on the bronchial smooth muscles to promote relaxation during asthmatic attacks. Synthetic ephedrine and another Ephedra compound, pseudoephedrine, are widely used safely in OTC medications, not only for the treatment of asthma, but hayfever and nasal congestion as well.

In addition, Ephedra is a powerful stimulant of the nervous system, increasing the force of contraction and output of the heart. It also increases blood pressure and amount of blood flow to the brain.

But, because certain amounts of ephedrine are being converted to methamphetamines ("speed" and "uppers") and being sold illegally, it has drawn the attention of sports drug-control officials. Some sports federations have determined that specific amounts of ephedrine in an athlete's system are grounds for disqualification, because of its use by certain persons who take it for a "speed-like" effect. The FDA has issued a warning statement against the conversion of Ephedra into the stimulant amphetamine.[68]

Persons with diabetes, hypertension, thyroid diseases, and cardiovascular disease should avoid this substance. There is a dangerous synergistic effect when combining Ephedra with cold and allergy medications containing ephedrine or pseudoephedrine, caffeine sources (coffee, green tea, aspirin), products containing kola nut (a CNS stimulant), or prescription medications that contain ephedrine.[69,70]

GAMMA-ORYZANOL

Gamma-oryzanol is one of four isomers derived from oryzanol (plant sterol), an extract from rice-bran oil. It has been purported to provide the same benefits as anabolic steroids, but without the side effects. However, oryzanol is not anabolic because it cannot be converted to testosterone by the human body. Due to poor absorption of oryzanol and other plant sterols (less than 5%), the risks for toxicity appear to be minimal.[71]

However, athletes take this product as an antioxidant to neutralize the free radicals released during intense exercise.[72] The concept of free radicals is not clearly understood, but many athletes believe that aerobic activity requires an extensive oxygen supply. Oxygen creates free radicals, which attach to and thereby damage cell membranes. Athletes believe that antioxidants compete with free radicals and prevent or eliminate cell damage, thus reducing recovery time after exertion. Many combine gamma-oryzanol with vitamin E. Like octacosanol (wheat-germ oil), little to no research data are available and all claims about gamma-oryzanol are therefore conjecture.

GINSENG

Ginseng is an herb that is popular among athletes. It is used primarily as an "adaptogen" on the basis of reports suggesting that it aids the body's response to stress and improves one's energy.

Although there are numerous forms of ginseng, the following three different types appear to have received most research attention about putative ergogenic effects on aerobic exercise performance in humans: Russian/Siberian ginseng or *Eleutherococcus senticosus* (*E. senticosus*); Ginsana and similar products containing the active ingredient G 115 (a standardized form of ginseng); and Panax ginseng, referred to as Chinese or Korean ginseng.[73] Other recognized varieties include Panax *quinquefolius* (American ginseng) and Panax *japonicus* (Japanese ginseng).

E. senticosus has been theorized to be the most potent of the various ginseng preparations, the effects being attributed to the glycosides called eleutherosides. Although substantial improvements in physical performance have been attributed to supplementation with *E. senticosus*,[74] few data in peer-reviewed scientific journals are available. In addition, there are few double-blind, cross-over, placebo-designed studies in the literature. In the study by McNaughton et al,[75] the authors note that although *E. senticosus* did tend to increase VO_{2max}, the increases were not significantly different from those noted in the placebo trial. In another study, Asano et al[76] reported a significant improvement in VO_{2max} in six male baseball players after 8 days of *E. senticosus* Maxim (2 mL twice a day). However, the investigators indicated a single-blind, placebo protocol. It appears that an order effect may have confounded the results. During a 5-day period, three control trials were followed by the placebo trial and then the ginseng trial, and analysis of the results indicates a stepwise increase in VO_{2max} over the 5-day period.

Several studies have shown that products containing G 115, a standardized ginseng extract, may improve physiologic functions or performance in aerobic exercise tasks. In a review article highlighting ergogenic aspects of ginseng, Sandberg[77] provided few details of the experimental protocol, but indicated that 12 weeks of Ginsana supplementation improved oxygen metabolism during and after a 15-minute step test. No specific data or statistical analyses were provided, but 29 of 30 subjects in the ginseng group showed improvement, whereas only about 10 subjects in the placebo group improved. The data are difficult to interpret because of the lack of information provided and the fact that they were published in international journals where the scientific process may have not been peer reviewed.

Forgo and Kirchdorfer[78] studied the effect of Ginsana supplementation (200 mg/day for 9 weeks) on heart rate, serum lactate, and predicted VO_{2max} in 20 boxers, wrestlers, and karate participants during or after an 8-minute progressive exercise task on a cycle ergometer, starting at 1.5 W kg and increasing every 2 minutes by 0.5 W kg. They reported ginseng supplementation induced significant decreases in heart-rate responses during the 20-minute recovery period after the exercise task, a significantly decreased serum lactate measured at the 6-minute point during exercise and throughout the recovery period, and a significant increase in the heart-rate predicted VO_{2max}. However, the experimental design simply involved a pretreatment and posttreatment protocol, so the results may be confounded by lack of a control or placebo group.

Only two studies have investigated the effect of Panax ginseng on aerobic exercise in humans, and the results contradict each other. McNaughton et al[75] reported a significant increase in VO_{2max}, after 6 weeks of supplementation with Chinese ginseng (1 g per day). Using a placebo, cross-over protocol, 30 subjects (15 males and 15 females) were randomly assigned to one of three groups and received either Chinese ginseng, Russian ginseng, or a placebo in a counterbalanced order for 6 weeks. Supplementation with the Chinese ginseng significantly increased VO_{2max} compared to the placebo, but not compared to the Russian ginseng. There was no washout period in this study, which could have confounded the results. However, in another study, Teves et. al[79] used a double-blind, placebo, two-group design to investigate the effect of 4 weeks' supplementation with Panax ginseng (2 g/day with a glycoside content

of 1.5%) on physiologic and performance parameters in 12 marathon runners. Before and after the supplementation period, the subjects completed a VO_{2max} test and three consecutive daily runs to exhaustion at 84% VO_{2max}. These investigators reported no significant effect either on VO_{2max}, heart rate, rating of perceived exertion (RPE), lactate, or time to exhaustion during the three consecutive runs.

Although the mechanism underlying the alleged ergogenicity of ginseng on physical performance has not been delineated, animal research has suggested ginseng may stimulate the hypothalamic-pituitary-adrenal cortex axis, increasing resistance to various stressors.[80,81] Additionally, other reports have theorized that ginseng may enhance myocardial metabolism,[79] increase oxygen extraction by muscles, and improve mitochondrial metabolism in the muscle,[82] all of which theoretically could enhance aerobic exercise performance.

Chong and Oberholzer[83] noted that although there is considerable in vitro evidence supportive of various physiologic roles of ginseng, further research should be directed to investigate to what extent in vitro evidence is reflected and confirmed in vivo. Research data about the ergogenic effects of ginseng supplementation on aerobic exercise performance in humans are, in general, limited and mixed, particularly data about *E. senticosus* supplementation.

Furthermore, after a recent review of the ergogenic properties of ginseng in general, Bahrke and Morgan[84] indicated that because of methodologic and statistical shortcomings, there is no compelling evidence to indicate ginseng supplementation enhances human physical performance and there remains a need for well-designed research to address this issue. These authors also concluded that there is no basis for banning ginseng per se by athletes because the substance has not been shown to improve performance.

Ciwujia is another popular herb that is being marketed extensively under the brand name Endurox. Ciwujia, a natural root grown in the northeast section of China, has been used continuously as part of traditional Chinese medicine for almost 1700 years. Varro Tyler[85] notes that ciwujia is another name for *E. senticosus*. But Wu et al point out that the genus *E. senticosus* includes about 20 species of shrubs from China, Russia, Korea, and Japan.[86]

The usual dose of ciwujia for humans is 9 to 27 g/day of the raw herb. In multiple studies, it has been administered to laboratory animals at doses ranging from 60 to 200 times the recommended human dose. Ciwujia does not contain caffeine and does not produce any stimulant or anabolic steroid side effects.[86]

Ciwujia has been used in traditional Chinese medicine to treat fatigue and to bolster the immune system. This root intrigued researchers because of published reports of mountain climbers using ciwujia.[87] These reports describe the use of ciwujia to improve work performance at high altitudes and low oxygen conditions. Additional studies showed that laboratory animals that received ciwujia survived longer under low oxygen conditions[88] and that ciwujia could increase oxygenation of heart muscle tissues.

Work completed at the Academy of Preventive Medicine, under the guidance of the Cornell Group, initially was conducted with laboratory animals; however, it was their human research that was most provocative.[89] In the first trial, 10 healthy male adults underwent an aerobic and anaerobic assessment using a stationary bicycle ergometer in which power was increased from 60 to 210 watts at 30-watt intervals. Each interval lasted 3 minutes. Subjects also had their heart monitored every minute. Energy expenditure, oxygen intake, carbon dioxide expiration, and lactic acid were measured at the end of each interval.

To assess anaerobic power, subjects were started at low resistance that increased to a specified load in 3 to 5 seconds. Subjects continued at their maximum strength for 30 seconds at which the maximum anaerobic power was recorded. After the initial assessment, each subject was administered 800 mg of ciwujia (Endurox) daily for 2 weeks. Subjects returned to the exercise physiology laboratory for a repeat of the aerobic and anaerobic assessments.

Mean increase in fat utilization [measured by respiratory quotient (RQ)] in the ciwujia group during the time of the study was 43.2%. By shifting the energy source from carbohydrate to fat during exercise, ciwujia increases fat metabolism and delays the build-up of lactic acid.

The anaerobic threshold was computed by plotting lactic acid levels versus power load for each group. The ciwujia group demonstrated a 12.4% increase in the anaerobic threshold over the control group.

After the administration of ciwujia, there was a decrease in lactic acid levels, which became more pronounced at higher energy loads. At higher workloads, for example, 150 to 180 watts, the decrease in lactic acid levels, when compared to that associated with the control group, ranged from 31% to 33%.

Ciwujia appears to be a safe herb. But, further research needs to be completed with subjects who train more intensely, including double-blind, cross-over, placebo-controlled studies to determine if it improves performance. Lastly, because many of the articles were published in the Chinese literature about ciwujia, the scientific process of peer review comes into question when reviewing the research on ciwujia.

GLANDULARS

Glandulars are extracts from animal glands such as the adrenals, thymus, pituitary, and testes. The claim is that they enhance the function of the same gland in the human body from which they were derived. For example, orchic extract from the testes supposedly enhances testosterone function.[90] However, glandular extracts are degraded during the digestive process and are inactive when they are absorbed; therefore, they do not exert pharmacological effect.[91] A word of caution—if the real hormone happens to be in the bottle (remember, these products are not regulated), it could have serious medical consequences.

GLUCOSAMINE/CHONDROITIN SULFATE

Health-nutrition stores, several new shows, and a new book, *The Arthritis Cure*, by Theodosakis promote the nutrition supplements glucosamine sulfate and chondroitin sulfate as a cure for osteoarthritis.[92,93] Glucosamine is synthesized by the body and plays a role in the maintenance and repair of cartilage. Glucosamine sulfate is an artificially synthesized salt of glucosamine. Chondroitin sulfate is also naturally present in cartilage and composed of repeating units of glucosamine with attached sugar molecules.

Based on animal studies of arthritis, glucosamine has been reported to have anti-inflammatory properties by inhibiting the activity of proteolytic enzymes that contribute to cartilage breakdown.[94] It is also thought that glucosamine stimulates cartilage cells to synthesize the glycosaminoglycans and proteoglycans that are the building blocks of cartilage.[94] Theodosakis claims that chondroitin sulfate and glucosamine supplements work synergistically to combat the enzymes that cause cartilage degeneration, and thus halt the progression of osteoarthritis. Theodosakis bases his claims on patient testimonials, which of course, are subjective and do not prove effectiveness. The reality is that a limited amount of research has been done that has focused on glucosamine, and no human research has evaluated the glucosamine/chondroitin combination.

Interest in glucosamine's potential as an arthritis treatment was initiated in the early 1980s when a number of human studies were conducted in Europe and Asia.[94–96] Although these studies were small and short-term, many patients reported relief from pain and ease of movement after taking 1.5 g of glucosamine in divided doses daily.

In one study, 68 athletes with cartilage damage in their knees were given 1500 mg of glucosamine sulfate daily for 40 days, and then 750 mg for 90 to 100 days. Of the 68 athletes, 52 ex-perienced complete resolution of symptoms and resumed full athletic training. After 4 to 5 months, athletes were able to train at rates that were possible before injury. Follow-up exams 12 months later showed no signs of cartilage damage in any of the athletes.[97]

More research is needed to assess the long-term benefits of glucosamine either symptomatically or on the underlying degenerative disease process. The important and unanswered question still remains of whether glucosamine can stop or retard the process of cartilage deterioration and stimulate cartilage growth in osteoarthritis patients. It is clear that glucosamine *cannot* influence the repair of cartilage when there is insufficient or no cartilage on joints.

However, recent analysis of 23 different products that supposedly contain glucosamine was performed by researchers at the University of Maryland. In *The Arthritis Cure*, 15 of these products are listed that Theodosakis says were tested and found to contain essentially what their labels claimed. However, the researchers were unable to test for N-acetyl glucosamine and therefore could not determine the total amount of glucosamine in three of the listed products. To make matters worse, the researchers noted that some of the products listed contained amounts of glucosamine that varied significantly from the amounts stated on their labels.

The Arthritis Foundation does not recommend glucosamine sulfate or chondroitin sulfate as treatments for osteoarthritis or any other form of arthritis.[98] While the studies conducted over the past 15 years show some promise, more long-term, rigorously controlled studies are needed to evaluate the effectiveness and safety of glucosamine sulfate and chondroitin sulfate as treatments for osteoarthritis.

GLUTAMINE

Glutamine is an amino acid important for many essential homeostatic functions and for the optimal functioning of a number of tissues in the body, particularly the immune system and the gut. However, during various catabolic states, such as infection, surgery, trauma, and acidosis, glutamine homeostasis is placed under stress, and glutamine reserves, particularly in the skeletal muscle, are depleted.[99,100]

Regarding glutamine metabolism, some believe that exercise stress may be viewed in a similar manner as other catabolic stresses. Plasma glutamine responses to both prolonged and high-intensity exercise are characterized by increased levels during exercise, followed by significant decreases during the recovery period after exercise with several hours of recovery required for restoration of levels that existed before exercise, depending on the intensity and duration of exercise. If recovery between exercise bouts is inadequate, the acute effects of exercise on plasma glutamine level may be cumulative, because overload training has been shown to result in low plasma glutamine levels, requiring prolonged recovery.[101]

Athletes suffering from the overtraining syndrome (OTS) appear to maintain low plasma glutamine levels for months or years. All these observations have important implications for organ functions in these athletes, particularly regarding the gut and the cells of the immune system, which may be adversely affected. It is easy to see that if a person trains intensely each day, he or she will start depleting his or her muscle glutamine stores before he or she has fully recovered from the workout. The result is that the amount of muscle glutamine lessens each day. Eventually, the muscle glutamine level goes below the critical amount needed to sustain an anabolic state and the athletes revert into a long-term catabolic state. The more a person works out to try and make his or her muscles grow, the more glutamine used and the greater the catabolic response. Some athletes have suffered from OTS for more than 2 years and have been shown to have low plasma glutamine levels for the entire time. This may be due to damage to the muscle's glutamine synthesizing system as a result of it being overtaxed from too much training.[102]

Persons suffering from OTS also are more susceptible to disease and infections as a result of decreased immunity. This may be due to the role of glutamine as a primary source of fuel for the cells of the immune system, particularly lymphocytes, macrophages, and killer cells.[103,104]

Finally, two studies by Varnier and associates have shown glutamine to have a stimulatory effect on glycogen resynthesis in human skeletal muscle.[105,106] Possible mechanisms include a direct effect of glutamine on muscle glycogen synthesis or a conversion of glutamine to alanine. Alanine is transaminated and converted into glucose in the liver and returned to the muscle cells, a mechanism called the glucose-alanine cycle and an example of gluconeogenesis.

GLYCEROL

Glycerol has gained popularity in recent years as an effective way to "hyperhydrate" before training and competition. Glycerol's chemical properties are said to be ideal for increasing a person's hydration status because it attracts and holds onto water like a sponge. It also is rapidly absorbed and evenly distributed throughout body fluids. Many athletes have heard about glycerol, and some are experimenting with it to avoid dehydration and boost performance.[107]

Scientific research on the beneficial effects of glycerol, however, is limited and somewhat conflicting. Studies have shown that subjects who drank a glycerol solution 2.5 hours before exercise in the heat had less urine output, lower body temperature, and increased sweat rate compared to subjects who drank water only.[108] However, a study by Murray and colleagues found no indication of hyperhydration in subjects consuming a glycerol solution during exercise.[109] Differences in how the studies were conducted may account for the discrepancies.

Two separate explanations have been provided for glycerol's effect on body-fluid regulation. The first is that glycerol initially expands total body water by increasing the volume of fluid between and within the cells. The excess water in those spaces is readily available to maintain plasma volume, thereby increasing sweat rate and reducing the increase of body temperature during exercise and thermal stress.

The second explanation may be related to glycerol's effect on antidiuretic hormone (ADH). ADH stimulates the kidneys to reabsorb more water and thus excrete less water. An increase in the release of ADH usually accompanies even small increases in plasma osmolality, which occurs with the absorption of glycerol.

Scientists at the U.S. Army Research Institute of Environmental Medicine proposed that ADH may be partly responsible for glycerol's effectiveness for improving fluid retention. ADH is a hormone produced by the pituitary gland in response to dehydration.[110] According to these scientists, even small changes in ADH concentrations can have marked effects on urine flow.

Can glycerol improve performance? The answer is, no one knows yet. Studies conducted at the University of New Mexico showed that subjects prehydrating with a glycerol solution increased endurance compared to those prehydrating with water alone.[111] Further research is needed to confirm this observation.

Glycerol is now available commercially. It is sold in premeasured packets that are to be mixed with a specific amount of water and consumed 1 to 2 hours before exercise. The dosage is based on body weight; using more than the recommended amount will not result in increased benefits.

Glycerol may be tolerated differently by different athletes. Headaches, bloating, nausea, vomiting, and dizziness have been reported by some users. Furthermore, persons with all types of diabetes, high blood pressure, or kidney disorders should not use glycerol because it may cause serious health problems.[109] Glycerol has recently been added to the International Olympic Committee's banned list as an infused product, but it is still legal as an oral supplement.

L-CARNITINE

L-carnitine is a short-chain carboxylic acid containing nitrogen that is synthesized in the body from the amino acids lysine and methio-nine. It is found in meat, specifically sheep and lamb, and in dairy products. Limited amounts of L-carnitine are found in fruits, vegetables, grains, and eggs.[112] Ninety-five percent of L-carnitine in the body is located in muscle. L-carnitine is not considered an essential nutrient because the body compensates for decreased intakes by increasing synthesis and reducing renal clearance of carnitine.[113] The following are two theories[34] about the potential ergogenic effect: (a) Increased L-carnitine may increase fatty acid oxidation, because it is needed to transport long-chain fatty acids across the mitochondrial membrane, and (b) L-carnitine may affect the acetyl CoA/CoA ratio.

L-carnitine has been found to have a favorable effect on blood lipids in the treatment of hypercholesterolemia.[114,115] L-carnitine may improve exercise tolerance in persons with peripheral vascular disease.[116] But, no ergogenic benefit was seen with L-carnitine supplementation (4 g for 7 days) during repeated bouts of high-intensity anaerobic exercise, despite increased serum carnitine levels.[117]

One study found an increase in lipid oxidation with L-carnitine supplemented intravenously, suggesting that hypercarnitemia slightly favors lipid oxidation over carbohydrate oxidation during recovery from intense exercise, and is associated with a faster recovery of heart rate. However, no effect of L-carnitine on VO_{2max} or total energy expenditure was observed.[118]

A review article discusses 13 studies on L-carnitine supplementation. Nine studies showed no effect of L-carnitine supplementation on increasing fatty acid levels, increasing VO_{2max}, or enhancing performance, whereas four studies did find some ergogenic benefit.[34]

MEDIUM-CHAIN TRIGLYCERIDES

The fat medium-chain triglyceride (MCT) oil was first synthesized during the early 1950s and has been commercially available in products appearing in the food, pharmaceutical, and medical fields.[119] Only recently has it been used in the athletic market.

MCTs are saturated fats that are composed of 6 to 12 carbons, whereas long-chain triglycerides (LCTs) are saturated and unsaturated fats with 14 to 24 carbons. Listed as generally recognized as safe (GRAS), MCT oil is clear, light-colored, has no flavor of its own, and has low viscosity.

MCTs are absorbed by the portal system and appear to be absorbed as fast as carbohydrate. They are not readily stored but are oxidized by the liver or sent to peripheral tissue for oxidation.

It has been speculated that MCTs can improve endurance athletic performance because they can enter the mitochondria without carnitine, unlike LCTs. Muscles produce most of their energy during exercise by breaking down fat and carbohydrate inside the mitochondria; because MCTs have the ability to enter the mitochondria rapidly, they have been speculated to increase energy production and help conserve muscle stores of carbohydrate.[120]

Recently, scientists have begun to investigate the role of MCTs in athletic performance. A study conducted by a team of researchers led by Noakes in South Africa[121] showed improved performance during a 40-km time trial. Six trained cyclists completed three endurance rides on separate days that began with a 2-hour ride at about 70% of their maximum heart rate. Each ride was then followed by a 40-km time trial that the cyclists were instructed to complete as quickly as possible. During the three rides, the cyclists consumed either a 4.3% MCT beverage, a 10% carbohydrate beverage, or a beverage containing both 4.3% MCTs and 10% carbohydrate. During all three rides, the cyclists began by consuming 14 oz of the drink at the beginning of the ride and then about 3.5 oz every 10 minutes of the ride.

After all the tests were completed, the MCT-carbohydrate drink produced the best performance in the 40-km time trial—just 65 minutes, versus 66 minutes and 45 seconds with carbohydrates and 72 minutes with just the MCTs.[121]

The researchers suggest that the addition of MCTs to the carbohydrate drink helped by resulting in decreased carbohydrate depletion in the cyclists' legs during the first 2 hours of the ride, replacing the carbohydrate as the primary fuel source during the 2 hours of riding. As a result, when the subjects increased their intensity during the time trial, the combined beverage spared more carbohydrate for the high-intensity effort. While the previous study offers promising results, other recent publications do not.

Horowitz et al[122] investigated the rate of muscle glycogen degradation during high-intensity exercise following ingestion of a carbohydrate and MCT mixture and compared it to an ingestion of only carbohydrates. Seven well-trained men cycled for 30 minutes at 85% VO_{2max}. One hour prior to the exercise bout, subjects consumed either carbohydrates or carbohydrates and MCT. Muscle biopsies were performed before and immediately after exercise. Results indicated that muscle glycogen utilization during exercise bouts was not different in the two trials. Furthermore, the rate of carbohydrate oxidation during the exercise was not different following the ingestion of carbohydrate or carbohydrate and MCT. The authors concluded that adding MCTs to a pre-exercise carbohydrate meal did not reduce the rate of glycogen utilization or the rate of carbohydrate oxidation during the exercise bout.

While the majority of scientific literature does not support the use of MCTs to spare muscle glycogen and thus improve performance, it will continue to be investigated. With the advances in technology and the coming of designer foods, the topic of MCTs will surely be revisited.

PHOSPHATIDYLSERINE

Research and clinical investigations have shown that phosphatidylserine (PS), a natural soy-derived phospholipid, may be effective in suppressing cortisol levels. PS helps stop the increase in adrenocorticotrophic hormone (ACTH) after exercise that leads to lower testosterone and increases in cortisol. Two human studies found that PS can actually eliminate exercise-induced increases in cortisol.

Unfortunately, cortisol, a catabolic stress hormone that increases in response to exercise, may interfere with training and athletic performance. Cortisol, at the cellular level, plays an important regulatory function in the metabolism of protein, fat, carbohydrate, sodium, and potassium. But, because cortisol is catabolic and is increased during and after training, decreasing cortisol levels may effectively help to improve performance and/or recovery from exercise.

The first study involved PS administered intravenously, which is impractical application for athletes.[123] The second study may be more relevant: It found that the oral administration of 800 mg of PS for 10 days significantly inhibited the exercise-induced increase in cortisol.[124] Long-term human studies using athletes must be undertaken to determine if this anticatabolic effect of PS could result in a true anabolic effect.

The researchers in the previous two studies hypothesize that PS might also blunt the body's production of cortisol in relation to exercise. PS is known to influence receptor-ligand interactions by interfering with lipid microviscosity in the cell membrane. The relative viscosities of phospholipids affect the position of membrane proteins with enzymatic activity, perhaps modifying their interactions with ligands. PS may affect the number of receptors in the cell membrane or interfere with the activity of protein kinase C, which controls hormone receptor transduction mechanisms. The researchers state that it is possible, therefore, that treatment with PS may alter corticotropin-releasing factor receptor interactions, and cause a reduced activation of the hypothalamo-pituitary-adrenal axis, both of which have a stimulatory action or permissive role on ACTH and cortisol responses.

Another reported potential benefit of PS supplementation may be improved mental performance. One study found that in just 3 weeks, PS supplementation reversed up to 12 years of memory decline that normally occurs between ages 25 and 65 years in normal adults.[125] The author states that when PS is given orally, it is rapidly absorbed and readily crosses the blood-brain barrier to reach the brain. There, it appears to act exclusively in cell membranes. Nerve-cell membranes are particularly high in PS. The PS helps activate and regulate proteins that play major roles in nerve function—the generation, storage, transmission, and reception of nerve impulses. More research is needed with regard to how this applies to athletes.

SODIUM BICARBONATE

Sodium bicarbonate buffers lactic acid in the blood. Claims have been made that sodium bicarbonate will help the body's buffer capacity and counteract the buildup of lactic acid in the blood, thereby improving anaerobic performance. Several studies have reported improved anaerobic performance (in 400- and 800-meter runs) with bicarbonate supplementation.[126] Taking 0.3 gm/kg of sodium bicarbonate with water over a 2- to 3-hour period may improve 800-meter run time by several seconds. However, as many as half of those individuals using sodium bicarbonate experience urgent and explosive diarrhea one hour after the loading. Effects of repeated ingestion are unknown, and caution is advised.

YOHIMBINE

Yohimbine is an alkaloid drug extracted from yohimbe bark that functions as an alpha 2-adrenoreceptor blocker (monoamine oxidase inhibitor)—thereby increasing serum levels of norepinephrine. It is marketed to increase serum testosterone levels to enhance muscle growth and strength and decrease body fat. It is also promoted as an aphrodisiac. Although yohimbine increases norepinephrine levels, there is no proof that it has anabolic effects. Its value as an aphrodisiac is inconclusive.

According to the FDA, documented health hazards include low blood pressure, weakness, and nervous stimulation, followed by paralysis, fatigue, stomach disorders, kidney failure, seizures, and death.[127] The FDA has declared yohimbine unsafe and ineffective for over-the-counter sale. Yohimbine is a monoamine oxidase inhibitor, which means that tyramine-containing foods (red wine, liver, cheese) and nasal decongestants or diet aids containing phenylpropranolamine should be rigorously avoided if it is used to prevent a hypertensive crisis.[128]

CONCLUSIONS AND RECOMMENDATIONS

As long as athletes push themselves to greater and greater physical performance, new nutritional ergogenic aids will be made available with the assumption that they will help produce record-breaking performance and aid in recovery. In addition to requiring strong scientific support, the effectiveness and health consequences of taking long-term nutritional supplementation should be documented by well-controlled research studies that are made available for review by both athletes and scientists.

Thanks to the 1994 Dietary Supplement and Health Education Act (DSHEA), dietary supplements don't have to be proven safe or effective to be sold.[5] There is also no guarantee that the product is what it says it is on the label.

While prescription and over-the-counter drugs and food additives must meet the FDA's safety and effectiveness requirements, supplements that are marketed with medical claims bypass these regulations. These products can go to market with no testing for efficacy, thus skipping the years-long process that drugs must undergo. The FDA is also prohibited from taking a product off the market unless the agency can prove that using the supplement will create a medical problem. Unfortunately, this law places the burden of proof of a supplement's safety on the over-taxed FDA rather than on the companies profiting from the sale of the supplement.

FDA approval is not required for package or marketing claims, so supplement manufacturers can put unsupported health claims on their labels. While the label does have to say that claims have not been reviewed or approved by the FDA, this caution is usually in small print. Lastly, supplements do not have to be manufactured according to any standards. Since supplements such as herbs are not regulated as drugs, no legal standard exists for their processing, harvesting, or packaging. In many cases contents and potency are not accurately listed on the label.

REFERENCES

1. Burke LM, Read RS. Dietary supplements in sports. *Sports Med*. 1993;15:43–65.
2. Grunewald KK, Bailey RS. Commercially marketed supplements for bodybuilding athletes. *Sports Med*. 1993;15:90–103.
3. Grandjean AC, Ruud JS. Olympic athletes. In: Wolinsky I, Hickson JF, eds. *Nutrition and Exercise and Sport*. Boca Raton, FL: CRC Press; 1994:447–454.
4. Clarkson PM. Nutrition for improved sports performance: current issues on ergogenic aids. *Sports Med*. 1996;21:393–401.
5. Bass IS, Young AL. *The Dietary Supplement Health and Education Act: A Legislative History and Analysis*. Washington, DC: Food and Drug Law Institute; 1996;5–100.
6. Abumrad N, Flakoll P. *The Efficacy and Safety of CaHMB (Beta-hydroxy-Beta-methylbutyrate) in Hu-*

mans. Memphis, TN: Vanderbilt University Medical Center, Annual Report: MTI; 1991.
7. Nissen S, Sharp R, Ray M, et al. Effect of leucine metabolite Beta-hydroxy-Beta-methylbutyrate on muscle metabolism during resistance training. *J Appl Physiol*. 1996;81:2095–2104.
8. Ostaszewski P, Kostiuk S, Balasinskia B, et al. The effect of leucine metabolite Beta-hydroxy-Beta-methylbutyrate (HMB) on muscle protein synthesis and protein breakdown in chick and rat muscle (abstract). *J Ani Sci*. 1996:1803.
9. Passwater R, Fuller J. *Building Muscle Mass, Performance and Health with HMB*. New Canaan, CT: Keats Publishing; 1997.
10. Nielsen F. Facts and fallacies about boron. *Nutrition Today*. 1992;27:6–12.
11. Ferrando A, Green N. The effect of boron supplementation on lean body mass, plasma testosterone levels, and

strength in bodybuilders. *Int J Sport Nutr.* 1993;3:140–149.

12. Bucci L. *Nutrients as Ergogenic Aids for Sports and Exercise.* Boca Raton, FL: CRC Press; 1993:14–18.

13. Lemon PWR. Do athletes need more dietary protein and amino acids? *Int J Sports Nutr.* 1995;5:S39–S61.

14. Newsholme EA, Acworth IN, Blomstrand E. Amino acids, brain neurotransmitters and a functional link between muscle and brain that is important in sustained exercise. In: Benzi G, ed. *Advances in Myochemistry.* London: John Libbey Eurotext; 1989:127–133.

15. Davis JM. Carbohydrate, branched-chain amino acids and endurance: the central fatigue hypothesis. *Sports Science Exchange.* Gatorade Sports Science Institute, Chicago, IL; 1996;9(2):1–6.

16. Davis JM, Bailey SP. Possible mechanisms of central nervous system fatigue during exercise. *Med Sci Sports Exerc.* 1996;29:45–57.

17. Kreider RB, Miriel V, Bertun E. Amino acid supplementation and exercise performance: an analysis of the proposed ergogenic value. *Sports Med.* 1993;16:190–209.

18. Costill DL, Dalsky GP, Fink WJ. Effects of caffeine ingestion on metabolism and exercise performance. *Med Sci Sports Exerc.* 1978;10:155–158.

19. Ivy JL, Costill DL, Fink WJ, et al. Influence of caffeine and carbohydrate feedings on endurance performance. *Med Sci Sports Exerc.* 1979;11:6–11.

20. Essig D, Costill DL, Van Handel RJ. Effects of caffeine ingestion on utilization of muscle glycogen and lipid during leg ergometer cycling. *Int J Sports Med.* 1980;1:86–90.

21. Knapik JJ, Jones BJ, Toner MM, et al. Influence of caffeine on serum substrate changes during running in trained and untrained individuals. In: Knuttgen HG, Vogel JA, Poortmans J, eds. *Biochem Exerc.* Champaign, IL: Human Kinetics; 1983:514–520.

22. Powers S, Byrd R, Tulley R, et al. Effects of caffeine ingestion on metabolism and performance during graded exercise. *Eur J Appl Physiol.* 1983;40:301–307.

23. Gaesser GA, Rich RG. Influence of caffeine on blood lactate response during incremental exercise. *Int J Sports Med.* 1985;6:207–211.

24. Fisher SM, McMurray RG, Berry M, et al. Influence of caffeine on exercise performance in habitual caffeine users. *Int J Sports Med.* 1986;7:276–280.

25. Casal DC, Leon AS. Failure of caffeine to affect substrate utilization during prolonged running. *Med Sci Sports Exerc.* 1985;17:174–179.

26. Cole K, Costill DJ, Starling R, et al. Effect of caffeine ingestion on perception of effort and subsequent work production. *Int J Sports Nutr.* 1996;6:14–23.

27. Spriet LL. Caffeine and performance. *Int J Sport Nutr.* 1995;5:S84–S99.

28. Dodd SL, Herb RA, Power SK. Caffeine and exercise performance. *Sports Med.* 1993;15:14–23.

29. Sandage BW, Sabounjian LA, White R, et al. Choline citrate may enhance athletic performance. *Physiologist.* 1992;35:236a.

30. Von Allworden HN, Horn S, Kahl J, et al. The influence of lecithin on plasma choline concentrations in triathletes and adolescent runners during exercise. *Eur J Appl Physiol.* 1983;67:87–91.

31. Conlay LA, Wurtman RJ, Blusztajn JK, et al. Decreased plasma choline concentrations in marathon runners (letter). *N Engl J Med.* 1986;175:892.

32. Spector SA, Jackman MR, Sabounjian LA, et al. Effects of choline supplementation on fatigue in trained cyclists. *Med Sci Sports Exerc.* 1995;27:669–673.

33. Wurtman RJ. Effects of dietary amino acids, carbohydrates and choline neurotransmitter synthesis. *Mt Sinai J Med.* 1988;55:75–86.

34. Kanter MM, Williams MH. Antioxidants, carnitine and choline as putative ergogenic aids. *Int J Sport Nutr.* 1995;5 (suppl 1991–1995):S120–S131.

35. Grunewald K, Bailey R. Commercially marketed supplements for bodybuilding athletes. *Sports Med.* 1993;15:90–103.

36. Berg F. *Weight Loss Quackery and Fads.* 2nd ed. Hettinger, ND: Healthy Weight Journal; 1996:16–17.

37. Coleman E. The chromium picolinate weight loss scam. *Sports Med Digest.* 1997(January):6–7.

38. Evans GW. The effect of chromium picolinate on insulin controlled parameters in humans. *Int J Biosocial Med Res.* 1989;11:163–180.

39. Clancy SP, Clarkson PM, DeCheke ME, et al. Effects of chromium picolinate supplementation on body composition, strength, and urinary chromium loss in football players. *Int J Sport Nutr.* 1994;4:142–153.

40. Hallmark MA, Reynolds TH, DeSouza CA, Dotson DO, Anderson RA, Rogers MA. Effects of chromium and resistive training on muscle strength and body composition. *Med Sci Sports Exerc.* 1996;28:139–144.

41. Federal Trade Commission. Companies advertising popular dietary supplement chromium picolinate can't substantiate weight loss and health claims, says FTC. FTC web page (http://www.ftc.gov) news release on commission actions. Nov. 7, 1996.

42. Schauss AG. Colloidal minerals: clinical implications of clay suspension products sold as dietary supplements. *Am J Natural Med.* 1997;4:5–10.

43. Schauss AG. *Trace Elements and Human Health.* 2nd ed. Tacoma, WA: Life Sciences Press; 1996.

44. Hurlbut CS. *Dana's Manual of Mineralogy.* New York: John Wiley & Sons; 1971:436.

45. Decker EA. The role of phenolics, conjugated linoleic acid, carnosine, and pyrroloquinoline quinone as nonessential dietary antioxidants. *Nutr Rev.* 1995;53:49–58.

46. Pariza M, Park Y, Cook M. Conjugated linoleic acid (CLA) reduces body fat. *FASEB J.* 1996;A560.

47. Chin SF, Storkson JM, Albright KJ, et al. Conjugate linoleic acid is a growth factor for rates as shown by enhanced weight gain and improved feed efficiency. *J Nutr.* 1994;124:2344–2349.

48. Furst P. New parenteral substrates in clinical nutrition, Part II. *Eur J Clin Nutr.* 1994;48:681–691.

49. Borg Magnusson IK, et al. Effects of a fat emulsion containing medium chain fatty acids and long chain fatty acids and energy metabolism in partially hepatectomized rats. *Clin Nutr.* 1995;14:23–28.

50. Harris RC, Soderlund K, Hultman E. Elevation of creatine in resting and exercised muscle of normal subjects by creatine supplementation. *Clin Sci.* 1992;83:367–374.

51. Balsom PD, Ekblom B, Soderlund K, et al. Creatine supplementation and dynamic high-intensity intermittent exercise. *Scand J Med Sci Sport.* 1993;3:143–149.

52. Volek JS, Kraemer WJ. Creatine supplementation: its effect on human muscular performance and body composition. *J Strength Cond Res.* 1996;10:200–210.

53. Greenhaff PL, Constatin-Teodosiu D, Hultman E. The effect of oral creatine supplementation on skeletal muscle ATP degradation during repeated bouts of maximal voluntary exercise in man. *Am J Physiol.* 1994;266 (SPTI):E725–E730.

54. Earnest CP, Snell PG, Rodrequez R, et al. The effect of creatine monohydrate ingestion on anaerobic power indices, muscular strength and body composition. *Acta Physiologica Scandinavia.* 1995;153:207–209.

55. Hultman E. Muscle creatine loading in men. *J Appl Physiol.* 1996;81:232–237.

56. Burke LM, Pyne DB, Telford RD. Effect of oral creatine supplementation on single-effort sprint performance in elite swimmers. *Int J Sport Nutr.* 1996;6:223–233.

57. Morales AJ, Nolan JJ, Nelson JC, et al. Effects of replacement dose of DHEA in men and women of advancing age. *J Endo and Metab.* 1994;78:1360–1367.

58. Regelson W, Kalimi M. Dehydroepiandrosterone (DHEA)—the multifunctional steroid. II. Effects on the CNS, cell proliferation, metabolic and vascular, clinical, and other effects. *Ann NY Acad Sci.* 1994;719:564–575.

59. Regelson W, Loria R, Kalimi M. Dehydroepiandrosterone (DHEA)—The "Mother Steroid" I. Immunological action. *Ann NY Acad Sci.* 1994;719:553–563.

60. Nestler JE, Usiskin KD, Barlascine CO, et al. Suppression of DHEAS levels by insulin: an evaluation of possible mechanisms. *J Clin Endocrinol Metab.* 1989; 69:1040–1046.

61. Clore JN. Dehydroepiandrosterone and body fat. *Obesity Res.* 1995; November 3 (suppl 4):613S–616S.

62. Labrie F, Belanger A, Simard J, et al. DHEA and peripheral androgen and estrogen formation: intracrinology. *Ann NY Acad Sci.* 1995;774:16–28.

63. Williams MH. The use of nutritional ergogenic aids in sports: Is it an ethical issue? *Int J Sports Nutr.* 1994;4:120–131.

64. Stanko RT, Robertson RJ, Spina RJ, et al. Enhancement of arm-exercise endurance capacity with dihydroxyacetone and pyruvate. *J Appl Physiol.* 1990;68:119–124.

65. Stanko RT, Robertson RJ, Galbreath RW, et al. Enhanced leg-exercise endurance with a high carbohydrate diet and dihydroxyacetone and pyruvate. *J Appl Physiol.* 1990;69:1651–1656.

66. Robertson RJ, Stanko RT, Goss Fl, et al. Blood glucose extraction as a mediator of perceived exertion during prolonged exercise. *Eur J Appl Physiol.* 1990;61:100–105.

67. Ephedrine. In: McEvoy GK, Litvak K, eds. *American Hospital Formulary Service Drug Information 93.* Bethesda, MD: American Society of Hospital Pharmacists; 1993;721–724.

68. Food and Drug Administration/Department of Health and Human Services Statement. FDA statement on street drugs containing botanical ephedrine. April 10, 1996.

69. Capwell R. Ephedrine-induced mania from a herbal diet supplement (letter). *Am J Psych.* 1995;152:647.

70. Bruno A, Nolte KB, Chapin J. Stroke associated with ephedrine use. *Neurology.* 1993;43:1313–1316.

71. Wheeler KB, Garleb KA. Gamma Oryzanol—plant sterol supplementation: Metabolic, endocrine, and physiologic effects. *Int J Sports Nutr.* 1991;1:178–191.

72. Woolley BH. Ergogenic aids. *Postgrad Med.* 1991; 89:195–205.

73. Dowling EA, Redondo DR, Branch JD. Effect of eleutherococcus senticosus on submaximal performance and maximal exercise performance. *Med Sci Sports Exerc.* 1996;28:482–489.

74. Talbert L, Pauly MM. *Eleutherococcus: king of the adaptogens.* American Institute of Health and Nutrition; 1991:1–16.

75. McNaughton LG, Egan G, Caelli G. A comparison of Chinese and Russian ginseng as ergogenic aids to improve various facets of physical fitness. *Internat Clin Nutr Rev.* 1989;9:32–35.

76. Asano KT, Takahashi T, Kugo H, et al. Effects of Eleutherococcus senticosus Maxim on physical performance and resources in maximal and submaximal work. In: *New Data on Eleutherococcus: Proceedings of the Second International Symposium on Eleutherococcus M. 1984.* Vladivostok: Far East Science Center, USSR Academy of Sciences; 1986: 229–239.

77. Sandberg F. Vitalitet och senilitet: effekten av ginsengglykosider pa prestationsformagan. *Sven Farm Tidskr.* 1980;84:499–502.

78. Forgo I, Kirchdorfer AM. Ginseng steigert die korperliche Leistung. *Artz Praxis.* 1981;33:1784–1786.

79. Teves MA, Wright JE, Welch MJ, et al. Effects of ginseng on repeated bouts of exhaustive exercise (abstract). *Med Sci Sports Exerc.* 1983;15:162.

80. Brekman II, Dardymov IV. New substances of plant origin which increase nonspecific resistance. *Ann Rev Pharmacol.* 1969;9:419–428.

81. Liu CX, Xiao PG. Recent advances on ginseng research in China. *J Ethnopharm.* 1992;36:27–38.

82. Asano KT, Takahashi T, Miyashita M, et al. Effect of Eleutherococcus senticosus extract on human physical working capacity. *Planta Med.* 1986;3:175–177.

83. Chong SKF, Oberholzer VG. Ginseng: is there a clinical use in medicine? *Postgrad Med J.* 1988;64:841–846.

84. Bahrke MS, Morgan WP. Evaluation of the ergogenic properties of ginseng. *Sports Med.* 1994;18:229–248.

85. Tyler VE. *Ginseng: The Honest Herbal.* Pharmaceutical Products Press, 1993.

86. Wu BC, Liu RM, Fang GX, et al. The pharmacology of ciwujia. *Acta Chinese Med Pharm.* 1985;2:29.

87. Heilongjiang Institute of Traditional Chinese Medicine and Materia Medica. Studies on Acanthopanax senticosus. In: *Proceedings of the Symposium on Pharmacology.* Shanghai, China: 1978.

88. Sui DY, Lu ZZ, Ma LN, Fan ZG. Effects of the leaves of Acanthopanax senticosus harms on myocardial infarct size in acute ischemic dogs. *Chung Kuo Chung Yao Tsa Chih.* 1994;19:746–747.

89. Wu YN, Wang XQ, Zhao YF, et al. Effects of ciwujia (Radix Acenthopanacis senticosu) preparation on human stamina. *J Hygiene Res.* (in Chinese). 1996;57–63.

90. Williams MH. Nutritional supplements for strength-trained athletes. *Sport Science Exchange.* 1993;6(6).

91. Newson M, ed. *U.S. Olympic Committee Handbook.* Colorado Springs, CO: U.S. Olympic Committee; 1989:49.

92. Coleman E. Nutrition update: A dietary "magic bullet" for articular cartilage? *Sports Med Digest.* 1997;19:(8).

93. *Tufts University Health & Nutrition Letter.* April 1997;15(2).

94. Bucci LR. *Nutrition Applied to Injury Rehabilitation and Sports Medicine.* CRC Press. 1994;195–203.

95. Vaz AL. Double-blind clinical evaluation of the relative efficacy of ibuprofen and glucosamine sulfate in the management of osteoarthrosis of the knee in outpatients. *Curr Med Res Opin.* 1981;7:104–114.

96. Brooks PM. Potter SR, et al. NSAID and osteoarthritis—help or hindrance? *J Rheumatol.* 1982;9:3–5.

97. Bohmer D, Ambrus P, et al. Treatment of chondropathia patellae in young athletes with glucosamine sulfate. In Bachl N, Prokop L, Suckert R, eds. *Current Topics in Sports Medicine.* Vienna, Austria: Urban and Schwarzenberg; 1984:799–900.

98. Arthritis Foundation. *An Answer to The Arthritis Cure.* May 14, 1997.

99. Lacey JM, Wilmore DW. Is glutamine a conditionally essential amino acid? *Nutr Rev.* 1990;48:297–309.

100. Wagenmaakers A. Amino acid metabolism, muscular fatigue and muscle wasting, speculations on adaptations to high altitude. *Int J Sports Med.* 1992;13:S110–S113.

101. Parry-Billings M, Budgett R, Koutedakis Y, et al. Plasma amino acid concentration in over training syndrome: possible effects on the immune system. *Med Sci Sports Exerc.* 1992;24 (12):1353–1358.

102. Rowbottom DG, Keast D, Morton AR. The emerging role of glutamine as an indicator of exercise stress and overtraining. *Sports Med.* 1996;21:80–97.

103. Castell LM, Poortman JR, Newsholme EA. Does glutamine have a role in reducing infections in athletes? *Eur J Appl Physiol.* 1996;73:488–490.

104. Rohde T, MacLean DA, Hartkopp A. The immune system and serum glutamine during a triathlon. *Eur J Appl Physiol.* 1996;74:428–434.

105. Varnier M, Leese GP, Rennie MJ, et al. Effect of glutamine on glycogen synthesis in human skeletal muscle. *Clin Nutr.* 1990;12:suppl 2.

106. Varnier M, Leese GP, Thompson J, Rennie MJ, et al. Stimulatory effect of glutamine on glycogen accumulation in human skeletal muscle. *Am J Physiol.* 1995;269:E309–E315.

107. Scheett TP, Webster MJ, Wagoner KD, et al. Effectiveness of glycerol as a rehydrating agent. *Med Sci Sport Exerc.* 1995;27:S19.

108. Riedesel ML, Allen DY, Peake GT, et al. Hyperhydration with glycerol solutions. *J Appl Physiol.* 1987;63:2262–2268.

109. Murray R, Eddy DE, Gregory LP, et al. Physiological responses to glycerol ingestion during exercise. *J Appl Physiol.* 1991;71:144–149.

110. Freund BJ, McKay JM, Laird JE, et al. Fluid hormone responses to glycerol hyperhydration during cold exposure. *Med Sci Sports Exerc.* 1995;27:S18.

111. Montner P, Stark DM, Riedesel ML, et al. Pre-exercise glycerol hydration improves cycling endurance time. *Int J Sports Med.* 1996;17:27–33.

112. Broquist HP. Carnitine. In: Shils ME, Olson JA, Shike M, eds. *Modern Nutrition in Health and Disease.* 8th ed. Philadelphia, PA: Lea & Febiger; 1994.

113. Stradler DD, Chernard CA, Rebouche CJ. Effect of dietary macronutrient content on carnitine excretion and

efficiency of carnitine reabsorption. *Am J Clin Nutr.* 1993;58:868–872.

114. Bahl JJ, Bressler R. The pharmacology of carnitine. *Annu Rev Pharmacol Toxicol.* 1987;27:257–277.

115. Nagao B, Kobayashi A, Yamazaki N. Effects of L-carnitine on phospholipids in the ischemic myocardium *Jpn Heart J.* 1987;28:243–251.

116. Brevetti G, Perna S, Sabba C, et al. Superiority of L-propionylcarnitine vs L-carnitine in improving walking capacity in patients with peripheral vascular disease: an acute, intravenous, double-blind crossover study. *Eur Heart J.* 1992;13:251–255.

117. Trappe SW, Costill DL, Goodpaster NB, et al. The effects of L-carnitine supplementation on performance during interval swimming. *Int J Sports Med.* 1994;15:181–185.

118. Natali A, Santoro L, Brandi D, et al. Effects of acute hypercarnitinemia during increased fatty substrate oxidation in man. *Metabolism.* 1993;42:594–600.

119. Babayan VK. Medium chain fatty acid esters and their medicinal and nutrition applications. *Journal of the American Oils Chemists Society.* 1991;58:49A.

120. Enig MG. Fat, calories and tropical oils in perspective. *Food Product Design.* 1991; May.

121. Van Zyle C, Lambert EV, Noakos TD, Dennis SC. Effects of ingestion on carbohydrate metabolism and cy-cling performance. *Biochem of Exerc.* 1994; Sept–Oct: 6.

122. Horowitz JF, Mora-Rodriguez R, Coyle EF. The effects of pre-exercise medium chain triglyceride ingestion on muscle glycogen utilization during high intensity exercise. *Med Science Sports Exerc.* 1995;27(supp 5): S203.

123. Monteleone P, Beinat L, Tanzillo L, et al. Effects of phosphatidylserine on the neuroendocrine response to physical stress in humans. *Neuroendocrinology.* 1990;52:243–248.

124. Monteleone P, Maj M, Beinat L, et al. Blunting by chronic phosphatidylserine administration of the stress-induced activation of the hypothalamo-pituitary adrenal axis in healthy men. *Eur J Clin Pharm.* 1992;41:385–388.

125. Crook TH, Tinklenber A, Yesavage J, et al. Effects of phosphatidylserine in age-associated memory impairment. *Neurology.* 1991;41:644–649.

126. Williams MH. Bicarbonate loading. *Sports Sci Exchange.* 1992;4(36).

127. *Unsubstantiated Claims and Documented Health Hazards in the Dietary Supplement Marketplace.* Washington, DC: Department of Health and Human Services, Public Health Service, Food and Drug Administration, 1993.

128. Tyler VE. *Yohimbe. The Honest Herbal.* Pharmaceutical Products Press, 1993.

CHAPTER 8

Fluid Needs of Athletes

Robert Murray

HISTORICAL OVERVIEW

It has long been recognized that body fluid balance is a critical factor in ensuring optimal health and performance. The value of adequate fluid consumption was likely self-evident to those who lived in tropical and desert environments centuries before scientists turned their attention to the topic. In fact, it wasn't until the late 1930s that researchers began to systematically investigate the physiologic responses to changes in hydration status. Before and during World War II, the ability of soldiers to withstand the stress of physical activity in the desert was of great interest to scientists. Knowing that the evaporation of sweat was of critical importance in temperature regulation, the researchers paid particular attention to the soldiers' drinking habits.[1] Not surprisingly, fluid intake failed to keep pace with the large sweat losses sustained by the soldiers, resulting in dehydration.[2,3] In fact, the researchers noted that, "In the course of experiments in both the desert and the hot room, we found that men failed to replace by ingestion all of the water they lost by sweating, even when adequate supplies of drinking water were available. In some cases this failure to maintain water balance resulted in considerable dehydration, even approaching dehydration exhaustion."[3] This "voluntary dehydration" is still common because voluntary fluid intake during physical activity usually replaces only about 50% of the sweat that is lost.[4–6]

SCIENTIFIC BACKGROUND

Regulation of Fluid Balance

Body-fluid balance is regulated by mechanisms that influence water and sodium excretion, and affect the sensation of thirst. When fluid is lost from the body in the form of sweat, plasma volume decreases and plasma osmolality increases (due to an increase in plasma sodium and chloride concentrations). These alterations are sensed by vascular pressure receptors and hypothalamic osmoreceptors, resulting in an increase in vasopressin (antidiuretic hormone) release from the pituitary gland and in renin release from the kidneys. These hormones (including the angiotensin II and aldosterone that result from an increase in plasma renin activity) serve to increase water and sodium retention by the kidneys and provoke an increase in thirst.[7] Under normal conditions, the resulting fluid intake eventually exceeds fluid losses,[8] plasma volume and osmolality return to normal levels, and water balance is restored by the kidneys (that is, excess fluid is excreted). However, for athletes, body-fluid balance is often compromised, because it is difficult for athletes to ingest enough fluid to offset the large volume of fluid that is lost during training and competition.

Daily Fluid Loss

The total volume of fluid lost from the body on a daily basis is determined by the environmental conditions, the size (and surface area) of the person, the person's metabolic rate, and the volume of excreted fluids. Fluid is periodically lost from the body by way of the kidneys (urine), gastrointestinal (GI) tract (feces), and eccrine sweat glands, and is constantly lost from the respiratory tract and the skin.[9]

Insensible water loss through the skin is relatively constant (Table 8–1), but insensible loss through the respiratory tract is affected by the ambient temperature, relative humidity, and ventilatory volume. Inhaled air is humidified during its passage through the respiratory tract such that exhaled air has a relative humidity of 100% (vapor pressure = 47 mm Hg). Inhaling warm, humid air slightly reduces insensible water loss because the inhaled air already contains substantial water vapor. As indicated in Table 8–1, athletes experience a greater insensible water loss through the respiratory tract merely because of the overall increase in ventilation that accompanies exercise. The air inhaled during cold-weather exercise contains relatively little water vapor, so as it is warmed and humidified during its transit through the respiratory tract, an additional water loss occurs. For this reason, it is important to keep in mind that even during cold-weather training and competition, fluid losses through the sweat glands and respiratory tract can be high.

Urine losses in athletes tend to be less than those in persons who are sedentary, a trend that is exacerbated by warm weather. Exercise causes a reduction in urine production as the kidneys attempt to conserve water and sodium to offset losses due to sweating.

Even in the absence of physical activity, daily fluid losses average about 2 to 3 L (Table 8–1). When athletes train and compete in warm environments, their daily fluid needs can be prodigious.[5] For example, an athlete who trains 2 hours each day can easily lose an additional 2 L of body fluid, resulting in a daily fluid requirement of more than 5 L. Many athletes train more than 2 hours each day, further increasing their fluid needs. Such losses can strain the capacity of the fluid-regulatory system such that thirst becomes an inadequate stimulus of fluid intake and dehydration results.

CURRENT RESEARCH

The deterioration in physiologic function that accompanies dehydration has been well-characterized by researchers (Table 8–2). Since 1990, research has focused less on the effects of dehydration and more upon how fluid intake influences physiologic and performance responses. This research has generated information of both scientific and practical importance. In recognition of these research findings, the American College of Sports Medicine (ACSM) published a position stand in January 1996 on exercise and fluid replacement.[10] The position stand includes

Table 8–1 Daily Fluid Losses (in mL) for an Athlete Weighing 70 kg

	Normal Weather (68°F)	Warm Weather	Exercise in Warm Weather (85°F)
Insensible loss			
Skin	350	350	350
Respiratory tract	350	250	650
Urine	1400	1200	500
Feces	100	100	100
Sweat	100	1400	5000
Total	2300	3300	6600

Source: Reprinted with permission from A.C. Guyton, *Textbook of Medical Physiology*, 8th ed., pp. 274–275, © 1991, WB Saunders Company.

Table 8–2 Physiologic Responses to Dehydration

Increased	*Decreased*
• Incidence of gastrointestinal distress	• Plasma volume
• Plasma osmolality	• Splanchnic and renal blood flow
• Blood viscosity	• Central blood volume
• Heart rate	• Central venous pressure
• Core temperature at which swe_ing begins	• Cardiac filling pressure
• Core temperature at which skin blood flow increases	• Stroke volume
• Core temperature at a given exercise intensity	• Cardiac output
• Muscle glycogen use	• Sweat rate at a given core temperature
	• Maximal sweat rate
	• Skin blood flow at a given core temperature
	• Maximal skin blood flow
	• Performance
	• Endurance capacity (exercise to exhaustion)

Source: Reprinted, by permission, from R. Murray, 1995, "Fluid Needs in Hot and Cold Environments," *International Journal of Sports Nutrition*, Vol. 5: S62–S73.

a number of practical recommendations for fluid intake for athletes. These guidelines emphasize the importance of an aggressive fluid-replacement plan designed to prevent even slight dehydration during training and competition.

Fluid Needs Before Exercise

Under normal circumstances, people usually consume more fluid than is lost in a given 24-hour period and the kidneys excrete the excess. However, athletes are not "normal" in this respect because their large sweat losses often make it difficult for them to ingest enough fluid to maintain normal hydration status. The large daily fluid needs of athletes necessitate that athletes pay close attention to their drinking habits so that they are adequately hydrated before and during training and competition. This is certainly true during periods of warm weather, when the sweat losses incurred during physical activity, plus the increased fluid loss associated with normal daily activities, can cause fluid needs to reach 10 L or more per day.[5] Under such circumstances, the thirst mechanism may not be responsive enough to ensure euhydration. This problem was demonstrated by Rico-Sanz et al,[11] who studied soccer players in Puerto Rico during 2 weeks of training. When the players were allowed to drink fluids ad libitum (average intake, 2.7 L/day), their total body water at the end of the week was about 1.1 L lower than when they were mandated to ingest 4.6 L of fluid per day. Monitoring changes in body weight before and after training is the easiest way to determine if an athlete has been successful at achieving normal hydration status, and for prescribing specific fluid-intake regimens for those athletes who find it difficult to rehydrate adequately.

The ACSM position stand[10] recommends that athletes ingest 500 mL (approximately 16 oz) of fluid 2 hours before exercise to help ensure adequate hydration and to provide enough time for the excretion of excess fluid. On warm days, athletes may be advised to drink an additional 250 to 500 mL (approximately 8 to 16 oz) of fluid (for example, sports drinks, fruit juice, water) 30 to 60 minutes before exercise. As a practical check on hydration status, athletes should pay attention to the color and volume of their urine. Well-hydrated athletes will normally void a light-colored urine of normal to above-normal volume within 60 minutes of exercise. If the urine is dark yellow in color, is of small volume, and has a strong odor, dehydration is likely and the athlete should continue drinking. Athletes who ingest vitamin supplements may produce a dark-yellow urine, so urine color, volume, and odor must all be considered as indicators of hydration status.

It has been hypothesized that ingesting a glycerol solution before exercise in the heat may confer cardiovascular and thermoregulatory advantages. In fact, ingesting glycerol solutions before exercise does result in a reduction in urine production and in the retention of fluid.[12] Glycerol-induced hyperhydration is accompanied by weight gain that is proportional to the amount of water retained (usually about 0.5 to 1 kg). After glycerol molecules are absorbed and distributed throughout the body water (with the exception of the aqueous humor and the cerebrospinal fluid compartments), their presence provokes a transient increase in osmolality, prompting a temporary reduction in urine production. As glycerol molecules are removed from the body water in the subsequent hours, plasma osmolality decreases, urine production increases, and the excess water is excreted.

There are a number of reasons why it is unwise to recommend glycerol-induced hydration to athletes, including the following: 1) Athletes pay a metabolic cost for carrying extra body weight. 2) There is no compelling evidence that glycerol-induced hyperhydration results in improved performance. 3) The side effects of ingesting glycerol can range from mild sensations of bloating and lightheadedness to more severe symptoms of headaches, dizziness, and nausea.[13]

Fluid Needs During Exercise—Temperature Regulation

The evaporation of sweat from the skin is the primary avenue for heat loss during vigorous exercise, a process that is particularly crucial during physical activity in warm environments. Approximately 0.58 kcal of heat is dissipated from the body with the evaporation of each gram of sweat, allowing for the dissipation of large quantities of heat.[14]

Individual sweating rates can vary widely depending upon the environmental temperature and humidity, the intensity of exercise, the type and amount of clothing worn by the athlete, the athlete's level of fitness and acclimation, and the athlete's genetic predisposition for sweating. For example, a sweat rate of as little as 250 mL per hour might be typical of a small person during light physical activity in a cool and dry environment, whereas the sweat rate of a well-acclimated, physically fit athlete can be 10-fold higher in hot and humid conditions.[14] The high sweat rates that are needed to sustain heat loss during the vigorous exercise that is most typical of sports training and competition inevitably lead to dehydration and hyperthermia unless fluid is ingested to match the volume of sweat that is lost.

Fluid Needs During Exercise—Physiologic Effects of Fluid Replacement

There is now no scientific doubt that adequate fluid intake during exercise is required to optimize performance and reduce the risk of heat-related illness. The fact that it is not possible for humans to adapt to dehydration[15] further underscores the necessity of drinking during exercise. Montain and Coyle studied the physiologic benefits of fluid replacement[16]; they demonstrated that closely matching sweat loss with fluid intake provided the greatest physiologic benefits. On four separate occasions, their subjects exercised in the heat for 2 hours. In one trial, no fluid was ingested and the subjects lost about 4% of their body weight. In the other trials, the subjects drank enough fluid during exercise to replace 20%, 50%, or 80% of their sweat loss, resulting in dehydration of 3%, 2%, and 1% of body weight. The increases in core temperature and heart rate, and the decrease in stroke volume, were directly influenced by dehydration, prompting the authors to note that, ". . . the optimal rate of fluid ingestion to attenuate hyperthermia and cardiovascular drift is the rate that most closely matches fluid loss through sweating, at least until the rate of fluid ingestion replaces 81% of sweat loss."[16]

The research of Walsh et al[17] corroborates this conclusion by illustrating the value inherent in avoiding even slight dehydration. Sixty minutes of cycling exercise resulted in a loss of 1.8% of body weight before the subjects exercised to exhaustion at 90% VO_{2max}. When dehydration was prevented by ingesting fluids throughout the 60 minutes of exercise, the subjects were able to complete about 10 minutes of exercise before experiencing exhaustion. When dehydrated by 1.8% of body weight, the subjects lasted only about 6 minutes. The authors concluded that the goal of fluid ingestion should be to fully replace sweat and urine losses.[17] This conclusion is echoed by the recommendations of the ACSM position stand on fluid replacement, including the following: "During exercise, athletes should start drinking early and at regular intervals in an attempt to consume fluids at a rate sufficient to replace all the water lost through sweating, or consume the maximal amount that can be tolerated."[10]

Fluid Needs During Exercise—Influence of Beverage Palatability

The ACSM guidelines also recommend that fluids be cool and flavored to enhance palatability and increase voluntary fluid intake, contain carbohydrate to enhance performance, and include sodium chloride to promote rehydration. Voluntary fluid consumption is influenced by beverage palatability. Altering beverage characteristics such as temperature, perceived sweetness, flavor type and intensity, beverage tartness, and mouthfeel can influence voluntary fluid intake.[2,18–20] This knowledge underscores the importance of providing athletes with beverages that will encourage voluntary fluid consumption. This effect was demonstrated by Wilk et al,[21] who reported that boys (ages 9 to 12 years) voluntarily ingested more of a sports drink than they did of plain water or a placebo during 3 hours of intermittent physical activity in the heat. The boys remained well-hydrated on the sports drink trial, but dehydrated when given access to the other two beverages, an effect attributed to the presence of flavor and sodium chloride in the sports drink.

Fluid Needs During Exercise—Effects on Performance

Consistent with the ACSM recommendation that fluids contain carbohydrate if performance improvement is desired, the research of Below et al[22] demonstrates the combined value of preventing dehydration and providing carbohydrate. In their study, subjects cycled for 50 minutes at 80% VO_{2max} before undertaking a "sprint to the finish" that required about 9 to 12 minutes to complete. Performance was improved by about 6% when subjects prevented dehydration by replacing 80% of sweat loss (versus replacing 13% of sweat loss). Performance was also improved by 6% when the subjects ingested 79 ± 4 g of carbohydrate (compared to no carbohydrate). When dehydration was prevented and carbohydrate was ingested, the performance benefits were additive (that is, a 12% performance improvement).

Fluid Needs During Exercise—The Timing of Fluid Ingestion

The timing of fluid ingestion during exercise directly influences physiologic response. Subjects in a study by Montain and Coyle[23] replaced 43% of sweat loss during 140 minutes of cycling exercise by ingesting a total of 1183 mL of a sports drink at the beginning of exercise, or in a bolus at either 40 or 80 minutes of exercise, or at 15-minute intervals throughout the exercise. The subjects experienced similar dehydration in each trial (–2.9% body weight). On all occasions, drinking attenuated the increase in serum osmolality and sodium concentration, increased forearm blood flow, maintained blood volume, and reduced the rate of heat storage. These responses lasted for about 40 minutes after bolus fluid intake (that is, at 0, 40, or 80 minutes). When the subjects ingested fluid at 15-minute intervals throughout exercise, the average values at the end of exercise for esophageal temperature, rectal temperature, heart rate, and rating of perceived exertion were all lower than when fluid was ingested at 80 minutes; however, the only statistically significant difference was with rectal temperature. Brown[24] reported similar findings for heart rate and rectal temperature when water was ingested at regular intervals throughout 165 minutes of exercise rather than when subjects waited until 135 minutes to drink.

One of the possible advantages of drinking at regular intervals is that the act of drinking stimulates heat loss by maintaining sweat rate.[16] For example, sweating is known to increase almost immediately after drinking in subjects who are dehydrated,[25] a response thought to be related to the oropharyngeal reflex. The act of swallowing fluids appears to initiate selected physiologic and hormonal responses,[26] some of which may help maintain sweat rate and heat loss during exercise. From a practical standpoint, the knowledge that drinking fluid in one large bolus confers transient benefits is valuable when it is not possible to ingest fluid at regular intervals during physical activity (for example, during a soccer match).

Fluid Needs after Exercise

When rapid rehydration is paramount (for example, when athletes train or compete more than once per day, or when athletes need to restore body weight quickly after weigh-ins), ingestion of plain water, fruit juices, and soft drinks provide an inadequate physiologic impetus for rehydration. Rapid and complete rehydration can be ensured only by the ingestion of adequate amounts of water *and* sodium chloride.[27–29] This normally occurs over the course of 12 to 24 hours, as the food and beverages that athletes ingest provide the water and sodium chloride required for euhydration. However, there are many circumstances during training and competition that prevent athletes from having 12 to 24 hours to rehydrate. During these occasions, drinking plain water, soft drinks, and fruit juice will be insufficient for promoting complete rehydration. The absorption of plain water into the bloodstream causes an abrupt decrease in plasma osmolality and partial restoration of plasma volume. These responses reduce the

drive to drink and increase urine production. The result is that athletes tend to drink too little and excrete too much fluid, prolonging dehydration.

It is common to recommend that athletes ingest two cups (16 oz) of fluid for every pound of body weight that has been lost during exercise.[30] Although this advice is well-intentioned, it fails to take into consideration the obligatory urine losses that occur during the period of rehydration. Such losses can represent 25% to 50% of the ingested fluid.[31] For this reason, athletes should be educated to ingest at least 20 oz of fluid for every pound of weight lost during exercise. This advice is particularly important during two-a-day training sessions and whenever rapid rehydration is desired. Mealtime provides an important opportunity for ensuring euhydration because substantial amounts of fluid and salt are normally consumed with meals. Athletes should be encouraged to take their time eating meals to help ensure adequate fluid intake.

Finally, when rapid rehydration is the goal, consumption of alcoholic and caffeinated beverages are contraindicated because of the diuretic properties of each. However, education efforts should reflect the fact that athletes will choose to consume such beverages. For athletes who do drink coffee, colas, beer, and similar beverages, the best advice is to do so in moderation and to take extra precautions to ensure adequate hydration before the next exercise session.

Practical Applications

Considering that dehydration is frequently experienced by virtually every athlete, and that even slight dehydration has a detrimental effect on health and performance, the need to educate coaches, athletes, and parents about the absolute necessity of remaining well hydrated should be obvious. In addition to increasing awareness of the dangers of dehydration, other practical steps can be taken to help athletes remain well hydrated. For example, cool fluids should be conveniently available at all times, and athletes should be trained to match fluid intake with sweat loss as closely as is practically possible

(Table 8–3).[32] This can be achieved by giving athletes ample opportunity to practice drinking during training sessions. When possible, athletes should be allowed to drink at frequent intervals (for example, every 10 to 20 minutes) throughout exercise. Plain water can be an acceptable fluid replacement beverage for some occasions, but because proper hydration and carbohydrate intake both improve performance, the ingestion of a sports drink can provide additional benefits, including an increase in voluntary fluid intake.[4,21]

Sports drinks usually contain a combination of carbohydrates and electrolytes in amounts substantially lower than fruit juices, soft drinks, and other beverages (Table 8–4). For example, well-formulated sports drinks usually contain 14 to 16 g of carbohydrate per 8-oz serving, providing a carbohydrate concentration of 6% to 7% (for example, 14 g/236 mL × 100 = ~6%). By comparison, soft drinks and fruit juices typically contain 35 to 42 g of carbohydrate per serving (12 oz; 355 mL), yielding a carbohydrate concentration of 10% to 12%. Beverage carbohydrate concentration has a direct impact upon the

rate at which ingested fluid is emptied from the stomach into the proximal small intestine. Whereas water and carbohydrate-electrolyte beverages containing up to 6% to 7% carbohydrate empty from the stomach at similar rates,[33,34] drinks containing greater carbohydrate concentrations result in significantly slower gastric emptying.[35,36] Dehydration complicates things further by reducing gastric emptying rate[34,37] and increasing the risk of GI distress.[37]

After the beverage has been emptied from the stomach into the small intestine (duodenum and jejunum), the composition of the beverage continues to have an important impact upon fluid absorption. Rapid fluid absorption from the intestinal lumen into the bloodstream requires the ingestion of carbohydrate (in the form of glucose, sucrose, or corn-syrup solids) and the presence of sodium. The presence of carbohydrate, particularly glucose, stimulates the cotransport of glucose and sodium from the intestinal lumen into the intestinal epithelial cell, an active process that stimulates water absorption.[38] The type and concentration of carbohydrate influences the rate of fluid absorption. Combinations of sucrose, glucose, fructose, and maltodextrins appear to promote similar rates of water flux, provided that the fructose and maltodextrin concentrations do not predominate. Also, carbohydrate concentrations less than 8% (fewer than 19 g of carbohydrate per 8 oz) appear to maximize fluid absorption.[39,40]

Table 8–3 Matching Fluid Intake with Sweat Loss[43]

Sweat Rate		Fluid Intake		Frequency
mL/h	lb/h	mL	oz	min
250	0.5	60	2	15
500	1.1	125	4	15
750	1.7	190	6.5	15
1000	2.2	250	8.5	15
1250	2.8	210	7	10
1500	3.3	250	8.5	10
1750	3.9	290	10	10
2000	4.4	330	11	10
2250	5.0	375	12.5	10
2500	5.5	415	14	10
2750	6.1	460	15.5	10
3000	6.6	500	17	10

Source: Reprinted, by permission, from R. Murray, 1995, "Fluid Needs in Hot and Cold Environments," *International Journal of Sports Nutrition*, Vol. 5: S62–S73.

Clinical and Therapeutic Applications

Fluid deficits can be life-threatening, whether caused by dehydration due to sweating or by the profuse fluid loss that can accompany diarrhea due to illness. In either case, the rapid replacement of fluid and electrolytes is required. This can be most easily accomplished by the ingestion of appropriately formulated carbohydrate-electrolyte beverages or by the intravenous infusion of similar fluids. The ingestion of a carbohydrate-electrolyte beverage [that is, oral rehydration solution (ORS)] has been promoted for decades by the World Health Organization

Table 8–4 Composition of Common Beverages (All Values per 8 oz; 236 mL)

Beverage	CHO (g)	PRO (g)	Fat (g)	Energy (kcal)	NA+ (mg)	K+ (mg)	Osmolality (mosm/kg H_2O)
Whole milk	11	8	8.2	150	120	370	~285
Skim milk	12	8.4	0.4	86	126	406	~275
Orange juice*	27	1.7	0.1	112	2	474	~1600
Apple juice**	29	0.2	0.3	116	7	296	~1300
Soft drink***	25	0	0	96	9	0	~650
Sports drink****	14	0	0	56	110	25	~280
WHO ORS	5	0	0	20	488	179	~330
Infant ORS*****	6	0	0	24	244	179	~270

CHO = carbohydrates; PRO = protein; WHO = World Health Organization; ORS = oral rehydration solution

* from concentrate

** bottled

*** Coca-Cola Classic, Coca-Cola Company, Atlanta, GA

**** Gatorade Thirst Quencher powder, Quaker Oats Company, Chicago, IL

***** Pedialyte, Ross Laboratories, Columbus, OH

for the treatment of diarrheal fluid losses caused by diseases such as cholera.[41] As noted in Table 8–4, ORS products are specifically formulated to replace the high sodium and potassium losses that occur with diarrhea, whereas sports drinks are formulated to replace the comparatively lower amounts of electrolytes lost in sweat. The carbohydrate content of ORS is kept low to reduce production and shipping costs but still ensure maximal stimulation of fluid absorption in the intestine.[42] Sports drinks contain higher amounts of carbohydrate to both stimulate rapid fluid absorption and provide ample exogenous carbohydrate to improve performance.[43]

Athletes suffering from heat exhaustion or heat stroke are usually dehydrated, a clinical challenge that is often addressed by intravenous infusion of glucose-saline solutions. Intravenous infusion of fluid quickly restores plasma volume, replaces some if not all of the fluid and sodium deficit, and provides a source of rapidly metabolizable energy. It should be remembered that administration of intravenous fluid indicates a *failure* on the part of the athlete to prevent dehydration. Oral consumption of fluids containing carbohydrates and electrolytes obviates the need for intravenous infusion of similar fluids and should always be the preferred route of administering fluids.

Key Study Illustrations

In October of 1995, veteran triathlete Paula Newby-Fraser prepared to defend her championship in the Ironman triathlon held annually in Kailua-Kona, Hawaii. Newby-Fraser had dominated the women's field in the Ironman event for almost a decade, but several women had begun closing the gap. Karen Smyers was one of those women. When the race began at 7 am with a 2.4-mile swim in the Pacific Ocean, it was already warm and sunny. After the competitors clambered out of the water and onto their bikes for a 112-mile ride along the hilly, lava-encrusted terrain of the Kona coast, the temperature climbed into the 80s, with a relative humidity ranging from 38% to 71%. Paula rode strongly throughout the bike leg, eventually taking and holding the lead as the riders headed into the bike-run transition area. Karen Smyers worked hard to stay close, but Paula was well ahead of the field at the beginning of the marathon run.

In past years, it was not unusual for Paula to walk through some of the aid stations during the run portion of the Ironman, because she understood the value of remaining well hydrated under such grueling conditions. However, with Karen Smyers steadily gaining on her, Paula ran through the aid stations, barely giving herself enough time to swallow a few mouthfuls of fluid. It was a competitive strategy that would have worked well had the finish line been 400 yards closer.

Although no on-the-spot measurements were made when Paula began to experience difficulty with less than a half mile to go, it is likely that her problems were precipitated by a combination of dehydration and mild hyperthermia. What was obvious was that Paula was no longer able to run. Exhausted and faltering, Paula paused in the middle of the road to try to collect herself, allowing Karen Smyers to pass and head on to victory. As Paula tried to will herself to the finish line, her staggering, uncoordinated gait appeared typical of the central nervous system dysfunction that can accompany dehydration and hyperthermia. Her ashen skin color indicated a decrease in skin blood flow, a reflexive response designed to shunt blood into the central circulation, the body's last ditch attempt to maintain central venous pressure at the expense of thermoregulation.

Within minutes, even slow walking proved to be too much, and Paula sat on the curb where medical personnel were able to observe her. After about 20 minutes of rest, during which time she drank some fluids, lay on her back in the street, and had buckets of water poured over her, Paula walked slowly to the finish line and then on to the medical tent where she received intravenous fluids.

Although Paula's plight was all the more sensational because of the nature of the event, she fell prey to perhaps the most common sports injury—dehydration. Most people have experienced the lightheadedness and fatigue that often accompany dehydration, whether in the middle of a difficult workout or in the middle of cutting the grass on a hot day. Fortunately, although dehydration may be the most common sports injury, it is also the most preventable. Decades of scientific research have established the incomparable value of adequate fluid replacement. The challenge for sports health professionals is to develop effective ways of translating science into practice to ensure that all athletes understand the benefits of remaining well hydrated.

REFERENCES

1. Adolph EF, Brown AH. Summary and conclusions. In: Adolph EF and associates, eds. *Physiology of Man in the Desert*. New York: Interscience Publishers, Inc; 1947:343.

2. Greenleaf JE. Environmental issues that influence intake of replacement beverages. In: *Fluid Replacement and Heat Stress*. Washington, DC: National Academy Press: 1991;XV:1–30.

3. Rothstein A, Adolph EF, Willis JH. Voluntary dehydration. In: Adolph EF and associates, eds. *Physiology of Man in the Desert*. New York: Interscience Publishers, Inc; 1947:254.

4. Broad E, Burke LM, Heely P, Grundy M. Body weight changes and ad libitum fluid intakes during training and competition sessions in team sports. *Int J Sport Nutr*. In press.

5. Maughan RJ, Shirreffs SM, Galloway DR, Leiper JB. Dehydration and fluid replacement in sport and exercise. *Sports Exerc Inj*. 1995;1:148–153.

6. Noakes TD, Adams BA, Myburgh KH, Greef C, Lotz T, Nathan M. The danger of an inadequate water intake during prolonged exercise. *Eur J Appl Physiol*. 1988;57:210–219.

7. Wade CE, Freund BJ. Hormonal control of blood flow during and following exercise. In: Gisolfi CV, Lamb DR, eds. *Perspectives in Exercise Science and Sports Medicine: Fluid Homeostasis during Exercise*. Indianapolis, IN: Benchmark Press; 1990;3:1–38.

8. Booth DA. Influences on human fluid consumption. In: Ramsay DJ, Booth DA, eds. *Thirst: Physiological and Psychological Aspects*. London: Springer-Verlag; 1991:56.

9. Guyton AC. *Textbook of Medical Physiology*. 8th ed. Philadelphia: WB Saunders Company; 1991:274–275.

10. American College of Sports Medicine. Position stand on exercise and fluid replacement. *Med Sci Sports Exerc.* 1996;28:i–vii.

11. Rico-Sanz J, Frontera W, Rivera M, Rivera-Brown A, Mole P, Meredith C. Effects of hyperhydration on total body water, temperature regulation and performance of elite young soccer players in a warm climate. *Int J Sports Med.* 1996;17:85–91.

12. Riedesel ML, Allen DY, Peake GT, Al-Qattan K. Hyperhydration with glycerol solutions. *J Appl Physiol.* 1987;63:2262–2268.

13. Murray R. Nutrition for the marathon and other endurance sports: environmental stress and dehydration. *Med Sci Sports Exerc.* 1992;24:S319–S323.

14. Sawka MN, Pandolf KB. Effects of body water loss on physiological function and exercise performance. In: Gisolfi CV, Lamb DR, eds. *Perspectives in Exercise Science and Sports Medicine: Fluid Homeostasis During Exercise.* Indianapolis, IN: Benchmark Press; 1990;3:1–38.

15. Sawka MN. Physiological consequences of dehydration: exercise performance and thermoregulation. *Med Sci Sports Exerc.* 1992;24:657–670.

16. Montain SJ, Coyle EF. The influence of graded dehydration on hyperthermia and cardiovascular drift during exercise. *J Appl Physiol.* 1992;73:1340–1350.

17. Walsh RM, Noakes TD, Hawkey JA, Dennis SC. Impaired high-intensity cycling performance time at low levels of dehydration. *Int J Sports Med.* 1994;15:392–398.

18. Boulze D, Monstruc P, Cabanao M. Water intake, pleasure and water temperature in humans. *Physiol Behav.* 1983;30:97–102.

19. Greenleaf JE. Problem: thirst, drinking behavior, and involuntary dehydration. *Med Sci Sports Exerc.* 1992;24:645–656.

20. Sohar E, Kaly J, Adar R. The prevention of voluntary dehydration. In: *Environmental Physiology and Psychology in Arid Conditions.* Paris, France: United Nations Educational, Scientific and Cultural Organizations; 1962:129–135.

21. Wilk B, Bar-Or O. Effect of drink flavor and NaCL on voluntary drinking and hydration in boys exercising in the heat. *J Appl Physiol.* 1996;80:1112–1117.

22. Below PR, Mora-Rodriguez R, Gonzalez-Alonso J, Coyle EF. Fluid and carbohydrate ingestion independently improve performance during 1 h of intense exercise. *Med Sci Sports Exerc.* 1994;27:200–210.

23. Montain SJ, Coyle EF. Influence of the timing of fluid ingestion on temperature regulation during exercise. *J Appl Physiol.* 1993;75:688–695.

24. Brown AH. Water storage in the desert. In: Adolph EF, ed. *Physiology of Man in the Desert.* New York: Interscience Publications, Inc. 1947:136–159.

25. Senay LC, Christensen ML. Cardiovascular and sweating responses to water ingestion during dehydration. *J Appl Physiol.* 1965;20:975–979.

26. Verbalis JG. Inhibitory controls of drinking: satiation of thirst. In: Ramsay DJ, Booth DA, eds. *Thirst: Physiological and Psychological Aspects.* London; Spring-Verlag; 1991:315–317.

27. Maughan R, Leiper JB, Shirreffs SM. Rehydration and recovery after exercise. *Sports Sci Exch.* 1996;9:1–4.

28. Nadel ER, Mack GW, Nose H. Influence of fluid replacement beverages on body fluid homeostasis during exercise and recovery. In: Gisolfi CV, Lamb DR, eds. *Perspectives in Exercise Science and Sports Medicine: Fluid Homeostasis During Exercise.* Indianapolis, IN: Benchmark Press; 1988:195.

29. Nadel ER. New ideas for rehydration beverages during and after exercise in hot weather. *Sports Sci Exch.* 1988;1:1–5.

30. Lyle BJ, Forgac T. Hydration and fluid replacement. In: Berning J, Nelson Steen S, eds. *Sports Nutrition for the 90s: The Health Professional's Handbook.* Gaithersburg, MD: Aspen Publishers, Inc; 1991:180.

31. Gonzalez-Alonso J, Heaps CL, Coyle EF. Rehydration after exercise with common beverages and water. *Int J Sports Med.* 1992;13:399–406.

32. Murray R. Fluid needs in hot and cold environments. *Int J Sport Nutr.* 1995;5:S62–S73.

33. Murray R, Eddy DE, Bartoli WP, Paul GL. Gastric emptying of water and isocaloric carbohydrate solutions consumed at rest. *Med Sci Sports Exerc.* 1994;26:725–732.

34. Neufer PD, Young AJ, Sawka MN. Gastric emptying during exercise: effects of heat stress and dehydration. *Eur J Appl Physiol.* 1989;58:433–439.

35. Bartoli WP, Horn MK, Murray R. Delayed gastric emptying during exercise with repeated ingestion of 8% carbohydrate solution. *Med Sci Sports Exerc.* 1995;27:S13.

36. Maughan R. Gastric emptying during exercise. *Sports Sci Exch.* 1993;5:1–5.

37. Rehrer NJ, Beckers EJ, Brouns F, Ten Hoor F, Saris WHM. Effects of dehydration on gastric emptying and gastrointestinal distress while running. *Med Sci Sports Exerc.* 1990;22:790–795.

38. Schedl HP, Maughan RJ, Gisolfi CV. Intestinal absorption during rest and exercise: implications for formulating an oral rehydration solution. *Med Sci Sports Exerc.* 1994;26:267–280.

39. Gisolfi CV, Summers RW, Schedl HP, Bleiler TL. Intestinal water absorption from select carbohydrate solutions in humans. *J Appl Physiol.* 1992;73:2142–2150.

40. Shi X, Summers RW, Schedl HP, Flanagan SW, Chang RT, Gisolfi CV. Effects of carbohydrate type and concentration and solution osmolality on water absorption. *Med Sci Sports Exerc.* 1995;27:1607–1615.

41. Banwell JG. Worldwide impact of oral rehydration therapy. In: Farthing MJG, ed. *Oral Rehydration Therapy: Past, Present, and Future.* Princeton, NJ: Excerpta Medical, Inc; 1990:29–37.

42. Schedl HP. Scientific rationale for oral rehydration therapy. In: Farthing MJG, ed. *Oral Rehydration Therapy: Past, Present, and Future.* Princeton, NJ: Excerpta Medical, Inc; 1990:14–21.

43. Murray R. The effects of consuming carbohydrate-electrolyte beverages on gastric emptying and fluid absorption during and following exercise. *Sports Med.* 1987;4:322–351.

CHAPTER 9

Body Composition Assessment and Relationship to Athletic Performance

Linda B. Houtkooper

The human body comprises more than 30 recognized major components at the atomic, molecular, cellular, tissue-system, and whole-body levels of body composition.[1] Direct measurement of body composition in living humans is not feasible. Thus, various models for indirect estimation of the constituents of the body have been developed.

The primary model used in the study of the relationship between body composition and athletic performance is the two-component chemical model. This model divides the body into fat mass (FM) and fat-free mass (FFM). Fat is a molecular-level component, not to be confused with fat cells or adipose tissue, which are cellular and tissue-system components of body composition. The terms fat and lipid are often confused and inappropriately interchanged.[2] Fat refers to the family of chemical compounds called triglycerides, whereas lipid is the more general term that includes triglycerides and many other compounds (for example, phospholipids and sphingolipids).[3] In the two-component chemical model, the fat component historically has included all lipids, and all other body constituents are included in the FFM. In more complex, three- or four-component chemical models, the FFM is subdivided into the following major constituents: water, mineral, and protein.[4]

BODY COMPOSITION MODELS AND ASSESSMENT METHODS

Criterion Models and Methods

Various methods are used for estimating body composition. The reference or criterion methods require expensive equipment and complex technical measurement skills. These factors limit the use of criterion methods to studies conducted in research laboratories. However, an understanding of these laboratory criterion methods and their limitations is important for the practitioner because field methods of body composition assessment can be no more accurate than the criterion methods used as the references for the development of the field methods.

Two-Component Models and Methods

The most widely applied criterion methods for dividing the body into FM and FFM are densitometry, hydrometry, and potassium (^{40}K) spectroscopy. These methods and others based on the two-component body composition model are similar in the sense that they rely upon a known and stable relationship between the body compartment of interest (FFM) and the measured body mass constituent. For example, FFM can be estimated using hydrometry by first estimating total body water (TBW) using isotopically labeled water dilution. FFM is then calculated from TBW on the basis of the average hydration of FFM, which is typically considered to be about 73%.[5] Similarly, FFM can be calculated from total body potassium (TBK), which can be estimated by ^{40}K counting[6,7] or measurements of total exchangeable potassium. Once TBK is known, FFM is calculated from the average concentration of potassium in FFM; in adult males, FFM = TBK, g/2.66 g, K per kg FFM and in adult females, FFM = TBK, g/2.55 g, K per kg FFM.[7] The validity and accuracy of both hydrometry and potassium spectroscopy depend largely on the appropriateness of the identified conversion constants for a person in which they are applied.

The most widely used criterion method for body composition assessment is densitometry. Using the densitometry method, underwater weighing is typically used to measure body volume. Whole body density (D_b) is then calculated using the following equation:

$$D_b = Body\ Weight/Body\ Volume \qquad (1)$$

The measured D_b value is then typically used in a prediction equation such as the Siri equation[8] to calculate percent body fat (%BF).

$$\%BF = \left[\frac{4.95}{D_b} - 4.50\right] 100 \qquad (2)$$

Densitometry is based on the relationship between D_b and the respective densities of the body compartments, regardless of how they are defined.[9] The general principle is that whole body density varies inversely with body fat, or

$$F = f(1/D_b) \qquad (3)$$

where F is the ether extractable lipid fraction of body mass and f, the function describing the relationship between fat and density. To derive simple, useful solutions for equation 3, an additional assumption is required [that is, the densities of the two compartments (FM and FFM) are constant]. The well-known Siri equation[8] and Brozek equation[5] used to predict relative body fat (%BF) represent the simplest solutions of

equation 1. In these equations, %BF is calculated from D_b, and densities of 0.9 g/cc and 1.1 g/cc for the fat[10] and fat-free constituents[5] are assumed according to the equation

$$1/D_b = F/d_F + FFM/d_{FFM} \qquad (4)$$

where $1/D_b$ is body mass, set equal to unity, divided by body density (D_b), and F/d_F and FFM/d_{FFM} are the fractions of body mass that are fat and fat-free divided by their respective densities. The density of adult human body fat is relatively constant within and among persons at 0.9 g/cc. In the simplest chemical model, FFM is composed primarily of water (W), protein (P), and mineral (M) compartments, and d_{FFM} (1.1 g/cc) is derived from the proportions of W, P, and M divided by constant values for their densities[11]:

$$d_{FFM} = W/d_W + P/d_P + M/d_M \qquad (5)$$

Thus, for d_{FFM} to be constant, the proportions of W, P, and M must be constant or they must vary in such a way that d_{FFM} does not change. In the densitometric approach, any deviation of D_b from the value of 1.1 g/cc is assumed to be due to the addition of body fat.

It is clear from a number of studies that the chemical composition of the FFM is not constant. Rather, there is considerable individual variation, and predictable changes in FFM constituents occur with growth, maturation, and aging.[11] Long-term specialized training such as regular resistance exercise may also alter FFM composition (for example, by increasing bone mass). Conversely, athletes in some sports may have less than average bone mass. Deviations from the assumed chemical composition of the FFM result in under- or overestimation of body fat using densitometry depending on whether the d_{FFM} is greater than or less than the assumed density of 1.1 g/cc. Thus, %BF may be overestimated in persons with lower than average bone mass and underestimated in persons with more than average bone mass. These errors in the densitometric criterion method for fat estimation are then passed on to simpler body composition field methods when they are validated against this criterion method. For example, in a female runner with lower than average bone mass, the predicted %BF value would be higher than her actual value.[12] If this runner's estimated %BF level was 15%, she may actually be at 10%BF, and attempts to further decrease her current relative body fat may decrease her body fat to an undesirably low level.

Multiple-Component Models and Methods

Because of the limitations in the two-component approach, new multi-component approaches have been developed where two or more constituents of the FFM are measured in the criterion method. Such approaches can provide a more accurate estimate of body composition than the two-component approach.[11,13]

Dual-energy X-ray absorptiometry (DXA) is a relatively new technology that is gaining acceptance as a criterion method for body composition assessment. The DXA methodology provides reliable estimates of bone mineral, fat, and lean soft-tissue masses in the body.[14] This methodology requires minimal subject cooperation compared to hydrodensitometry (underwater weighing methodology) and accounts for variability in bone mineral in the body. Additional research is needed to establish DXA as an acceptable criterion method for body composition assessment.[15]

A four-component (4C) chemical model of body composition has been derived by dividing the FFM into its primary constituents of water (W), protein (P), and mineral (M), as depicted by the following:

$$1/D_b = F/d_F + W/d_W + P/d_P + M/d_M \quad (6)$$

where W/d_W, P/d_P, and M/d_M are the fractions of water, protein, and mineral divided by their respective densities and the fraction of F is divided by its density, F/d_F.

Three-component (3C) models can also be derived by combining two constituents of the FFM into one component. For example, if the protein and mineral fractions of FFM are combined, then

$$1/D_b = F/d_F + W/d_W + S/d_S \quad (7)$$

where S/d_S represents the nonaqueous (solids) fraction of FFM divided by its density. This approach is useful as a criterion method when it is expected that the body water fraction of the FFM varies from the designated biologic constant of 0.73. Variation in body water accounts for the largest proportion of variance in d_{FFM} in the general population.[12] A second 3C model can be derived by combining water and protein to form the lean soft tissue (LST) fraction of FFM, depicted in the following:

$$1/D_b = F/d_F + M/d_M + LST/d_{LST} \quad (8)$$

This approach is useful when it is expected that the mineral fraction of FFM deviates from the designated constant of 6.8%,[5] which is possible in some athletic groups (for example, swimmers, runners with amenorrhea, bodybuilders).

Multiple component models are useful to minimize the potential errors in estimates of %BF associated with variability in FFM composition. The ideal laboratory procedure is to combine measures of D_b with measures of body water and bone mineral and to then estimate body composition using an equation based on a 4C model of body composition. This approach eliminates the need for assumptions about the proportionalities among the constituents of the FFM and provides the best criterion estimate of body composition against which to validate field methods. A recent study of weight trainers by Modlesky et al[16] used a 4C model as the criterion method for estimation of body composition and calculation of %BF. These investigators demonstrated that in young, white, male weight trainers with high musculoskeletal development, d_{FFM} is lower than the assumed values of 1.1 g/cc and that the Siri equation overestimated %BF compared to the %BF criterion value estimated from the Lohman 4C equation.[11] The lower d_{FFM} for the weight trainers was due primarily to higher water and secondarily to lower mineral and protein fractions of the FFM than those found in white men with average musculoskeletal development.

Alternatively, D_b can be combined with measures of body water or bone mineral, and estimates of body fat based on 3C models can be derived. Although more accurate than the 2C equations, these equations do assume a constant protein-to-mineral (equation 7) or protein-to-water (equation 8) ratio, and individual deviations from the assumed ratios introduce error, albeit less than the 2C model. Whether body water or bone mineral is measured depends on which constituent is likely to vary most within the population being studied.

Validation of New Methods

Historically, new methods of body composition assessment have been primarily validated against a criterion method based on a hydrodensitometric two-component (2C) approach using underwater weighing techniques or volume measurements based on air displacement.[17,18] As discussed earlier in this chapter, historically underwater weighing, or more recently air displacement, has been used to determine body volume, and whole body density (D_b) is then estimated using body mass (weight) measured on a scale divided by the measured value for body volume. Body density (D_b) can also be accurately estimated from skinfold equations.[19–21] Thus, accurate estimates of D_b can be made using three different methods. However, as discussed earlier, substantial errors can occur when a D_b value is converted to %BF using prediction equations based on 2C models such as the Brozek or Siri equations.[5,8]

Anthropometric measurements include height, weight, skinfold thicknesses, circumferences, and skeletal widths. Body composition prediction equations, based on 3C or 4C models, which estimate %BF directly from anthropometric measurements, can provide a means to accurately estimate relative body fat. Unfortunately, few such equations have been published with the notable exception of the Slaughter et al[22] equations for children and adolescents and the Williams et al equations[23] for older men and women.

An alternative approach is to estimate %BF from D_b alone using modifications of the Siri

equation derived from estimates of FFM composition in the population of interest. Using average estimates of water and mineral fractions of the FFM for a given age to estimate d_{FFM}, Lohman[24] has derived 2C equations for use in children and adolescents. These equations make it possible to use densitometry as a criterion method in children. However, it is important to note that, at any age, children and adolescents of the same gender differ to some extent from the average water and mineral fraction of the FFM, which leads to increased errors in %BF estimation when the Lohman[11] equations are used to estimate %BF. Unfortunately, there has been no systematic attempt to define the average water and mineral fractions in different groups of athletes, and thus estimation of %BF from measured D_b can be confounded by variability in FFM composition and density. A better description of these parameters in different groups of athletes is an important focus for future research.

Clinical Field Methods

Field methods are relatively simple techniques for estimating body composition often used in clinical applications outside of a laboratory setting. An understanding of the strengths and limitations of the major field methods for estimating body composition can enable practitioners to improve the accuracy and reliability of their measurements and estimations of body composition.

Anthropometry

As has been previously discussed, measurements of skinfold thicknesses at various sites, bone dimensions, and limb circumferences can be used in equations to predict %BF or to predict D_b, which can then be used in an equation to predict %BF.[25,26] The skinfold method is based on the assumptions that the thickness of the adipose tissue directly under the skin reflects a constant proportion of the total FM and the sites selected for measurement represent the average thickness of the adipose tissue under the skin.[27] Accurate estimation of body composition from skinfolds depends on selecting a prediction equation appropriate for the person being assessed, using an appropriate skinfold caliper, and accurately measuring the same skinfold sites used in the development of the prediction equation. Heyward and Stolarczyk[28] have published an excellent reference guide that provides directions for accurately measuring skinfolds and step-by-step instructions for selecting appropriate skinfold prediction equations based on the age, gender, ethnicity, and activity level of a client or group of subjects.

Measurement of skinfold thicknesses, without conversion to %BF, can also be used to track changes in body fat of athletes. Carefully measuring a set of skinfolds at specific body sites at regular intervals can indicate if the thicknesses (that is, body fat levels directly under the skin) are changing.

Bioelectrical Impedance

Bioelectrical impedance analysis (BIA) is based on the relationship between the volume (the body) and length of the conductor (height), and its impedance, which reflects the resistance to the flow of an electric current. Impedance measurements are made with a person lying flat on a nonconducting surface with electrodes attached to specific sites on the wrist and ankle. A low-dose (800 μamp), single frequency (50-KHz) current is passed through the person and the value for resistance is measured. Selected equations are then used to estimate FFM. In turn, %BF is calculated using the following equations:

$$Body\ Weight\ (BM) - FFM = FM \qquad (9)$$
$$\%BF = FM/BM \qquad (10)$$

The accuracy of prediction equations derived from BIA is improved when population-specific equations (age-, gender-, and fatness-level specific) are used to predict FFM.[10,29,30] Prediction equations derived from impedance analysis have prediction errors of 3% to 5% when measurements are made using a standard technique, which includes controlling for fluid intake and physical activity before measurements. Validity

of BIA measurements for athletes will be significantly affected if measurements are not made using standard technique.[29,31] Bioelectric impedance analyses also tend to overestimate FM in persons who are lean and underestimate FM in persons who are obese.[29] BIA measurements made using standard techniques and appropriate prediction equations provide relatively accurate estimates of body composition for groups of people but are less accurate for providing estimates of body composition for a person.[29] Heyward and Stolarczyk[28] have published directions for accurately measuring BIA and clear instructions for selecting a BIA prediction equation that is appropriate for the age, gender, ethnicity, and activity level of a group of subjects.

Near Infrared Reactance

This method is based on the principles of light absorption and reflection. A fiber optic probe is positioned at mid-biceps, and an electromagnetic radiation wave (infrared light beam) is emitted. Reflected energy or light absorption is monitored as the light beam penetrates subcutaneous fat and muscle, and is reflected off the bone and conducted to the optical detector in the probe. Limited validation research has been conducted using this method. More studies are needed to validate and cross-validate this technique for both the general population and athletes.[28,32]

Prediction Errors for Body Composition Methods

Prediction errors are a combination of the error associated with variations in FFM composition and the technical measurement errors associated with the criterion and field techniques. The total error when estimating %BF from body density estimated from skinfolds, for example, includes the errors associated with variations in body water and mineral from their assumed fractions of the FFM and the technical errors associated with the measurement of skinfolds. Additional inaccuracies in skinfold measurements occur if the measured skinfold sites are not representative of the subjects' fat distribution and if the ratio of external to internal fat is different from the group in which the skinfold equation for prediction of body composition was developed. The errors in predicting body composition from skinfolds can be minimized by selecting a method based on an appropriate model that has been validated for the group of interest, and by careful measurements following standardized measurement techniques.

Despite the potential for errors with body composition estimation methods, it is possible to measure %BF, FFM, or FM with sufficient accuracy to assess body composition and to monitor changes in body composition that are larger than the prediction errors for the methods. With carefully used measurement methods, it is possible to estimate %BF with an error of approximately 3% to 4% fat and FFM with an error of 2 to 2.5 kg.[11,27] This means that if %BF is actually 15%, predicted values may be as high as 19% or as low as 11%, and if the actual FFM value is 60 kg the predicted values could range from 62.5 to 57.5 kg. With inappropriate methods and poor measurement technique, prediction errors will be much larger.

It is important to interpret all body composition estimation results with consideration for the magnitude of the inherent prediction error when making recommendations for athletes. Thus, recommending a range for the %BF or FFM goal for an athlete is more appropriate than making a single point recommendation. A follow-up assessment is warranted for persons whose body composition value is the low or high end of the recommended range to confirm estimates by more than one technique.

BODY COMPOSITION STATUS OF ATHLETES

A concern in athletics is the determination of the ideal body weight or ideal body composition for peak performance in a sport. The term ideal weight or body composition implies a known optimal combination of body FM and FFM. The ideal relative FM or FFM for an athlete in a spe-cific sport is difficult to define because all aspects of physique, plus many other factors, contribute to successful performance. Recommendations for body weight and body composition goals for athletes are usually based on average %BF and FFM values obtained from measurements of samples of elite athletes in a sport.[26,33]

Figures 9–1 and 9–2 summarize reported %BF values of elite female and male athletes in various sports.[33–40]

Little data have been published characterizing the body composition of athletes younger than 18 years. Malina and Bouchard[41] and Fleck[37] reported %BF values for young athletes and nonathletes based on 2C densitometric estimates. The data indicated that young athletes, as a group, have lower %BF levels than nonathletes of the same age and gender. These studies included age-group swimmers, runners, gymnasts, tackle football players, and wrestlers. The range of %BF values for girls was 13% to 23% and for boys was 4% to 15%. The published values of %BF for all athletes need to be interpreted with consideration for the prediction error inherent in their measurement. Heyward and Stolarczyk[28] recently published a review of recommended body composition methods and prediction equations for estimation of body composition for persons who are physically active and athletes.

BODY COMPOSITION AND PHYSICAL PERFORMANCE

Although ranges of %BF for athletes are related to successful performance within a sport, athletic performance cannot be accurately predicted solely on the basis of body composition. All the components of physique—body size, structure, and composition—are significant determinants of athletic success. Each is related to performance in a logical and predictable way. Persons who are heavier, for example, have an advantage over their lighter counterparts when an activity demands that the inertia of another body or an external object must be overcome. Persons who are lighter have the advantage when the goal is to propel the body, especially

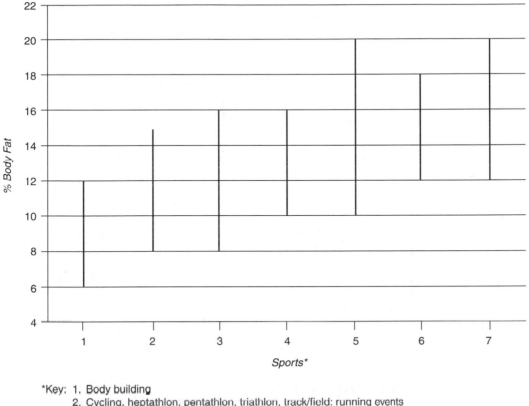

*Key: 1. Body building
2. Cycling, heptathlon, pentathlon, triathlon, track/field: running events
3. Ballet, gymnastics, orienteering, rowing, skating
4. Basketball, canoeing, kayaking, fencing, horse racing
5. Racquetball, skiing, soccer, swimming, synchronized swimming, tennis, volleyball, weight lifting
6. Baseball, softball, ice hockey, field hockey
7. Golf, track/field: field events

Figure 9–1 Reported Ranges of %Body-Fat Levels Measured in Female Athletes from Various Sports

over moderate to long distances. Persons who are taller, with longer levers (limbs) and a higher center of gravity, have the advantage in jumping and throwing events, whereas persons who are shorter have the advantage when the body must be rotated around an axis such as in diving and tumbling events.

Fat Mass and Performance

Evidence from athletes in various age groups has indicated that there is an inverse relationship between FM and performance of physical activi-

ties requiring translocation of the body weight either vertically, such as in jumping, or horizontally, such as in running.[4,42,43] Excess fatness is detrimental to these types of activities because it adds non-force-producing mass to the body. Because acceleration is proportional to force, but inversely proportional to mass, excess fat at a given level of force application can result in slower changes in velocity and direction.[4,44] Excess fatness increases the metabolic cost of physical activities requiring movement of the total body mass.[45] This indicates that one would expect that in most types of performances in-

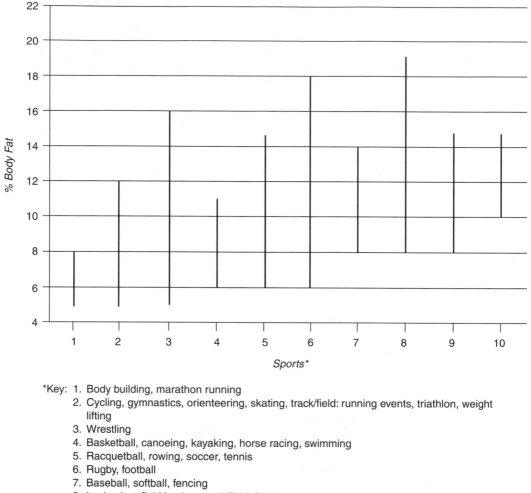

Figure 9–2 Reported Ranges of %Body-Fat Levels Measured in Male Athletes from Various Sports

*Key: 1. Body building, marathon running
    2. Cycling, gymnastics, orienteering, skating, track/field: running events, triathlon, weight lifting
    3. Wrestling
    4. Basketball, canoeing, kayaking, horse racing, swimming
    5. Racquetball, rowing, soccer, tennis
    6. Rugby, football
    7. Baseball, softball, fencing
    8. Ice hockey, field hockey, track/field: field events
    9. Skiing, ski jumping, volleyball
    10. Golf

volving movement of the body mass a relatively low %BF would be advantageous both mechanically and metabolically.[4]

Cross-sectional data indicate that %BF is inversely related to aerobic capacity (VO$_{2max}$) expressed relative to body weight and to distance running performance.[46] Only a few experimental studies have investigated the effect of altered body composition on physical performance. Cureton and coworkers conducted three studies investigating the effects of experimental alter-ation in excess weight on physiologic response to exercise and on physical performance capabilities.[47–49] Data from these experimental studies demonstrated that running performance of persons who are fit and of normal weight decreased with increasing weight added by a weight belt and shoulder harness. Their performances were similar to those of persons who are obese of similar FFM but greater body weight.

In contrast, in some sports in which absorbing force or momentum is important, such as contact sports, adequate amounts of appropriately distributed FM are advantageous. Long-distance swimmers also benefit from a relatively high FM compared to other athletic groups because of the role fat plays in thermal insulation and its contribution to buoyancy.[50]

Fat-Free Mass and Performance

Performance of activities that require the application of force, particularly against external objects, such as throwing, pushing, and weight lifting, are positively related to the absolute amount of FFM and therefore body size.[4,44] However, a large absolute amount of FFM and large body size may have a negative influence on performance requiring translocation of the body weight such as in running, jumping, or rotation of the body about an axis, as in gymnastics or diving. It is obvious that an elite gymnast would not perform well as an offensive lineman in football or vice versa.

The data are clear that the best positive correlations of physical performance of military-related physical tasks are with FFM rather than %BF. In investigations of the relationship of body composition to performance of military tasks, FFM was the best predictor of performance capability as assessed by maximal aerobic capacity, treadmill run time, 12-minute run distance, and the ability to push, carry, and exert torque.[44] Based on their data, Harman and Frykman suggested that military recruits should be required to meet standards for both minimum FFM and maximum %BF. For most sports, high ratios of FFM to FM at a given body weight are associated with better performances, although too little body fat results in deterioration in both health and physical performance.[33]

Problems of Extreme Leanness

Athletes in sports such as gymnastics, dancing, diving, body building, distance running, and track are typically lean. They follow rigorous training programs but often also restrict their dietary intake to control their weight. For male athletes, concerns about attaining low FM center around sports in which participants must "make weight" such as wrestling, boxing, and horse racing. The potential advantage of a low %BF for successful performance of athletes in these types of sports is evident. However, there are negative health and performance implications related to extreme weight cutting. The levels of %BF considered to be minimal levels compatible with health are 5% for males and 12% for females.[10]

When an athlete's body weight decreases below a certain critical level, decrements in performance and increases in both minor and major illnesses and injuries are likely to occur.[33,50] Currently, this critical level of weight is poorly defined. The magnitude of weight reduction typically attained by wrestlers through dehydration and starvation has been shown to have little effect on laboratory tests of exercise performance lasting less than 30 seconds but impairs performance of longer durations.[51] There is no consistent evidence that dehydration causes poor performance in wrestling or increases the incidence of acute or long-term illness or injury.[51]

Athletes who constantly strive to reach or maintain a weight or %BF goal that is inappropriate are also at risk for developing eating disorders. At the elite or world-class level, the prevalence of eating disorders in females is approximately 50% in several sports.[33] The female athlete prone to an eating disorder is also at high risk of developing a triad of interrelated disorders that include anorexia nervosa or bulimia nervosa, menstrual dysfunction, and bone demineralization.[33]

CONCLUSION

A considerable amount of research has focused on the development of methods to more accurately and reliably measure the body composition and to describe %BF levels of athletes. Little experimental research effort has been directed at investigating the relationship of body composition to athletic performance and long-term health status. Data indicate that excess body fat negatively influences performance, high ratios of FFM to FM at a given body weight are generally positively related to performance, and very low levels of body fat result in deterioration in health and physical performance.

Given the available body composition assessment methods and their inherent errors, as well as the influence of factors other than body composition that contribute to athletic success, it is not reasonable to define exact levels of optimal %BF or FFM levels for individual athletes in different sports. It is feasible, however, to define ranges associated with top performance in a sport and to use these ranges to establish training goals for body weight and body composition that are also compatible with good performance and health. Considering the strong positive relationship between a high FFM-to-FM ratio at a given body weight and physical performance, more emphasis should be placed on defining the ranges for these relationships to performance in athletic groups.

REFERENCES

1. Wang Z, Pierson RN, Heymsfield SB. The five level model: a new approach to organizing body composition research. *Am J Clin Nutr*. 1992;56:19–28.
2. Heymsfield SB, Wang Z. Measurement of total-body fat by underwater weighing: new insights and uses for old method. *Nutrition*. 1993;9:472–473.
3. Gurr MI, Harwood JL. *Lipid Biochemistry*. 4th ed. London: Chapman and Hall; 1991.
4. Boileau RA, Lohman TG. The measurement of human physique and its effect on physical performance. *Orthop Clin of North Am*. 1977;8:563–581.
5. Brozek J, Grande F, Anderson JT, Keys A. Densitometric analysis of body composition: revision of some quantitative assumptions. *Ann NY Acad Sci*. 1963;110:113–140.
6. Flynn MA, Nolph GB, Baker AS, Martin WM, Krause G. Total body potassium in aging humans: a longitudinal study. *Am J Clin Nutr*. 1989;50:713–717.
7. Forbes GB. *Human Body Composition: Growth, Aging, Nutrition and Activity*. New York: Springer-Verlag; 1987.
8. Siri WE. The gross composition of the body. *Adv Biol Med Physiol*. 1956;4:239–280.
9. Behnke AR, Wilmore JH. *Evaluation and Regulation of Body Build and Composition*. Englewood Cliffs, NJ: Prentice Hall; 1974.
10. Fidanza FA, Keys A, Anderson JT. Density of body fat in man and other animals. *J Appl Physiol*. 1953;6:252–256.
11. Lohman TG. *Advances in Body Composition Assessment*. Champaign, IL: Human Kinetics; 1992:1–6, 7–24, 37–56, 109–118.
12. Bunt JC, Going SB, Lohman TG, Heinrich CH, Perry CD, Pamenter RW. Variation in bone mineral content and estimated body fat in young adult females. *Med Sci Sports Exerc*. 1990;22:564–569.
13. Siri WE. Body composition from fluid spaces and density: analysis of methods. In: Brozek J, Henschel H, eds. *Techniques for Measuring Body Composition*. Washington, DC: National Academy of Science; 1961:223–244.
14. Mazess RB, Barden HS, Bisek JP, Hanson J. Dual-energy absorptiometry for total-body and regional bone-mineral and soft-tissue composition. *Am J Clin Nutr*. 1990;51:1106–1112.
15. Roubenoff R, Kehayias JJ, Dawson-Hughes B, Heymsfield SB. Use of dual-energy x-ray absorptiometry in body-composition studies: not yet a "gold standard." *Am J Clin Nutr*. 1993;58:589–591.
16. Modlesky CM, Cureton KJ, Lewis RD, Prior BM, Sloniger MA, Rowe DA. Density of the fat-free mass and estimates of body composition in male weight trainers. *J Appl Physiol*. 1996;80:2085–2096.
17. McCrory MA, Gomez TD, Bernauer EM, Mole PA. Evaluation of a new air displacement plethysmograph for measuring human body composition. *Med Sci Sports Exerc*. 1995;27:1686–1691.
18. Dempster P, Aitkens S. A new air displacement method for determination of human body composition. *Med Sci Sports Exerc*. 1995;27:162–197.
19. Jackson AS, Pollock ML. Generalized equations for predicting body density in men. *Br J Nutr*. 1978;40:497–504.
20. Jackson AS, Pollock ML, Ward A. Generalized equations for predicting body density of women. *Med Sci Sports Exerc*. 1980;12:175–182.
21. Jackson AS, Pollock ML. Practical assessment of body composition. *Phys Sports Med*. 1985;13:76–84.

22. Slaughter MH, Lohman TG, Boileau RA, et al. Skinfold equations for estimation of body fatness in children and youth. *Hum Biol.* 1988;60:709–723.

23. Williams DP, Going SB, Lohman TG, Hewitt MJ, Haber AE. Estimation of body from skinfold thicknesses in middle-aged and older men: a multiple component approach. *Am J Human Biol.* 1992;4:595–605.

24. Lohman TG. Assessment of body composition in children. *Pediatr Exerc Sci.* 1989;1:19–30.

25. Sinning WE, Dolny DG, Little KD, et al. Validity of "generalized" equations for body composition analysis in male athletes. *Med Sci Sports Exerc.* 1985;17(1):124–130.

26. Sinning WE, Wilson JR. Validity of "generalized" equations for body composition analysis in women athletes. *Res Q Exerc Sport.* 1984;55(2):153–160.

27. Lukaski HC. Methods for the assessment of human body composition traditional and new. *Am J Clin Nutr.* 1987;46:537–556.

28. Heyward VH, Stolarczyk LM. *Applied Body Composition Assessment.* Champaign, IL: Human Kinetics; 1996

29. Houtkooper LB, Going SB, Lohman TG, Howell W. Why bioelectrical impedance analysis should be used to estimate adiposity. *Am J Clin Nutr.* 1996;64:436S–448S.

30. Segal KR, Van Loan M, Fitsgerald PI, Hodgedon JA, Van Itallie TB. Lean body mass estimation by bioelectrical impedance analysis: a four-site cross-validation study. *Am J Clin Nutr.* 1988;47:7–14.

31. Lukaski HC, Bolonchuk WW, Siders WA, Hall CB. Body composition of athletes using bioelectrical impedance measurements. *J Sports Med Phys Fitness.* 1990;30:434–440.

32. Manore M, Benardot D, Love P. Body measurements. In: Benardot D, ed., *Sports Nutrition: A Guide for the Professional Working with Active People.* 2nd ed. Chicago: American Dietetic Association; 1993:88.

33. Wilmore JH. Body weight standards and athletic performance. In: Brownell KD, Rodin J, Wilmore JH, eds. *Eating, Body Weight, and Performance in Athletes.* Philadelphia: Lea & Febiger, 1992:315–329.

34. Berg K, Latin RW, Baechle T. Physical and performance characteristics of NCAA Division I football players. *Res Q Exerc Sport.* 1990;61(4):395–401.

35. Clarkson PM, Freedson PS, Keller B, Carney D, Skrinar M. Maximal oxygen uptake, nutritional patterns and body composition of adolescent female ballet dancers. *Res Q Exerc Sport.* 1985;56(2):180–184.

36. DeGaray AL, Levine L, Carter JEL. *Genetic and Anthropological Studies of Olympic Athletes.* New York: Academic Press; 1974.

37. Fleck SJ. Body composition of elite American athletes. *Am J Sports Med.* 1983;11:398–403.

38. Hirata K. Physique and age of Tokyo Olympic champions. *J Sports Med Phys Fitness.* 1996;6:207–222.

39. Houtkooper L, Aldag L, Hall M, Myers B, Going S, Lohman T. Nutritional status of elite female heptathletes. *Med Sci Sports Exerc.* 1992;24:S184.

40. Thorland WG, Johnston GO, Housh TJ, Refsell MJ. Anthropometric characteristics of elite adolescent competitive swimmers. *Hum Biol.* 1983;55:735–748.

41. Malina RM, Bouchard C. Characteristics of young athletes. In: *Growth, Maturation and Physical Activity.* Champaign, IL: Human Kinetics; 1991;443–463.

42. Malina RM. Physique and body composition: effects on performance and effects on training, semistarvation, and overtraining. In: Brownell KD, Rodin J, Wilmore JH, eds. *Eating, Body Weight, and Performance in Athletes.* Philadelphia: Lea & Febiger; 1992:94–114.

43. Pate RR, Slentz CA, Katz DP. Relationships between skinfold thickness and performance of health related fitness test items. *Res Q Exerc Sport.* 1989;60:183–189.

44. Harman EA, Frykman PN. The relationship of body size and composition to the performance of physically demanding military tasks. In: Marriott BM, Grumstrup Scott J, eds. *Body Composition and Physical Performance: Applications for the Military Services.* Washington, DC: National Academy Press; 1992:105–118.

45. Buskirk E, Taylor IIL. Maximal oxygen intake and its relation to body composition with special reference to chronic physical activity and obesity. *J Appl Physiol.* 1957;11:72–78.

46. Cureton KJ. Effects of experimental alterations in excess weight on physiological responses to exercise and physical performance. In: Marriott BM, Grumstrup-Scott J, eds. *Body Composition and Physical Performance: Applications for the Military Services.* Washington, DC: National Academy Press; 1992:71–78.

47. Cureton KJ, Sparling PB, Evans BW, Johnson SM, Kong UD, Purvis JW. Effect of experimental alterations in excess weight on aerobic capacity and distance running performance. *Med Sci Sports Exerc.* 1978;15:218–223.

48. Cureton KJ, Sparling PB. Distance running performance and metabolic responses to running in men and women with excess weight experimentally equated. *Med Sci Sports Exerc.* 1980;12:288–294.

49. Sparling PB, Cureton KJ. Biological determinants of sex difference in 12 min run performance. *Med Sci Sports Exerc*. 1983;15:218–222.

50. Tipton CM. Making and maintaining weight for interscholastic wrestling. *Sports Sci Exchange*. 1990;2:22.

51. Horswill CA. Physiology and nutrition for wrestling. In: Lamb DR, Knuttgen HG, and Murray R, eds. *Perspective in Exercise Science and Sports Medicine, Vol 7: Physiology and Nutrition for Competitive Sport*. Carmel, IN: Cooper Publishing; 1994:131–179.

CHAPTER 10

Energy Balance

Janice L. Thompson and Melinda Manore

HISTORICAL OVERVIEW

A person is said to be in energy balance when energy intake is equal to energy expenditure. Energy intake comprises all foods and beverages consumed, whereas energy expenditure includes the components of resting metabolic rate (RMR), the thermic effect of food (TEF), and the energy expended through physical activity. The RMR is defined as the energy expended due to resting physiologic functions including ventilatory and cardiovascular activity, protein, glycogen, and triglyceride synthesis, and cellular electrical activity. The TEF is the increase in energy expenditure resulting from digestion, absorption, transport, and storage of nutrients. The energy cost of physical activity accounts for all activities done above resting level.

The contributions of RMR, TEF, and energy cost of physical activity to total daily energy expenditure (TDEE) have been reported to be 60% to 75%, 10% to 15%, and 10% to 30%, respectively.[1] The contribution of exercise energy expenditure to TDEE in the athlete can be high, especially for those engaging in endurance and ultraendurance events. In these cases, RMR can account for less than 50% of TDEE.[2] Maintaining energy balance is critical to the athlete, because it contributes to the adequate intake of necessary energy and nutrients and to achieving a body weight and body composition that result in optimal performance.

Maintaining optimal energy balance in male athletes has traditionally been believed to be easy, especially in male endurance athletes. However, recent evidence of energy efficiency in male and female athletes[2-4] suggests that achieving energy balance may not be as simple for the athlete as previously assumed. It is well-recognized that many male wrestlers and female athletes participating in distance running, gymnastics, dancing, and figure skating consume relatively low energy intakes to maintain competitive body weights.[5] In addition to needing adequate energy intake to maintain nitrogen balance and fat-free mass, many athletes must consume large amounts of carbohydrate to maintain adequate glycogen stores. It has been suggested that an endurance athlete needs a minimum of 500 g (or 2000 kcal) of carbohydrate per day to adequately maintain glycogen stores.[6,7] Meeting this goal may be easy for a male athlete consuming 5000 kcal/day, but is impossible for a female athlete who is attempting to maintain a low body weight and percentage of body fat by consuming 1800 kcal/day.

Energy intake has traditionally been estimated using 24-hour dietary recalls, diet histories, food frequency questionnaires, and weighed food records. Sources of error inherent in the estimation of energy intake include the day-to-day variation of energy intake of a person, the disturbance of normal dietary intake due to the recording and measuring of food intake, and errors related to analyzing reported intakes.[8] The accuracy of energy intake reflecting total daily energy need is questionable, with errors reported as high as ±30% of actual energy need.[9-12] If an athlete's actual energy need is 3000 kcal/day, his or her reported energy intake could range from 2100 to 3900 kcal/day. Recommendations to meet the extremes of this range could result in significant weight loss or weight gain, and ultimately prove detrimental to performance.

Predicting whether a person will either over- or underreport energy intake is difficult. The assessment method used, the activity level of the subject, and the degree of obesity all appear to play a role in the direction of error in reporting dietary intake.[12,13] Although many persons who are obese and do not train consistently underreport dietary intake,[14,15] and females who are heavier and train have been shown to report lower energy intakes than females who have a lower body weight and train,[16] it is impossible to predict whether any person will overreport, underreport, or accurately report energy intake. It has been shown that the number of days required to estimate the true average energy intake of a person is 14 days, and the number necessary to estimate this same value for a group of persons is 3 days.[17]

The practicality of having anyone, including an athlete, report at least 14 days of dietary intake is questionable and highlights the limitations of using energy intake data to estimate total daily energy need. However, there are many athletes for whom estimating energy intake may be more convenient and accurate than for persons who are inactive. This is true for those athletes who keep detailed diet and activity records for personal reasons. Because the act of record-keeping is part of these persons' daily routine, the errors due to interruption of daily energy intake may be minimized or absent. In addition, many athletes eat similar foods over long periods, and also consume foods that are simple to measure and record, such as yogurt, bagels, fruit, and sports beverages and snack bars. These foods are easier to record and analyze than mixed recipes and foods from restaurants.

Total daily energy expenditure can also be estimated using reports of physical activity. The most commonly used methods to estimate activity level include published activity questionnaires or self-reported activity records. The estimation of RMR, which is then multiplied by an appropriate energy factor (usually determined using reported activity level), is another method used.[9] There are a number of errors inherent in the estimation of activity, including the person's ability to accurately report activities, the accuracy of estimating RMR, the large variability of energy cost among persons doing similar activities, and the accuracy of using energy tables and/or equations to estimate the energy cost of an activity.[8,18]

The accuracy of using activity records to estimate total daily energy expenditure is highly variable, with errors for various methods reported to range from 6% to 30% of actual energy need.[9,10] It is critical to note that there appear to be no studies validating the use of various energy intake and energy expenditure methods in estimating the total daily energy needs of athletes. Thus, it is not known which, if any, of the methods currently available are more accurate, more practical, and therefore, more appropriate for an athletic population.

The doubly labeled water technique is a promising method developed to estimate energy expenditure in a free-living environment over a prolonged period.[19] A person's energy expenditure is determined from an estimation of carbon dioxide production calculated by comparing the different turnover rates of isotopically labeled oxygen (^{18}O) and hydrogen (^{2}H). Exhibit 10–1 contains a review of some advantages and limitations of this technique. Because of these limitations, most practitioners attempting to estimate the energy balance of an athlete at the present time will need to rely upon the alternative assessment methods of energy intake and expenditure previously discussed.

CURRENT RESEARCH

A review of the recent research on energy balance in humans highlights many of the chal-

Exhibit 10–1 Advantages and Limitations of Using the Doubly Labeled Water Technique To Determine Energy Expenditure of Athletes

---

Advantages
- Noninvasive
- Less restrictive (persons are in free-living situation)
- Only a few urine samples necessary for analyses
- Can estimate total body water, fat-free mass, and energy expenditure

Limitations
- Relatively expensive
- Limited availability of labeled water
- High precision mass spectrometer needed for analysis
- Need to get an average respiratory quotient (RQ) from an assessment of dietary intake; if a general RQ (based on the average U.S. food intake) is used for an athlete, the error in calculating energy expenditure could be as high as 5%

---

lenges of attempting to estimate energy balance in active persons. Genetic influences on energy expenditure and substrate utilization,[20] highly variable training regimens, and seasonal fluctuations in energy intake and expenditure all contribute to the complexity of determining energy balance in athletes.

One of the primary areas of controversy in estimating energy balance in athletes is whether highly active persons have a higher RMR. Cross-sectional studies comparing the RMR values of active and inactive subjects report equivocal results.[21–24] Poehlman et al[22] have suggested that there may be some training threshold one must reach to result in an increase of RMR. Whereas some longitudinal studies have shown that training can result in a significant increase in RMR,[25,26] others have shown no change in RMR or 24-hour energy expenditure with exercise training.[27,28]

The length of time between the last exercise bout and the measurement of RMR appears to be critical, as it has been shown that RMR significantly decreases in male and female athletes with a 3-day interruption of training.[29,30] Although these findings suggest that athletes have an increased RMR due to physical training, other cross-sectional studies have shown highly variable RMR values for male endurance athletes of similar body size, fat-free mass, and activity levels (Figure 10–1).[2,3]

These data present an interesting dilemma for the practitioner attempting to predict RMR in an athlete. Although it is most desirable to measure RMR, the majority of facilities do not have the equipment to do this measurement. Thus, most practitioners must rely upon the use of published equations to predict RMR. A recent study assessed the accuracy of a number of published RMR prediction equations in male and female endurance athletes.[31] The actual RMR of 24 male and 13 female endurance athletes was compared to values predicted using equations by Harris and Benedict,[32] Mifflin et al,[33] Owen et al,[34] Owen et al,[35] and Cunningham.[36] Only the equation by Cunningham was not significantly different from measured RMR. As shown in Figure 10–2, the RMR values predicted by the Cunningham and Harris and Benedict equations were within approximately 200 kcal of measured RMR.

There appear to be no other studies available comparing the accuracy of published prediction equations to measured RMR in other athletic populations. In addition, there have been no RMR prediction equations specifically developed for elite or recreational athletes. Until this information is available to the practitioner, one must use those equations presently available to predict RMR of the athlete if a direct measurement cannot be taken. Practitioners and athletes need to be aware of the magnitude of error possible when using these equations.

Another controversial issue is whether some athletes have an increased energy efficiency at rest and during various activities. The term energy efficiency is used in the present context to represent a state of metabolic adaptation that allows for a person to maintain body weight on an

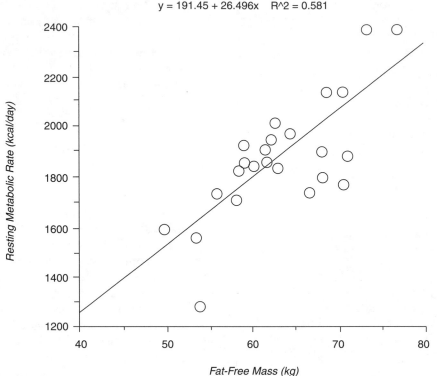

$$y = 191.45 + 26.496x \quad R^2 = 0.581$$

Figure 10–1 Regression of Resting Metabolic Rate on Fat-Free Mass for 24 Male Endurance Athletes of Similar Body Size, Fat-Free Mass, and Activity Levels. *Source:* Adapted, by permission, from J. Thompson, M. Manore, and J.S. Skinner, 1993, "Resting Metabolic Rate and Thermic Effect of a Meal in Low– and Adequate–Energy Intake Male Endurance Athletes," *International Journal of Sports Nutrition*, Vol. 3(2): 200; and from J.L. Thompson et al., Daily Energy Expenditure in Male Endurance Athletes with Differing Energy Intakes, *Medicine and Science in Sports and Exercise*, Vol. 27, No. 3, p. 351, © 1995, Williams & Wilkins.

energy intake that would appear inadequate when compared to his or her activity level. A number of male and female athletes report energy intakes that appear to be inadequate to maintain energy balance based upon reported activity levels.[2,3,37,38] Despite these low energy intakes, the athletes are weight-stable. It has been suggested that the existence of energy efficiency in certain athletes could account for the low energy intakes reported, and may also contribute to the menstrual dysfunction observed in many female athletes.[5]

The few studies of energy efficiency in male athletes have shown a lower RMR and spontane-

ous physical activity level (measured in a respiratory chamber) in the athletes reporting relatively low energy intakes.[2,3] The majority of data available in female athletes do not support energy efficiency in those females reporting relatively low energy intakes and/or those with menstrual dysfunction.[13,16,39] It is important to note, however, that there are few studies of male and female athletes available that used more accurate assessments of energy balance such as a respiratory chamber, feeding subjects to nitrogen balance and body weight maintenance, or using doubly labeled water to estimate free-living energy expenditure.

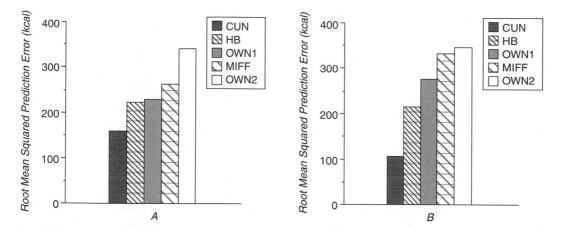

Figure 10–2 Root Mean Squared Prediction Errors for Each Resting Metabolic Rate (RMR) Prediction Equation Compared with Actual RMR Values in 24 Male (Panel A) and 13 Female (Panel B) Highly Trained Endurance Athletes. CUN = Cunningham[36]; HB = Harris and Benedict[32]; OWN1 and OWN2 for men = Owen et al.[35]; OWN1 and OWN2 for females = Owen et al.[34]; MIFF = Mifflin et al.[33] *Source:* J. Thompson and M. Manore: Predicted and Measured Resting Metabolic Rate of Male and Female Endurance Athletes. Copyright The American Dietetic Association. Reprinted by permission from *Journal of the American Dietetic Association*, Vol. 96, No. 1, p. 33, © 1996.

Recently reported results of an eloquent study of energy balance and responses to overfeeding in monozygotic twins may help explain the variability in energy intake and increased energy efficiency observed in some athletes.[20] The results of this study showed that genetics plays a significant role in a person's response to overfeeding. Twelve pairs of identical twins were overfed 1000 kcal/day, 6 days/week, under highly controlled conditions. As expected, significant increases in body weight and body fat were observed over the course of overfeeding. There was a highly individual change in weight for each of the twins, with the range in weight gain equal to 4 to 13 kg for the same overfeeding stimulus. There was also a large degree of variation in the proportion of fat and fat-free mass gained, with those gaining the most body weight also gaining a much higher proportion of body weight as fat mass. Genetics appear to play an important role in the degree of body weight and body fat gained, because the gain in body weight was similar within each twin pair. It was theorized that those who gained less weight had expended more of the excess energy intake through increasing RMR, TEF, and spontaneous activity (as voluntary physical activity was controlled), and they had higher obligatory costs of fat and protein gains.

This study has important implications for the maintenance of energy balance in athletes. Contrary to popular belief, being highly active may not guarantee one's ability to achieve and maintain a competitive body weight. Many persons, despite their high activity level, may be more predisposed to gaining body weight and storing body fat at a given energy intake. It would follow that a person with these characteristics could be more energy efficient, and would need to consume less energy than expected from reported activity levels. Studies need to be conducted on athletes from various sports using more sophisticated energy balance assessments before the existence of energy efficiency in athletes reporting low-energy intakes can be supported or refuted with confidence.

Another explanation of the increased RMR observed in some athletes involves the total energy flux through the body.[40,41] Many athletes are in energy balance, but have a high energy expenditure, and must have a high energy intake to meet the energy demands. These athletes would be considered to be in a state of high energy flux. It has been recently shown that this state of energy flux increases RMR in athletes.[41] Being in a state of negative or positive energy balance (under- or overfeeding in relation to energy expenditure), or in low energy flux (being less active with an energy intake sufficient to meet energy demands) does not appear to affect RMR (Figure 10–3). Energy intake has been shown to account for a large proportion of the variance in RMR in male and female endurance athletes;[31] the contribution of intake to RMR may be a result of its relationship with total energy flux in the athlete.

CLINICAL/THERAPEUTIC APPLICATIONS

The most affordable, practical, and accurate way to estimate energy balance in athletes is not known. The maintenance of body weight over time is one practical measure that can be used to determine whether an athlete is in energy balance. To counsel athletes on making appropriate dietary changes or healthy adjustments in body composition, a reasonable estimation of energy balance needs to be done. Because few practitioners have the opportunity to directly assess energy balance using highly sophisticated techniques, one must rely upon self-reported energy intake and activity data and published prediction equations to estimate RMR. Although it is important to recognize the limitations of these assessment tools, they are still useful when trying to get a general idea of energy balance in the athlete.

It is difficult to determine which energy intake and energy expenditure assessment tool is most appropriate for athletes, because the validity of these tools in an athletic population has not been adequately studied. Many practitioners are asked to determine energy balance for individual athletes, and it is important to stress that most assessment tools are not as representative of true energy intake in an individual as they are for groups of persons.[12,17] One major limitation of the available energy expenditure assessment tools is the assumption that persons with similar body weights will have similar energy expenditures for any given activity. This assumption has been questioned,[8] and in light of recent evidence, it appears that genetics plays a significant role in the amount of energy expended during performance of some activities.[42]

When attempting to estimate energy balance in an athlete, it is important to understand the potential sources of error in the methods used, and to attempt to minimize these errors. It does appear that the Cunningham equation[36] (Table 10–1) can be used with confidence in predicting RMR in endurance athletes. Although this equation is simple to use, it does require the measurement of fat-free mass. If methods are not available to determine fat-free mass, the equation of Harris and Benedict[32] (see Table 10–1) has been shown to predict RMR to within 200 kcal/day in male and female endurance athletes.[31]

From the information presented in this chapter, it is obvious that studies need to be done to determine the most accurate field assessments of energy balance in athletes. In addition, RMR prediction equations need to be developed from and for active persons. It is also important to be able to distinguish between when an athlete is underreporting energy intake and when an athlete may have a lower energy need due to the presence of some degree of energy efficiency.

CASE STUDY ILLUSTRATION

The following is an example of determining energy balance in a male endurance athlete (Athlete #1). Athlete #1, a marathon runner, was a volunteer in a study of energy balance in low– and adequate–energy intake male athletes.[3] He had been training for and competing in marathons for 2 years before participation in this study. He reported no concerns with body weight or any previous history of eating disor-

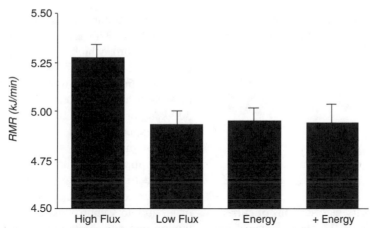

Figure 10–3 Average Resting Metabolic Rate (RMR) for Each of Four Different Energy Balance/Flux Conditions in Eight Highly Trained Men (x ± SEM). High flux is significantly different from all other conditions, $P <$ .05. *Source:* Reprinted with permission from R.C. Bullough et al., Interaction of Acute Changes in Exercise Energy Expenditure and Energy Intake on Resting Metabolic Rate, *The American Journal of Clinical Nutrition*, Vol. 61, No. 3, p. 477, © 1995, American Society of Clinical Nutrition.

ders, and he had been weight-stable (experienced a change in weight no greater than +/– 3.5 kg) for at least 2 years. Table 10–2 contains descriptive characteristics of Athlete #1.

The RMR of Athlete #1 was measured on two occasions, separated by no more than 10 days. The RMR was measured as previously described.[3] The week after the RMR measurements were completed, Athlete #1 was asked to complete 7 days of weighed food records and activity records. He was provided with a calibrated household scale, and was asked to weigh

or measure (with measuring cups and spoons) all foods consumed over seven consecutive 24-hour periods. He also included labels from any packaged foods consumed. During this same period, Athlete #1 was asked to record all activities done. Appendix 10–A contains samples of instructions and recording sheets for food intake and activities.

After 1 day of recording, Athlete #1 reviewed his diet and activity records with the study investigator. This meeting served to ensure that he was completing the records in a clear and complete

Table 10–1 Equations for Predicting Resting Metabolic Rate (RMR) in Healthy Athletes

Reference	Equation
Cunningham[36]	RMR (kcal/day) = 500 + 22(FFM)
Harris and Benedict[32]	Males: RMR (kcal/day) = 66.47 + 13.75(wt) – 5(ht) – 6.76(age)
	Females: RMR (kcal/day) = 655.1 + 9.56(wt) – 1.85(ht) – 4.68(age)

Note: FFM = fat-free mass (kg); wt = body weight (kg); ht = height (cm); and age = age (years).

Source: J. Thompson and M. Manore, Predicted and Measured Resting Metabolic Rate of Male and Female Endurance Athletes. Copyright The American Dietetic Association. Reprinted by permission from *Journal of the American Dietetic Association*, Vol. 96, No. 1, p. 31, © 1996.

Table 10–2 Descriptive Characteristics of an Athlete (Athlete #1) Participating in the Assessment of Energy Balance

Age (yrs)	27
Height (cm)	177.8
Weight (kg)	61.9
Body fat (%)	4.6
Fat-free mass (kg)	59.1
Treadmill VO$_{2max}$ (ml·kg-1·min-1)	64.0
Resting metabolic rate (kcal/d)	1918

manner. Any necessary clarifications or corrections were executed at this time, because his memory of the foods eaten and activities done over the previous 24 hours would most likely be better than after the entire 7-day period. Once all records were completed, Athlete #1 returned them to the study investigator for analysis.

This case study illustration will provide an example of estimating energy balance for Athlete #1 for 1 day. Exhibit 10–2 contains a diet record for 1 day of the study. The record was analyzed using the Food Processor Plus nutrient analysis program (version 6; ESHA Research, Salem, OR). As shown in Exhibit 10–3, the estimated energy intake for Athlete #1 for 1 day was 4042 kcal. The percentage of total energy provided by carbohydrates, fat, and protein were 66%, 19%, and 15%, respectively.

The energy expenditure of Athlete #1 was estimated using the energy expenditure factors summarized by Mulligan and Butterfield.[38] The activity record completed by Athlete #1 is included in Figure 10–4. A spreadsheet was used to document the amount of time spent at various activities. The total time spent at each activity was calculated (Exhibit 10–4). The estimated energy expenditure for Athlete #1 for this day was 4364 kcal. This value compares closely with his diet record, which estimated his energy intake at 4042 kcal. Considering the error inherent in estimating energy intake and expenditure, these records compare within approximately 300 kcal, or less than 10% of energy intake or energy expenditure.

Although the values obtained from these records appear reasonable, there is no gold standard of comparison. The methods illustrated here can give a good general indication of an athlete's approximate energy needs. Although one may have more confidence in the results if both intake and activity records match closely, it is important to remember that over- and underestimations of energy intake and expenditure can occur. Efforts to minimize errors should include the following: 1) encouraging the athlete to record his or her food intake and activity level as accurately as possible (using scales and measuring cups/spoons); 2) recording as one is cooking and just after eating (to prevent one from forgetting the consumption of various foods); 3) including labels from foods and calling restaurants for details of food amounts and preparation; 4) recording one's activities every 15 to 30 minutes. Although this can be tedious, it should be a better indicator of the details of one's daily life than when one attempts to remember the various activities done over the previous 24-hour period; 5) directly measuring RMR; and 6) when estimating energy balance in female athletes, it is important to obtain records over the various phases of the menstrual cycle, because energy needs have been reported to fluctuate during the menstrual cycle.[43,44]

Exhibit 10–2 Diet Record for Athlete #1

Date ___/___/___   Day of the week _____

Food Intake Diary   NAME: _____

Time (AM/PM)	FOODS AND BEVERAGES INCLUDE: fresh, frozen, lowfat, etc.	AMOUNT	METHOD OF PREPARATION (baked, fried, broiled, etc.)	Food Exchanges
9:45 am	Gatorade	8 fl oz		
10 am	Bagel—oat bran	110 grams	Plain	
10:30 am	Bagel—whole wheat	120 grams	Plain	
12:45 pm	Taco Bell bean burritos	2	As sold	
	Slice soft drink	25 fl oz	With ice (very little)	
3 pm	Bagel—whole wheat	120 grams	Plain	
6 pm	Tortilla chips—light Mi Ranchito nacho chips	60 grams		
9:30 pm	Bread—whole wheat—oat 'n honey	2 slices—80 grams/slice	Plain	
	Cheese—lowfat Frigo mozzarella	60 grams		
	Turkey—smoked, sliced lunch meat	75 grams		
	Lettuce—iceberg	2 leaves		
	Nonfat milk	1 cup		
	Cereal—Cracklin' Oat Bran—Quaker	120 grams	With milk (see above)	
10:30 pm	Nonfat milk	1 3/4 cups		
	Grandma's oatmeal raisin cookies	6 each	Dipped in milk (see above)	

Exhibit 10–3 Nutrient Analysis of Diet Record for Athlete #1

Analysis: Athlete #1

Amount	Item	Code
8 fl oz	Gatorade sports drink	20053.
110 g	Oat bran bagel	42103.
120 g	Whole wheat bagel	42092.
2 each	Taco Bell bean burrito w/red sauce	56519.
25 fl oz	Lemon lime soda pop	20032.
120 g	Whole wheat bagel	42092.
60 g	Light nacho tortilla chips (lower fat)	44054.
160 g	Whole wheat bread	42014.
60 g	Lowfat mozzarella cheese—shredded	1020.
75 g	Turkey/chicken breast—smoked lunchmeat	13064.
2 piece	Iceberg/crisphead lettuce leaves	5084.
1 cup	Nonfat skim milk	6.
120 g	Cracklin' Oat Bran cereal	40039.
1.75 cup	Nonfat skim milk	6.
6 each	Oatmeal raisin cookie	47003.

(Need Profile for Comparison)   Weight: 3035 g (107 oz)
Cost: Water: 67%

Calories	4042	Pantothenic	7.57 mg
Protein	159 g	Vitamin C	76.2 mg
Carbohydrates	697 g	Vitamin D	11.7 mcg
Fat—total	88.4 g	Vitamin E—alpha E	6.68 mg
Saturated fat	26.7 g	Calcium	2141 mg
Mono fat	32.2 g	Copper	2.66 mg
Poly fat	18.8 g	Iron	36 mg
Omega 3 FA	.473 g	Magnesium	903 mg
Omega 6 FA	7.46 g	Manganese	17.4 mg
Cholesterol	113 mg	Phosphorus	3235 mg
Dietary fiber	97.6 g	Potassium	5027 mg
Total vitamin A	3069 RE	Selenium	124 mcg
A—Retinol	2224 RE	Sodium	8858 mg
A—Carotenoid	30.2 RE	Zinc	24 mg
Thiamin—B1	3.96 mg	Complex carbohydrates	259 g
Riboflavin—B2	8.87 mg	Sugars	202 g
Niacin—B3	55.5 mg	Mono-saccharide	84.6 g
Niacin equiv.	17.7 mg	Di-saccharide	33.7 g
Vitamin B6	4.91 mg	Alcohol	0 g
Vitamin B12	4.7 mcg	Caffeine	0 mg
Folate	818 mcg	Water	2037 g

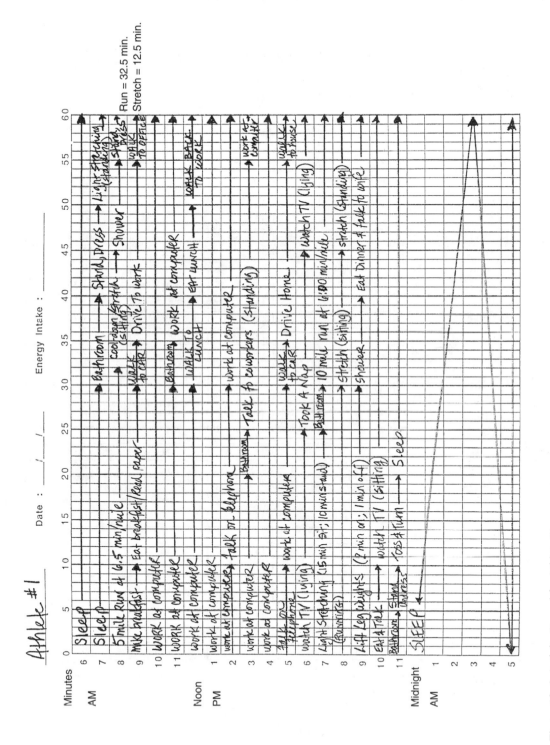

Figure 10-4 Activity Record for Athlete #1

Exhibit 10–4 Spreadsheet Analysis of Daily Energy Expenditure for Athlete #1

Subject Name					
	Activity	*Efactor*	*RMR (kcal/min)*	*Minutes*	*Total Energy*
Lie	Sleeping		1.33	510	610.47
	Rest		1.33		0
	Read		1.33		0
	Write		1.33		0
	Sex		1.33		0
	Toss/turn		1.33	10	14.63
	Watch TV		1.33	40	53.2
	Talk		1.33		0
Sit	Inactive		1.33	10	15.96
	Active		1.33		0
	Read		1.33	10	15.96
	Talk		1.33	45	71.82
	Write		1.33		0
	Type		1.33	350	791.35
	Eat		1.33	35	65.17
	Drive		1.33	40	111.72
	Games		1.33		0
	TV/movie		1.33	50	79.8
	Stretch/yoga		1.33	42.5	79.135
	Office		1.33		0
	Sing		1.33		0
	Piano		1.33		0
	Dress		1.33		0
Stand	Dress		1.33	20	77.14
	Inactive		1.33		0
	Active		1.33		0
	Talk		1.33	30	55.86
	Write		1.33		0
	Cook		1.33	10	25.27
	Dishes		1.33		0
	Eat		1.33		0
	Mill around		1.33		0
	Personal care		1.33	50	192.85
	Shopping		1.33		0
	Office		1.33		0
	Party		1.33		0
	Housework		1.33		0
	Stretch/yoga		1.33	35	65.17
Walk	Flat		1.33	40	154.28
	Downhill		1.33		0

continues

Exhibit 10–4 continued

Subject Name					
	Activity	*Efactor*	*RMR (kcal/min)*	*Minutes*	*Total Energy*
	Uphill		1.33		0
	Upstairs		1.33		0
	Fast		1.33		0
	With load		1.33		0
	Eating		1.33		0
	Hike		1.33		0
	Tennis		1.33		0
	Bicycle		1.33		0
	Dance, exercise		1.33		0
	Dance, social		1.33		0
	Swim		1.33		0
Sit	Row		1.33		0
Stand	Calisthenics		1.33		0
	Aerobics		1.33		0
Run	6.0–6.9 min/mi		1.33	92.5	1697.745
	7.0–7.9 min/mi		1.33		0
	8.0–8.9 min/mi		1.33		0
	9.0–9.9 min/mi		1.33		0
	10–10.8 min/mi		1.33		0
	> 10.8 min/mi		1.33		0
	Hilly run		1.33		0
Stand	Gardening		1.33		0
	Lift weights		1.33	20	186.2
	Move furniture		1.33		0
Sit	Motorcycle		1.33		0
Stand	Pet care		1.33		0
	Drafting		1.33		0
Run	Upstairs		1.33		0
Stand	Child care		1.33		0
Kneel	Kneel		1.33		0
					4363.73 total

Note: Total energy can be calculated using the appropriate energy factors, such as those found in K. Mulligan and G. Butterfield, *British Journal of Nutrition*, Vol. 64, 1990.

REFERENCES

1. Ravussin E, Bogardus C. Relationship of genetics, age, and physical fitness to daily energy expenditure and fuel utilization. *Am J Clin Nutr*. 1989;49:968–975.

2. Thompson JL, Manore MM, Skinner JS. Resting meta-bolic rate and thermic effect of a meal in low- and adequate-energy intake male endurance athletes. *Int J Sport Nutr*. 1993;3:194–206.

3. Thompson JL, Manore MM, Skinner JS, Ravussin E,

Spraul M. Daily energy expenditure in male endurance athletes with differing energy intakes. *Med Sci Sports Exerc*. 1995;27:347–354.

4. Myerson M, Gutin B, Warren MP, et al. Resting metabolic rate and energy balance in amenorrheic and eumenorrheic runners. *Med Sci Sports Exerc*. 1991; 23:15–22.

5. Brownell KD, Steen SN, Wilmore JH. Weight regulation practices in athletes: analysis of metabolic and health effects. *Med Sci Sports Exerc*. 1987;19:546–556.

6. Hoffman CJ, Coleman E. An eating plan and update on recommended dietary practices for the endurance athlete. *J Am Diet Assoc*. 1991;91:325–330.

7. Coyle EF. Substrate utilization during exercise in active people. *Am J Clin Nutr*. 1995;61:968S–979S.

8. Garrow JS. Resting metabolic rate as a determinant of energy expenditure in man. In: Garrow JS, Halliday D, eds. *Substrate and Energy Metabolism*. London: John Libbey; 1985;102–106.

9. Mahalko JR, Johnson LK. Accuracy of predictions of long-term energy needs. *J Am Diet Assoc*. 1980;77:557–561.

10. Todd KS, Herdes M, Calloway DH. Food intake measurement: problems and approaches. *Am J Clin Nutr*. 1983;37:139–146.

11. de Vries JHM, Zock PL, Mensink RP, Katan MB. Underestimation of energy intake by 3-d records compared with energy intake to maintain body weight in 269 nonobese adults. *Am J Clin Nutr*. 1994;60:855–860.

12. Sawaya AL, Tucker K, Tsay R, et al. Evaluation of four methods for determining energy intake in young and older women: comparison with doubly labeled water measurements of total energy expenditure. *Am J Clin Nutr*. 1996;63:491–499.

13. Beidleman BA, Puhl JL, De Souza MJ. Energy in female distance runners. *Am J Clin Nutr*. 1995;61:303–311.

14. Romieu I, Willett WC, Stampfer MJ, et al. Energy intake and other determinants of relative weight. *Am J Clin Nutr*. 1988;47:406–412.

15. Prentice AM, Black AE, Coward WA, et al. High levels of energy expenditure in obese women. *Br Med J*. 1986;292:983–987.

16. Edwards JE, Lindeman AK, Mikesky AE, Stager JM. Energy balance in highly trained female endurance runners. *Med Sci Sports Exerc*. 1993;25:1398–1404.

17. Basiotis PP, Welsh SO, Cronin FJ, Kelsay FL, Mertz W. Number of days of food intake records required to estimate individual and group nutrient intakes with defined confidence. *J Nutr*. 1987;117:1638–1641.

18. Acheson KJ, Campbell IT, Edholm OG, Miller DS, Stock MF. The measurement of daily energy expenditure—an evaluation of some techniques. *Am J Clin Nutr*. 1980;33:1155–1164.

19. Schoeller DA, van Santen E. Measurement of energy expenditure in humans by doubly labeled water. *J Appl Phys Respir Environ Exerc Phys*. 1982;53:955–959.

20. Bouchard C, Tremblay A, Després JP, et al. The response to long-term overfeeding in identical twins. *N Engl J Med*. 1990;322:1477–1482.

21. Poehlman ET, Melby CL, Badylak SF. Resting metabolic rate and postprandial thermogenesis in highly trained and untrained males. *Am J Clin Nutr*. 1988;47:793–798.

22. Poehlman ET, Melby CL, Badylak SF, Calles J. Aerobic fitness and resting energy expenditure in young adult males. *Metabolism*. 1989;38:85–90.

23. Broeder CE, Burrhus KA, Svanevik LS, Wilmore JH. The effects of aerobic fitness on resting metabolic rate. *Am J Clin Nutr*. 1992;55:795–801.

24. Schulz LO, Nyomba BL, Alger S, Anderson TE, Ravussin E. Effect of endurance training on sedentary energy expenditure measured in a respiratory chamber. *Am J Physiol*. 1991;260:E257–E262.

25. Tremblay A, Fontaine E, Poehlman ET, Mitchell D, Perron L, Bouchard C. The effect of exercise-training on resting metabolic rate in lean and moderately obese individuals. *Int J Obesity*. 1986;10:511–517.

26. Campbell WW, Crim MC, Young VR, Evans WJ. Increased energy requirements and changes in body composition with resistance training in older adults. *Am J Clin Nutr*. 1994;60:167–175.

27. Broeder CE, Burrhus KA, Svanevik LS, Wilmore JH. The effects of either high-intensity resistance or endurance training on resting metabolic rate. *Am J Clin Nutr*. 1992;55:802–810.

28. Buemann B, Astrup A, Christensen NJ. Three months aerobic training fails to affect 24-hour energy expenditure in weight-stable, post-obese women. *Int J Obesity*. 1992;16:809–816.

29. Herring JL, Molé PA, Meredith CN, Stern JS. Effect of suspending exercise training on resting metabolic rate in women. *Med Sci Sports Exerc*. 1992;24:59–65.

30. Tremblay A, Nadeau A, Fournier G, Bouchard C. Effect of a three-day interruption of exercise-training on resting metabolic rate and glucose-induced thermogenesis in trained individuals. *Int J Obesity*. 1988;12:163–168.

31. Thompson JL, Manore MM. Predicted and measured resting metabolic rate of male and female endurance athletes. *J Am Diet Assoc*. 1996;96:30–34.

32. Harris JA, Benedict FG. *A Biometric Study of Basal Metabolism in Man* (Vol 279). Philadelphia: J.B. Lippincott Co; 1919.

33. Mifflin MD, St Jeor ST, Hill LA, Scott BJ, Daugherty SA, Koh YO. A new predictive equation for resting energy expenditure in healthy individuals. *Am J Clin Nutr.* 1990;51:241–247.

34. Owen OE, Kavle E, Owen RS, et al. A reappraisal of caloric requirements in healthy women. *Am J Clin Nutr.* 1986;44:1–19.

35. Owen OE, Holup JL, D'Alessio DA, et al. A reappraisal of the caloric requirements of men. *Am J Clin Nutr.* 1987;46:875–885.

36. Cunningham JJ. A reanalysis of the factors influencing basal metabolic rate in normal adults. *Am J Clin Nutr.* 1980;33:2372–2374.

37. Dahlström M, Jansson E, Nordevang E, Kaijser L. Discrepancy between estimated energy intake and requirement in female dancers. *Clin Physiol.* 1990;10:11–25.

38. Mulligan K, Butterfield GE. Discrepancies between energy intake and expenditure in physically active women. *Br J Nutr.* 1990;64:23–36.

39. Wilmore JH, Wambsgans KC, Brenner M, et al. Is there energy conservation in amenorrheic compared with eumenorrheic distance runners? *J Appl Physiol.* 1992;72:15–22.

40. Goran MI, Calles-Escadon J, Poehlman ET, O'Connell M, Danforth Jr E. Effects of increased energy intake and/or physical activity on energy expenditure in young healthy men. *J Appl Physiol.* 1994;77:366–372.

41. Bullough RC, Gillett CA, Harris MA, Melby CL. Interaction of acute changes in exercise energy expenditure and energy intake on resting metabolic rate. *Am J Clin Nutr.* 1995;61:473–481.

42. Bouchard C, Tremblay A, Nadeau A, et al. Genetic effect in resting and exercise metabolic rates. *Metabolism.* 1989;38:364–370.

43. Barr SI, Janelle KC, Prior JC. Energy intakes are higher during the luteal phase of ovulatory menstrual cycles. *Am J Clin Nutr.* 1995;61:39–43.

44. Bisdee JT, James WPT, Shaw MA. Changes in energy expenditure during the menstrual cycle. *Br J Nutr.* 1989;61:187–199.

Food Record Instructions

1. Record your *name and date* at the head of each page.

2. In the column marked "TIME" indicate the time that you started eating each meal or snack. Keep the record with you (or a small notepad), and record things directly after consuming them.

3. In the column marked "FOODS AND BEVERAGES" record a description of *all* the food eaten. *Use as much detail as possible in describing the food or drink.* For instance,

   a) SPECIFY   NOT JUST
   - *low-fat* milk   milk
   - *canned tomato* soup   soup
   - chicken *breast* with *skin* chicken
   - fresh broccoli   broccoli
   - sole   fish

   b) Remember to record *all condiments or additions to foods*: mayonnaise on a sandwich, gravy or sauce on vegetables or meats, butter or margarine on bread, salad dressings on salads, or sugar and creamer added to coffee or tea. Include all your snacks and nibbles, no matter how small!

   c) When describing mixed casserole-type dishes, be specific about the individual ingredients. If home prepared, write down the exact recipe, recording the total number of portions in the recipe and the number of portions you consumed of the total. If you consume store-bought, prepackaged items, please attach food labels.

4. In the column labeled "AMOUNT" record the weight or amount of food eaten.

   a) Standard units can be used for foods like bread (1 slice of whole wheat bread), fruits (1 large banana), and some vegetables (1 small carrot).

   b) For other foods measured more easily by volume (beverages, cooked vegetables, rice, etc.) or consumed in small amounts, *regular household measurements* (cups, teaspoons, tablespoons) should be used, for example:
   - 1 c (or 8 fl oz) nonfat milk
   - 3/4 c broccoli, steamed
   - 1 c cantaloupe, cubed
   - 2 tbsp peanut butter

   c) If you have a *food scale*, items such as meat, cheese, cookies, and cake should be weighed and recorded on the form as ounces or grams. Remember to make sure that you don't include the weight of the container as food weight.

5. In the column labeled "METHOD OF PREPARATION" include the details of how your food was cooked. For example, specify the following for the items listed above:
   - Chicken breast with skin, *batter-baked*
   - fresh broccoli, *steamed, with butter*
   - sole, *breaded* and *pan-fried*

6. When *eating out*, approximate the sizes by listing the width, length, and thickness, or by drawing the size of the portion on the

back of the food record. Although it is not ideal to eyeball-estimate portions of food, frequent use of measuring utensils at home will also lead to greater familiarity with food quantities. Waiters can also provide information about the serving sizes and ingredients.

7. **Most Important:** We want you to continue eating your normal diet during the recording days. It is important that you not change your eating habits during this time.

Exhibit 10–2 is an example of a completed food record form. We have included a blank form in this Appendix.

Be accurate and detailed. Our nutrition analysis will only be as precise as the information you give us.

ACTIVITY RECORD PROCEDURE

Collection of Data

1. The record begins at 6:00 AM. Subjects receive a labeled and dated sheet the previous evening so that time of rising in the morning can be recorded.

2. Subject carries a watch with minute intervals, the diary sheet, and a pen and pencil throughout the day.

3. The time at which an activity begins is recorded to the minute. For most activities, the code letter (see below) can be used to minimize writing. Others will require more description. For unusual activities a subject participates in, a code letter can be agreed upon. *Both position and activity* should be recorded unless obvious. The following are examples:

Position	Activity	Obvious Position
Sitting	Reading	Walking
Standing	Watching TV	Ping Pong
Lying	Talking	Bicycling

4. The length of time of the activity is marked with an arrow until the beginning of the next activity.

5. If the subject rises during the night, the times of rising and going back to bed and activity are noted on the back of the previous day's record sheet.

6. Comments can be noted on the back of the sheet about emotional state that may affect energy level, etc.

Date __/__/__

Day of the week _____

Food Intake Diary   NAME: _____

Time (AM/PM)	FOODS AND BEVERAGES INCLUDE: fresh, frozen, lowfat, etc.	AMOUNT	METHOD OF PREPARATION (baked, fried, broiled, etc.)	Food Exchanges

CODES

Position	Code	Activity	Code
Standing	ST	Eating, drinking	E
Sitting	Si	Reading	R
Lying	L	Personal care, showering	PC
Walking	W	Dressing	Dr
		Talking	T
		Writing	Wr
		Watching TV	TV
		Driving a car	D
		Office	O
		Sleeping	S
		Rest	Rs
		Toss/turn	Tt
		Sex	Se
		Cooking	Co
		Dishes	Di
		Housework	HW
		Shopping	Sho
		Mill around	MA
		Games; cards	Gm
		Gardening	G
		In class	C
		Bicycle	B
		Playing pool	P
		Treadmill	TM
		Others (list):	

Name : _____

Date : ____ / ____ / ____

Energy Intake : _____

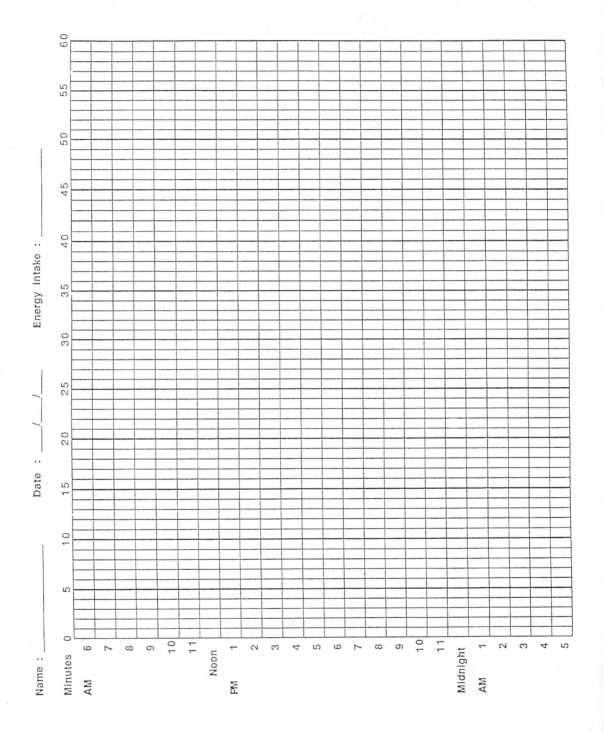

CHAPTER 11

Eating Disorders

Jorunn Sundgot-Borgen

A number of athletes are suffering from disturbed eating behavior and clinical eating disorders such as anorexia nervosa and bulimia nervosa. Existing studies indicate that eating disorder problems are more common among athletes than nonathletes, and even more prevalent among those athletes representing weight-related sports than among those representing sports in which leanness is considered less important. Psychological, biologic, and social factors interrelate to produce the clinical picture of eating disorders. Specific risk factors for the development of eating disorders occur in some sport settings.

The role of the sport nutritionist in working with athletes with weight and eating disorders is crucial. Therefore, nutritionists should have good knowledge of the symptomatology of eating disorders, how to approach the athlete, and how to establish trust that can lead to effective treatment.

This chapter reviews the definitions, diagnostic criteria, prevalence, and risk factors for the development of eating disorders in sport. Practical implications for the identification and treatment of eating disorders in athletes are also discussed.

HISTORICAL OVERVIEW

During the second half of the 19th century, detailed case reports of self-starvation began to surface. Gull[1] emphasized the clinical findings of starvation and did not concern himself, as did Lasegue, with the illness' emotional aspects. Thus, Gull simply noted the occurrence of amenorrhea, constipation, loss of appetite, decreased vital signs, and emaciation. Gull's recommended treatment is simple, but perhaps a bit heavy-handed and authoritarian: "The treatment required is obviously that which is fitted for persons of unsound mind: The patient should be fed at regular intervals, and surrounded by persons who would have moral control over them; relations and friends being generally the worst attendants."[1, p 26]

During the 20th century, two major events occurred that led to a revolution in our understanding of eating disorders. The first came from Dr. Hilde Bruch. She delved into the psyche of patients with anorexia. The 20th century brought forth a second contribution of extreme importance: the report by Gerald Russell.[2] Russell listed the following criteria: 1) The patients suffer from powerful and intractable urges to overeat. 2) They seek to avoid the fattening effects of food by inducing vomiting or abusing purgatives or both. 3) They have a morbid fear of becoming fat.[2, p 445]

A number of years ago, concerns were raised about the rapid, frequent, and severe weight loss and regain cycles in male wrestlers.[3] Both the American College of Sports Medicine[4] and the American Medical Association[5] have issued position stands warning against the dangers of these practices in wrestlers. Since the beginning of the 1980s, a number of papers have focused on eating disorders and athletes.[6–14]

DEFINITIONS AND DIAGNOSTIC CRITERIA

Eating disorders are characterized by gross disturbances in eating behavior. They include anorexia nervosa, bulimia nervosa, and eating disorders not otherwise specified.[15] Athletes constitute a unique population, and special diagnostic considerations should be made when working with this group.[6,16,17] Even if mild variants of eating disorders are observed in athletes (that is, only some symptoms required for a formal diagnosis), they should be given immediate attention because they may severely compromise health and performance. An attempt has been made to identify the group of athletes who show significant symptoms of eating disorders, but who do not meet the standard criteria.[6] These athletes have been classified as having a subclinical eating disorder termed anorexia athletica. Health care professionals working with athletes should be aware of the needs, expectations, and performance demands of athletes because this awareness and experience may be helpful in both diagnosis and treatment.[17] It is assumed that many cases of anorexia nervosa and bulimia nervosa begin as subclinical variants of these disorders. Early identification may prevent development of the full disorder.[18] Finally, subclinical cases are more prevalent than those meeting the formal diagnostic criteria for eating disorders.

Anorexia Nervosa

Anorexia nervosa is characterized by a refusal to maintain body weight over a minimal level considered normal for age and height, a distorted body image, an intense fear of fatness or weight gain, while being underweight and having amenorrhea (Exhibit 11–1). Persons with anorexia nervosa "feel fat," while in reality they are underweight.[16]

Exhibit 11–1 Diagnostic Criteria for Anorexia Nervosa

A. Refusal to maintain body weight at or above a minimally normal weight for age and height (for example, weight loss leading to maintenance of body weight less than 85% of that expected; or failure to make expected weight gain during period of growth, leading to body weight less than 85% of that expected)
B. Intense fear of gaining weight or becoming fat, even though underweight
C. Disturbance in the way in which one's body weight or shape is experienced, undue influence of body weight or shape on self-evaluation, or denial of the seriousness of the current low body weight
D. In postmenarcheal females, amenorrhea (that is, the absence of at least three consecutive menstrual cycles). [A woman is considered to have amenorrhea if her periods occur only after hormone (for example, estrogen) administration.]

Specify type:
  Restricting type: During the episode of anorexia nervosa, the person has not regularly engaged in binge eating or purging behavior (that is, self-induced vomiting or the misuse of laxatives, diuretics, or enemas).
  Binge eating/purging type: During the current episode of anorexia nervosa, the person regularly engages in binge eating or purging behavior (that is, self-induced vomiting or the misuse of laxatives, diuretics, or enemas).

Source: Adapted with permission from *Diagnostic and Statistical Manual of Mental Disorders*, 4th ed., pp. 1–2, © 1994, American Psychiatric Association.

Bulimia Nervosa

Bulimia nervosa is characterized by binge eating (rapid consumption of a large amount of food in a discrete period) and purging. This typically involves consumption of high-energy foods, usually eaten inconspicuously or secretly. By relieving abdominal discomfort through vomiting, the person can continue the binge.[16] The *Diagnostic and Statistical Manual of Mental Disorders* (DSM-IV) criteria for bulimia nervosa include the following: recurrent episodes of binge eating, inappropriate behavior to prevent weight gain, the occurrence of binge eating and inappropriate compensatory behaviors at least twice a week for at least 3 months, and self-evaluation based on body shape and weight[19] (Exhibit 11–2).

Eating Disorders Not Otherwise Specified

The eating disorders not otherwise specified category is for eating disorders that do not meet the criteria for any specific eating disorder. Examples of eating disorders not otherwise specified are listed in Exhibit 11–3, and this category acknowledges the existence and importance of a variety of eating disturbances.[17]

Anorexia Athletica

The main feature of anorexia athletica is an intense fear of gaining weight or becoming fat, even though an affected person is already lean (at least 5% less than expected normal weight for age and height for the general population). Weight loss is accomplished by a reduction in energy intake, often combined with extensive or compulsive exercise. The restrictive energy intake is below that required to maintain the energy requirements of the high training volume.[20] In addition to normal training to enhance performance in sport, athletes with anorexia athletica exercise excessively or compulsively to purge their bodies of the effect of eating. These athletes frequently report binge eating and the use of vomiting, laxatives, or diuretics. The binge eating is usually planned and included in a strict training and study schedule. It is important to note that the definition of a binge used by an athlete with anorexia athletica is usually within the usual daily caloric requirements for unaffected athletes. Because it is often difficult for elite athletes to have time for more than two meals, some

Exhibit 11–2 Diagnostic Criteria for Bulimia Nervosa

A. Recurrent episodes of binge eating. An episode of binge eating is characterized by both of the following: (1) eating, during a discrete period (for example, within any 2-hour period), an amount of food that is larger than what most people would eat during a similar period in similar circumstances, and (2) a sense of lack of control over eating during the episode (for example, a feeling that one cannot stop eating or control what or how much one is eating).

B. Recurrent inappropriate compensatory behavior to prevent weight gain, such as self-induced vomiting; misuse of laxatives, diuretics, or other medications; fasting; or excessive exercise.

C. The binge eating and inappropriate compensatory behaviors both occur, on average, at least twice a week for 3 months.

D. Self-evaluation is unduly influenced by body shape and weight.

E. The disturbance does not occur exclusively during episodes of anorexia nervosa.

Specify type:

Purging type: The person regularly engages in self-induced vomiting or misuses laxatives, diuretics, or enemas.

Nonpurging type: The person uses other inappropriate compensatory behaviors, such as fasting or excessive exercise, but does not regularly engage in self-induced vomiting or the misuse of laxatives, diuretics, or enemas.

Source: Adapted with permission from *Diagnostic and Statistical Manual of Mental Disorders*, 4th ed., pp. 1–2, © 1994, American Psychiatric Association.

do not meet the caloric requirements.[20] The binges reported by typical anorexia athletica patients are often due to a decreased glucose level. Like other eating disorder patients, these athletes are trying to save calories and delay their meals

Exhibit 11–3 The Eating Disorders Not Otherwise Specified Category

1. All of the criteria for anorexia nervosa are met except the person has regular menses.
2. All of the criteria for anorexia nervosa are met except, despite significant weight loss, the person's current weight is in the normal range.
3. All of the criteria for bulimia nervosa are met except binges occur at a frequency of less than twice a week or a duration of less than 3 months.
4. A person of normal body weight regularly engages in inappropriate compensatory behavior after eating small amounts of food (for example, self-induced vomiting after the consumption of two cookies).
5. A person repeatedly chews and spits out, but does not swallow, large amounts of food.
6. Recurrent episodes of binge eating occur in the absence of inappropriate compensatory behaviors characteristic of bulimia nervosa.

Source: Adapted with permission from *Diagnostic and Statistical Manual of Mental Disorders*, 4th ed., pp. 1–2, © 1994, American Psychiatric Association.

until after training. The criteria for anorexia athletica listed in Exhibit 11–4 include a modification of the original criteria introduced by Pugliese et al.[21]

Some athletes with anorexia athletica also meet the criteria of eating disorders not otherwise specified. Most athletes have a higher percentage of lean body mass than age-matched nonathletes. Body weight more than 5% lower than expected could indicate that an athlete is too lean. Athletes with anorexia athletica usually indicate that they need to lose weight because of the requirements of their sport often motivated by directions from their coach.

PREVALENCE OF EATING DISORDERS IN ATHLETES

Data on the prevalence of eating disorders in athletic populations is limited and equivocal. Most studies have looked at obsessive preoccupation with weight and food, disturbed body image, or the use of pathogenic weight control methods. Only a few have looked at clinical eating disorders. There are a number of methodologic weaknesses in the studies. Most investigators have used self-developed questionnaires without giving information about validity and reliability; the populations investigated are not clearly defined, there is a lack of control groups, and different measures are used.

Female Athletes

Estimates of the prevalence of the symptoms of clinical eating disorders and eating disorders among female athletes range from less than 1% to as high as 62%.[7,8,22,23] Estimates vary greatly depending on whether they are based on self-reports or clinical interviews, and on the athletic population investigated. Only one study has used clinical evaluation and the American Psychiatric Association criteria applied across athletes and controls.[23] Data from that study showed that the prevalence of DSM-III-R diagnosed anorexia nervosa is 1.3%, which is somewhat higher than the prevalence reported for nonathletes. Diagnosed bulimia nervosa was 8.2% among female elite athletes. Above 8% also met the criteria for anorexia athletica. The prevalence within each sport category, however, was significantly different.[23] Eating disorders were significantly more prevalent in aesthetic (34%) and weight-dependent sports (27%) compared to endurance sports (20%), technical sports (13%), and ball-game sports (11%). The prevalence of anorexia nervosa seems to be within the same range as that reported for nonathletes,[24] whereas bulimia nervosa and subclinical eating disorders seem to be more prevalent among female athletes.[23]

Exhibit 11–4 Diagnostic Criteria for Anorexia Athletica

1. Weight loss >5% of expected body weight	+
2. Delayed puberty (no menstrual bleeding at age 16 years—that is, primary amenorrhea)	(+)
3. Menstrual dysfunction (primary amenorrhea, secondary amenorrhea, and oligomenorrhea)	(+)
4. Gastrointestinal complaints	(+)
5. Absence of medical illness or affective disorder explaining the weight reduction	+
6. Distorted body image	(+)
7. Excessive fear of becoming obese	+
8. Restriction of food (<1200 kcal/day)	+
9. Use of purging methods (self-induced vomiting, laxatives, diuretics)	(+)
10. Binge eating	(+)
11. Compulsive exercise	(+)

+: Absolute criteria, (+): relative criteria

Source: Adapted with permission from J Sundgot-Borgen, Risk and Trigger Factors for the Development of Eating Disorders in Female Elite Athletes. *Medicine and Science in Sports and Exercise*, Vol. 4, pp. 414–419, © 1994, Williams and Wilkins.

Male Athletes

Most of the studies on male athletes that have attempted to determine the prevalence of pathologic weight control methods and eating disorders have involved athletes competing in weight-dependent or weight-class sports.

Anorexia nervosa is approximately one-tenth as common in males as it is in females.[24] Studies of the prevalence of bulimic behavior in college students indicate a prevalence of 0% to 5% in males as compared with 5% to 10% in females.[24] However, Andersen[24] argues that more males are afflicted than previously assumed. It is not clear whether the gender differences observed in the general population also exist among athletes, because most studies deal with female athletes only.

Results from existing studies on male athletes indicate that the frequency of eating disturbances and pathologic dieting practices varied from none to 57%, depending on the definition used and the population studied.[8,9,13,25,26]

No studies on male athletes and eating disorders have used the American Psychiatric Association criteria to diagnose male athletes with different degrees of eating disturbances. Therefore, the true prevalence of clinically diagnosed eating disorders is not known. In a study by Blouin and Goldfield,[27] body builders reported significantly greater body dissatisfaction, a high drive for bulk, a high drive for thinness, and increased bulimic tendencies when compared with runners and martial artists. They also reported frequent use of anabolic steroids. The most liberal attitudes toward using steroids were held by body builders with symptoms of an eating disorder.

Sykora et al[13] compared eating, weight, and dieting disturbances among male and female lightweight and heavyweight rowers. Females displayed more disturbed eating and weight-control methods than did males. Male rowers were more affected by weight restriction than were female rowers, probably because they gained more during the off-season. Males of lighter weight showed greater weight fluctuation during the season and gained more weight during the off-season than did females of lighter weight and males and females of heavier weight.

There are many similarities between male athletes and males with eating disorders, including the preoccupation with body size and shape.[28] However, data suggest that male athletes with eating disorders are special cases, even when compared with other male athletes.[28] A number of male athletes tend to have temporary, situation-related symptoms that improve during off-season. For example, those competing in weight-class sports experience frequent and large cycles of weight loss that can have enduring medical consequences. However, most tend to normalize these behaviors when their sport is not in season.[24]

As is true for female athletes, there are insufficient data on male athletes to establish the prevalence of specific problems across sports or across levels of ability within sports. The studies necessary to define causal relationships between athletic participation, personality variables, and eating disturbances in athletes have not been done. Studies are needed in which prevalence is defined in males and females in the same sports at equivalent levels of training and competition. A summary of the studies conducted to date have been presented previously.[29]

Despite the methodologic weaknesses, existing studies are consistent in showing that symptoms of eating disorders and pathogenic weight control methods are more prevalent in female athletes than nonathletes, and more prevalent in sports in which leanness or a specific weight are considered important, than among athletes competing in sports where these factors are considered less important.[6,9–12,14,30–32]

RISK FACTORS FOR THE DEVELOPMENT OF EATING DISORDERS

Psychological, biologic, and social factors are implicated in the development of eating disorders.[33,34] Personality, hunger intensity, and activity level contribute to the psychological predisposition. Social factors, especially the cultural phenomenon of equating thinness with success in women, may also contribute.[35] It has been claimed that female athletes appear to be more vulnerable to eating disorders than the general female population, because of additional stresses associated with the athletic environment.[14,36] There are some factors within the sport

setting that seem to function as risk or trigger factors for the development of eating disorders.

The Attraction to Sport Hypothesis

It has been suggested that sport or specific sports attract persons who are anorexic before commencing their participation in sports.[17] These persons seem to use or abuse exercise to expend extra calories or to justify their abnormal eating and dieting behavior. Others have suggested that many persons who are anorexic are attracted to sports in which they can hide their illness.[37] Those athletes are representing the recreational part of athletics and will rarely be found among the elite athletes.

Exercise and the Inducement of Eating Disorders

A bio-behavioral model of activity-based anorexia nervosa was proposed in a series of studies by Epling and Pierce[38] and Epling et al.[39] They suggest that dieting and exercising initiate the anorexic cycle. Specifically, they contend that strenuous exercise tends to suppress appetite, which serves to decrease the value of food reinforcement. As a result, food intake decreases, while the motivation for more exercise increases.

A recent study reported that some elite endurance athletes with eating disorders could not give any specific reason why they developed an eating disorder.[23] However, many reported that with a sudden increase in training volume, a significant amount of weight was lost, and anorexia nervosa or anorexia athletica developed.[23] Costill[40] found that some athletes who increased their training volume experienced caloric deprivation. Furthermore, it has been claimed that appetite may be truly diminished, in part as a result of changes in endorphin levels.[41] Thus, it has been speculated that the increased training load may induce a caloric deprivation in endurance athletes, which in turn may elicit biologic and social reinforcements leading to the development of eating disorders.[23] Data from a study by

Brownell et al[29] indicated that the degree of training intensity plays a significant role in the development of eating disorders for male runners. However, not all persons with anorexia nervosa exercise. Thus, longitudinal studies with close monitoring of the volume, type, and intensity of the training of athletes representing different sports are needed before the question about the role played by different sports in the development of eating disorders can be answered.

Early Start of Sport-Specific Training

It is claimed that a person's natural body type inherently steers the athlete to an appropriate sport.[42] However, a number of athletes start sport-specific training at prepubertal age and may, therefore, not be able to choose the sport most suitable for their adult body type. Athletes with eating disorders have been shown to start sport-specific training at an earlier age than athletes who do not meet the criteria for eating disorders.[23]

Hamilton et al[30] suggested that dancers who have undergone a stringent process of early selection (girls who are enrolled during late childhood and where rigid standards for weight, body shape, and technique must be constantly met) may be more naturally suited to the thin body image demanded by ballet directors, and, therefore, are less at risk.

Dieting and Body-Weight Cycle

Athletes reduce body weight for several reasons, including to compete in a lower weight class, to improve aesthetic appearance, or to increase physical performance.[23] Most athletes in weight-class events compete in a class below their natural body weight. Reduction of body weight is considered necessary, because failure to "make weight" results in disqualification from competition. Also, a reduction of body weight and fat mass is considered advantageous in the aesthetic sports. Extra weight is thought to impair performance and detract from appearance

in the eyes of judges. Finally, a reduced body weight and relative fat mass are expected to increase physical performance capacity. This is the predominant reason for body-weight reduction in endurance sports such as running, cross-country skiing, road cycling, and jumping events for height or distance. Improved physical ability might also be an additional argument behind body-weight reduction in weight-class and aesthetic sports.

Weight cycling usually occurs in athletes who wish to keep weight at a certain level, but have difficulty accomplishing this. An example may be a gymnast who wishes to have a low weight to get the best score from the judges. During the off-season, weight increases and restricted eating or additional exercise may be necessary to restore the desired weight. Such athletes frequently engage in cycles where they keep their body weight low for periods, but then gain weight because of their restraint weakness or when physiologic processes seek to restore a higher body weight.[29] In addition to the pressure to reduce weight, athletes are often pressed for time and they have to lose weight rapidly to make or stay on the team. As a result, they often experience frequent periods of restrictive dieting or weight cycling.[23] Such periods have been suggested as important risk or trigger factors for the development of eating disorders in athletes.[23,42] Little information is available on the physiologic adaptation of athletes who have restricted their diet or have experienced weight cycling over a period.

Personality Factors

The characteristics of a sport (for example, emphasis on leanness or individual competition) may interact with the personality traits of the athlete to start and perpetuate an eating disorder.[43] Some of the personality traits exhibited by athletes in general are similar to traits manifested by many patients with eating disorders. For example, both groups tend to be characterized by high self-expectation, perfectionism, persistence, and independence.[44] It may be that these qualities, which enable these persons to succeed in sports, also place athletes more at risk of developing eating disorders.[44] Williamson et al[45] concluded that eating disorders in collegiate athletes are multidetermined, and several risk factors must occur during the same time to cause overconcern with body size and shape, which in turn leads to pathologic eating, dieting, and purgative habits.

Traumatic Events

Some athletes with eating disorders who experience a significant weight loss without intending to lose weight report that they had lost their coach or changed coaches before the weight-loss period.[23] These athletes describe their coaches as being vital to their future athletic career. Other athletes have reported that they developed eating disorders as a result of an injury or illness that left them temporarily unable to continue their normal level of exercise, as previously described by Katz.[41]

Injured athletes are also likely to become depressed. If they are predisposed to have an eating disorder, this depression can play a role in the development of the disorder in at least two ways. First, depression often changes a person's eating patterns by increasing or decreasing appetite and caloric intake. Second, the athlete could use the eating disorder in an attempt to manage depression.[17]

Thus, the loss of a coach or unexpected illness or injury can probably be regarded as traumatic events similar to those described as trigger mechanisms for eating disorders in non-athletes.[18]

The Impact of Coaches and Trainers

Pressure to reduce weight has been the general explanation for the increased prevalence of eating disorders among athletes. When an athlete is not performing as well as a coach believes he or she should, the coach will look for an explanation and a solution. Unfortunately, many coaches decide to have an athlete lose weight

based only on how the athlete looks and what the scale reads when the athlete is weighed. In this case, the athlete may lose weight, but not increase performance.[17,20] A number of investigations report that athletes started dieting after coaches had advised a reduction in weight.[12] Many of these athletes are young and extremely impressionable. For them such a recommendation could be seen as a necessary step to achieve success in their sport. Rosen and Hough[11] reported that 75% of young athletes who were told by their coaches that they were too heavy started using pathologic weight loss methods. However, they did not report how many of these young athletes actually developed eating disorders. In a study comparing athletes with eating disorders with those not suffering from eating disorders, results showed that among those who had been told to lose weight, but had not developed eating disorders, 75% had received guidance during the weight loss, as compared with 10% of those who had developed eating disorders.[23] Therefore, it is not necessarily dieting per se, but whether the athlete receives guidance or not, that is important.

A few studies have examined the educational level among athletes, coaches, and athletic trainers.[19,46,47] Findings indicate that too few of the coaches have a formal education in sport and that they lack knowledge in the area of weight control and nutrition.[19,46,47]

Rules

Health care personnel and representatives of those sports-governing bodies where eating disorders are known to be a problem should examine the rules and regulations of their sport. Age for participation in international competitions, a certain percent body fat, rules, judging procedures, and coaching standards should be evaluated to determine if changes could diminish the pressure on athletes to strive for unrealistic and dangerously low body weights. Coaches and athletes should be educated about the dangers of eating disorders and the importance of good nutrition, and the rigorous weight standards imposed on athletes in some sports needs to be addressed. Eating disorders will always be a problem in young athletes involved in sports where weight and leanness are considered important for performance, unless age and body-fat limits for participation are introduced.

MEDICAL ISSUES

Eating disorders can result in serious medical problems and even be fatal. Often, signs and symptoms of eating disorders are ignored until serious medical damage has occurred.[17] Whereas most complications of anorexia nervosa occur as a direct or indirect result of starvation, complications of bulimia nervosa occur as a result of binge-eating and purging.[17] Hsu,[48] Johnson and Connor,[49] and Mitchell[50] provide information about the medical problems patients with eating disorders encounter. Studies have reported mortality rates from less than 1% to as high as 18% in persons with anorexia nervosa in the general population.[17] Regardless of how mortality is measured, death is usually attributable to fluid and electrolyte abnormalities or suicide.[79] Mortality in bulimia nervosa is less well-studied, but deaths do occur, usually secondary to the complications of the binge-purging cycle or from suicide. Mortality rates of athletes with eating disorders are not known.

For years, athletes have used and abused drugs to control weight.[17] Some athletes use dieting, bingeing, vomiting, sweating, and fluid restriction for weight control. It is clear that many of these behaviors exist on a continuum and may present health hazards for the athlete. Laxatives are probably the type of drug most commonly abused by athletes with weight and eating disorders. From 4% to 75% of athletes[23] reportedly abuse laxatives. Abuse of laxatives is an ineffective method of weight loss, because the weight loss that occurs is due to temporary fluid loss rather than prevention of caloric absorption.[29] Long-term high-dose abuse of various diet pills is infrequently reported among athletes. The normal fluctuation in weight during the menstrual cycle or a pressure to reduce

weight fast can lead to initiation of diuretic use.[23] It should be noted that diet pills often contain drugs in the stimulant class, and that both these and diuretics are banned by the International Olympic Committee (IOC) as doping agents.

IDENTIFYING ATHLETES WITH EATING DISORDERS

Most persons with anorexia nervosa or anorexia athletica do not realize that they have a problem, and, therefore, do not seek treatment on their own. These athletes might consider seeking help only if they see that their performance is leveling off. Usually, a coach or parent will call and ask how to approach the problem. Physical and psychological characteristics listed in Exhibits 11–5 and 11–6 may indicate the presence of anorexia nervosa or anorexia athletica.

Most athletes suffering from bulimia nervosa are at or near normal weight. Athletes with bulimia usually try to hide their disorder until they feel that they are out of control, or when they realize that the disorder negatively affects sport performance. Therefore, the team staff must be able to recognize the physical symptoms and psychological characteristics listed in Exhibits 11–7 and 11–8. The presence of some of these characteristics does not necessarily indicate the presence of the disorder. However, the likelihood of the disorder being present increases as the number of characteristics increases.[17]

THE EFFECT OF EATING DISORDERS ON ATHLETIC PERFORMANCE

The effect of eating disorders on athletic performance is influenced by the severity and chronicity of the eating disorder and the demands of the sport. For example, anorexia nervosa will probably have different effects on an endurance athlete such as a distance runner than on an athlete in a less aerobic sport such as gymnastics.

A number of studies have shown that both athletic control subjects and athletes suffering from eating disorders who need to keep lean to improve performance consume surprisingly low

Exhibit 11–5 Physical Symptoms of Athletes with Anorexia Nervosa or Anorexia Athletica

1. Significant weight loss beyond that necessary for adequate sport performance
2. Amenorrhea or menstrual dysfunction
3. Dehydration
4. Fatigue beyond that normally expected during training or competition
5. Gastrointestinal problems (for example, constipation, diarrhea, bloating, postprandial distress)
6. Hyperactivity
7. Hypothermia
8. Bradycardia
9. Lanugo
10. Muscle weakness
11. Overuse injuries
12. Reduced bone mineral density
13. Stress fractures

Source: Adapted with permission from RA Thompson and R Trattner-Sherman, *Helping Athletes with Eating Disorders,* © 1993, Human Kinetics.

Exhibit 11–6 Psychological and Behavioral Characteristics of Athletes with Anorexia Nervosa and Anorexia Athletica

1. Anxiety, both related and unrelated to sport performance
2. Avoidance of eating and eating situations
3. Claims of "feeling fat" despite being thin
4. Resistance to weight gain or maintenance recommended by sport support staff
5. Unusual weighing behavior (for example, excessive weighing, refusal to weigh, negative reaction to being weighed)
6. Compulsiveness and rigidity, especially about eating and exercise
7. Excessive or obligatory exercise beyond that required for a particular sport
8. Exercising while injured despite prohibitions by medical and training staff
9. Restlessness—relaxing is difficult or impossible
10. Social withdrawal from teammates and sport support staff, as well as from people outside sports
11. Depression
12. Insomnia

Source: Data from RA Thompson and R Trattner-Sherman, *Helping Athletes with Eating Disorders,* © 1993, Human Kinetics; and J Sundgot-Borgen, Risk and Trigger Factors for the Development of Eating Disorders in Female Elite Athletes, *Medicine and Science in Sports and Exercise,* Vol. 4, pp. 414–419, © 1994, Williams & Wilkins.

amounts of calories.[50–52] Athletes with eating disorders, except for some of the athletes with bulimia nervosa, consume diets low in energy and key nutrients.[20]

Athletes know that the quickest way to lose weight is by losing body water. Water is essential for the regulation of body temperature, and a dehydrated athlete becomes overheated and fatigued more easily. It has been shown that loss of endurance and coordination due to dehydration impairs exercise performance.[18,20]

Reduced plasma volume, impaired thermoregulation and nutrient exchange, decreased glycogen availability, and decreased buffer capacity in the blood are plausible explanations for reduced performance in aerobic, anaerobic, and muscle endurance work, especially after rapid weight reduction.

Absolute maximal oxygen uptake (measured as 1 per minute) is unchanged or decreased after rapid body-weight loss, but maximal oxygen uptake expressed in relation to body weight (mL per kg body weight per minute) may increase after gradual body-weight reduction.[53,54] Anaerobic performance and muscle strength are typically decreased after rapid weight reduction with or without 1 to 3 hours of rehydration. When tested after 5 to 24 hours of rehydration, performance is maintained at euhydrated levels.[55,56]

The long-term effects of body-weight reduction and eating disorders in athletes are not clear. Biologic maturation and growth have been studied in female gymnasts before and during puberty: There are sufficient data to conclude that young female gymnasts are smaller and mature

Exhibit 11–7 Physical Symptoms of Athletes With Bulimia Nervosa

1. Callus or abrasion of back of hand from inducing vomiting
2. Dehydration, especially in the absence of training or competition
3. Dental and gum problems
4. Edema, complaints of bloating, or both
5. Electrolyte abnormalities
6. Frequent and often extreme weight fluctuations
7. Gastrointestinal problems
8. Low weight despite eating large volumes
9. Menstrual irregularity
10. Muscle cramps, weakness, or both
11. Swollen parotid glands

Adapted with permission from RA Thompson and R Trattner-Sherman, *Helping Athletes with Eating Disorders*, © 1993, Human Kinetics.

Exhibit 11–8 Psychological and Behavioral Characteristics of Athletes with Bulimia Nervosa

1. Binge eating
2. Agitation when bingeing is interrupted
3. Depression
4. Dieting that is unnecessary for appearance, health, or sport performance
5. Evidence of vomiting unrelated to illness
6. Excessive exercise beyond that required for the athlete's sport
7. Excessive use of the restroom
8. Going to the restroom or "disappearing" after eating
9. Self-critical, especially concerning body, weight, and sport performance
10. Secretive eating
11. Substance abuse—legal, illegal, prescribed, or over-the-counter drugs, medications, or other substances
12. Use of laxatives, diuretics (or both) that is unsanctioned by medical or training staff

Source: Adapted with permission from RA Thompson and R Trattner-Sherman, *Helping Athletes with Eating Disorders*, © 1993, Human Kinetics.

later than similar females from sports that do not require extreme leanness (for example, swimming).[57,58] It is, however, difficult to separate the effects of physical strain, energy restriction, and genetic predisposition to delayed puberty.

Besides increasing the likelihood of stress fractures, early bone loss may prevent achievement of normal peak bone mass. Thus, after the typical period after menopause, former athletes who once had frequent or longer periods of amenorrhea may again be at high risk of sustaining fractures.

The psychological and medical features and consequences of eating disorders among athletes and nonathletes have been described and discussed in detail elsewhere.[17,29,41] Abnormal laboratory findings and characteristic endocrine abnormalities of eating disorders are discussed by Katz.[41]

A drawback in studies on body-weight reduction in athletes is that the relationship between performance test results and actual competitive performance are not clear.[53] Most investigators have used athletes in weight-class events as study participants. More longitudinal data on gradual body-weight reduction in endurance athletes and aesthetic sports are clearly needed.

CASE HISTORIES

Female Athlete with Anorexia Nervosa

Anne was a 22-year-old international-level cross-country skier (168 cm, 47 kg, 8% body fat). She initially presented for treatment with menstrual dysfunction (amenorrhea for the last 2 years). She met all the DSM-IV[19] criteria for anorexia nervosa. When asked in the initial session about her eating, she denied any difficulty, but she was thin and claimed that the weight loss was related to an increase in training volume during the last year. When asked to do a 7-day-weight registration, she admitted that she was following a restricted regimen of vegetables and grains, about 800 kcal daily. She ate only at specific times, usually the same three or four foods each day. During this period, she trained 4 hours each day, skiing, running, and weight-training. She and her coach both believed that she could perform better at her present weight. She had started dieting 3 years earlier, and Anne enhanced her performance level during the first season despite the restricted eating, and used her sport to rationalize her training and eating regimens the following years. She developed a stress fracture 1 month before consultation (possibly due to 3 years of menstrual dysfunction), and had difficulty following the alternate training plan designed by the team's physical therapist. The coach was informed that his athlete was actually suffering from an eating disorder, and therefore not allowed to compete. The reason Anne developed an eating disorder was the intense wish to enhance performance. Because no deep psychological trauma could explain her eating disorder, a psychologist was not included in the treatment team from the beginning. The nutritionist, her coach, and Anne carefully planned her eating and training schedule. To resume menses and reduce the risk of further loss of bone mass, a gynecologist prescribed oral contraceptives. Anne reduced her training from 12 hours a week to 6 hours, using non-weight-bearing activities. After 2 months, her energy intake was above 1300 kcal, and she gradually increased weight. At present, 6 months after the initial consultation, she is still improving, but struggling with the reduced training load and her fear of losing control of her eating behavior.

Male Athlete with Bulimia Nervosa

Erik was an 18-year-old ski jumper (172 cm, 60 kg). He sought treatment, reporting that he had been bingeing and purging 3 to 16 times a week for the last 2 years. He met all the DSM-IV[19] criteria for bulimia nervosa. He had no doubt that the demand to "make ideal weight" for ski jumping was the precipitating factor in his disorder. Before his involvement in competitive ski jumping, he had no concerns about his weight and had never dieted. To make weight,

Erik usually restricted his diet to about 800 kcal, induced vomiting, and used extreme amounts of laxatives. The reason for seeking treatment was that he had experienced fatigue and cramps during the last season, and his coach claimed that he was not as focused as usual. Because his eating behavior was extremely chaotic, he was referred to a cognitive treatment therapist who worked closely with the sports nutritionist. Erik had to relearn what, how much, and when to eat. The nutritionist followed the treatment plan suggested by Clark.[59] Erik is still in treatment. He has learned how to be more at peace with himself and with food. He still fights the urge to binge, but he is improving.

TREATMENT OF EATING DISORDERS

Once coaches, teammates, or health care staff members suspect that an athlete has an eating problem, questions about referral and arrangement for treatment, implementation of the therapeutic regimen, monitoring of specific therapeutic strategies, and arranging for follow-up should arise.[17] Qualified health care professionals should treat athletes with eating disorders. Ideally, these persons should also be familiar with, and have an appreciation for, the sport environment.[17,59] Because most patients suffering from eating disorders are female, the patient will be referred to as she.

It is more threatening for athletes with bulimia nervosa or bulimic symptoms to admit they have an eating disorder than for those suffering from anorexia nervosa or anorexia athletica. Many athletes with bulimic symptoms have binged and purged for years, and regard their disorder as a disgusting habit.

Athletes with eating disorders usually resist treatment until they reach a point of despair.[59] Usually, athletes are more likely to accept the idea of receiving a consultation than committing to ongoing treatment. An appointment for an evaluation should be made as soon as possible because the athlete's fear and ambivalence about treatment may make her change her mind if given the opportunity.[17] Getting the athlete to accept a referral for an evaluation is sometimes a significant accomplishment in itself, but getting her to then participate in formal treatment may be another challenge. However, if the presence of an eating disorder is confirmed during the evaluation, then the specialist providing the evaluation can play a major role in convincing the athlete of the need for treatment and can begin to motivate her to get treatment.[17]

The success of the treatment plan must be based on establishing a trusting relationship between the athlete and the care providers. This includes respecting the athlete's desire to be lean for athletic performance, and expressing a willingness to work together to help the athlete be lean and healthy. The treatment team needs to listen to the athlete's fears and irrational thoughts about food and weight, then present a rational approach for achieving self-management of healthy diet and weight.[59]

Refusal of Medical Examination

If the athlete does not accept the initial referral or does not even admit that a problem exists, it is probably best not to push too hard at this point unless you believe the athlete is at risk medically. At this point, it is important to schedule a medical examination. If she continues to refuse this examination, close observation is required until she is willing to undergo a medical examination. If the athlete is underweight, give her information concerning a healthier weight. Ask her if she is having difficulty sleeping; if she is feeling depressed, weak, tired, or irritable; if her menstrual cycle has ceased; and if her performance level has decreased. If she admits to these problems, suggest that they may all be related to her eating or weight-control behavior. The consequence of refusing medical examination must be decided for each athlete depending on the severity and the athlete's situation.

Suspension from sports is a good solution only for a few cases. Those athletes who really want to continue at a competitive level in their sport will often, if denied, train on their own, which in some cases may be more dangerous because no one will be monitoring their exercise. Denying the athlete participation in her

sport may further reduce her self-esteem. She may view the suspension as an attempt by others to control.[17]

The athlete's family may be involved in the process of getting the athlete to receive treatment. One factor affecting this involvement is the athlete's age—the younger the athlete, the more the family's involvement is recommended. Certainly, one would anticipate more involvement with younger athletes.[17]

Treatment for an eating disorder can involve either inpatient or outpatient treatment, or both. The decision about the appropriate treatment mode for the athlete is usually made by the professional health care providers involved in her care. Generally, most persons with anorexia nervosa require at least some inpatient treatment, although the health care provider may try outpatient treatment if the person's weight is stable and not extremely low and she is not purging.[48] Conversely, most persons with anorexia athletica and bulimia nervosa can and should be treated on an outpatient basis.[50]

Types of Treatment

Typically, treatment regimens include individual psychotherapy and group and family therapy. Nutritional counseling and, for some cases, pharmacotherapy are often included as adjuncts to the treatment regimen. The combination of cognitive behavior treatment and nutritional counseling is effective for motivated athletes.

Group treatment can benefit the athlete in many ways. An athlete often discovers that she is not alone, that others have a similar problem. It gives her a support group that understands her feelings and eating problem. Group therapy provides a safe environment for the athlete to practice the new skills and attitudes she has learned.[17]

Nutritional Counseling

Nutritional counseling is often part of a multimodal treatment approach. Most athletes and nonathletes with eating disorders report that the onset of their eating disorder was preceded by a period of dieting. Apart from the binge eating, most of the patients with bulimia as well as patients with anorexia athletica and anorexia nervosa show a restrictive eating pattern: 80% of nonathletes with bulimia and 29% of athletes with eating disorders eat one meal or less a day.[20] Most of the athletes with eating disorders have practiced abnormal eating behaviors, and their attitudes about eating are often based on myths and misconceptions. Persons with eating disorders do not remember what constitutes a balanced meal or "normal" eating. Therefore, the major roles for the nutritionist seem to be an evaluator, nutrition educator and counselor, behavior manager, and active member of the treatment team.

The aims of a nutritional counseling program should be the following: 1) to enable the patient to understand principles of good nutrition, her nutritional needs as an athlete, and the relationships between restrictive eating and overeating and 2) to learn regular eating and maintain a regular pattern of eating through meal planning.

Treatment Goals and Expectations

Athletes have the same general concerns as nonathletes about increasing their weight, but they also have concerns from a sport standpoint. What they think is an ideal competitive weight, one that they believe helps them be successful in their sport, may be significantly lower than their treatment goal weight. As a result, athletes may have concerns about their ability to perform in their sport after treatment.

It may take months or years to recover from an eating disorder. Generally, anorexia nervosa requires a longer treatment time than bulimia nervosa. For athletes to complete treatment successfully, they must be able to trust the persons involved in managing and treating their difficulties.

Most athletes with eating disorders are willing to allow a coach or other support staff only minimal contact with the therapist. Others want the coach involved and view this as evidence of caring and concern on the part of the coach.

Teammates of an athlete with an eating disorder are often aware of the problem and may also know that the athlete is receiving treatment. However, information about the athlete with an eating disorder should be handled as the athlete desires. Some athletes may not want their parents to know about their disorder. Therapists cannot release information even to parents without the athlete's consent, except under special circumstances and in the case of minors.

Training and Competition

Once an athlete has been evaluated and the health care professionals have determined that she needs treatment, several issues that relate to training and competition arise. The most important question is whether the athlete should be allowed to continue to train and compete while recovering from the disorder. The athlete who is being considered for continuing training and competition while in treatment must undergo extensive medical and psychological evaluations. These evaluations must indicate that the athlete is not at risk medically and that competition will not increase her risk either medically or psychologically.[17] According to Thompson and Trattner-Sherman,[17] athletes should maintain a weight of no less than 90% of health-related "ideal" weight. The athlete should eat at least three balanced meals a day, consisting of enough calories to sustain the preestablished weight standard the dietitian has proposed. Females who have been amenorrheic for 6 months or more should undergo a gynecologic examination for hormone-replacement therapy to be considered. In addition, bone mineral density should be assessed and results should be within normal range.

Usually, training needs to be restricted and competition not allowed. However, this will also depend on the type of sport, the competitive level, and the athlete's general situation.

Health Maintenance Standards

If the athlete meets the criteria just mentioned, the bottom-line standards about health maintenance must be imposed to protect the athlete. The treatment staff determines these and individually tailors them according to the athlete's particular condition. These standards may vary among athletes or by sport.

The following list represents the minimal criteria for the athlete to continue competition and training: (1) The athlete must agree to comply with all treatment strategies as best she can. (2) The athlete must genuinely want to compete. (3) The athlete must be closely monitored on an ongoing basis by the medical and psychological health care professionals handling her treatment and by the sport-related personnel who are working with her in her sport. (4) Treatment must always take precedence over sport. (5) If any question arises at any time about whether the athlete is meeting or is able to meet the preceding criteria, competition is not to be considered a viable option while the athlete is receiving treatment.[17]

Athletes Receiving Treatment

Continuing training and competition could have advantages for some athletes. Some athletes will be motivated to receive treatment by the opportunity to continue training. Being allowed to train or compete is a source of wellbeing or self-esteem for these athletes.[17]

However, sport may play such a significant role in the eating disorder that the athlete's participation in sport may help to maintain or perpetuate it. In addition, allowing an athlete to compete while affected by an eating disorder may give her the message that sport performance is more important than her health.

PREVENTION OF EATING DISORDERS IN ATHLETES

Early intervention is important, because eating disorders are more difficult to treat the longer they progress. However, most important of all is the prevention of circumstances or factors that could lead to an eating disorder. Therefore, professionals working with athletes should

be informed about the possible risk factors for the development, early signs, and symptoms of eating disorders; the medical, psychological, and social consequences of these disorders; how to approach the problem if it occurs; and what treatment options are available. This improves awareness and facilitates early detection and intervention.

Coaches should realize that they can strongly influence their athletes. Coaches or others involved with young athletes should not comment on an athlete's body size, or require a young athlete who is still growing to lose weight. Without further guidance, dieting may result in unhealthy eating behavior or eating disorders in athletes who are highly motivated but uninformed.

Weight-Loss Recommendation

Most athletes have an ideal body composition for their sport. A change in body composition and weight loss can be achieved safely if the weight goal is realistic and based on body composition rather than weight-for-height standards. Use of the skinfold appraisal techniques is recommended, because of the large time and equipment demands required when using hydrostatic weighing. Coaches should not be involved in the weight or nutrition issues. Coaches should not have access to the results of the different measures included in the evaluation of the athlete's body composition and documentation of the possible need for changes. One person who specializes in this area should be the one responsible for determining the suggested range of percent body fat that would be ideal for the athlete in question. Recommendations for safe weight loss in athletes have been discussed elsewhere.[60]

CONCLUSION

The prevalence of subclinical and clinical eating disorders is higher among athletes than nonathletes, but the relationship to performance or training level is unknown. Additionally, athletes competing in sports where leanness and a specific weight are considered important are more prone to eating disorders than athletes competing in sports where these factors are considered less important. Therefore, it is necessary to examine anorexia nervosa, bulimia nervosa, and subclinical eating disorders and the range of behaviors and attitudes associated with eating disturbances in athletes to learn how these clinical and subclinical disorders are related.

Only qualified health care professionals should treat athletes with eating disorders. Ideally, these persons should also be familiar with, and have an appreciation for, the sport environment.

Sport nutritionists have an important role in the prevention and treatment of subclinical and clinical eating disorders.

REFERENCES

1. Gull W. Anorexia nervosa (apepsia hysterica, anorexia hysterica). *Trans Clin Soc Lond.* 1874;7:22–28.
2. Russell G. Bulimia nervosa: an ominous of anorexia nervosa. *Psychol Med.* 1979;9:429–448.
3. Tipton CM, Theng TK, Paul WD. Evaluation of the Hall methods for determining minimal wrestling weights. *J Iowa Med Soc.* 1969;59:571-574.
4. American College of Sports Medicine. Position stand on weight loss in wrestlers. *Med Sci Sports Exerc.* 1976;8:XI–XIII.
5. American Medical Association. Committee on the Medical Aspects of Sports. Wrestling and weight control. *JAMA.* 1967;201:541-543.
6. Sundgot-Borgen J. Prevalence of eating disorders in female elite athletes. *Int J Sport Nutr.* 1993;3:29–40.
7. Gadpalle WJ, Sandborn CF, Wagner WW. Athletic amenorrhea, major affective disorders and eating disorders. *Am J Psychiatry.* 1987;144:939–943.
8. Burckes-Miller ME, Black DR. Male and female college athletes. Prevalence of anorexia nervosa and bulimia nervosa. *Athletic Training.* 1988;2:137–140.
9. Dummer GM, Rosen LW, Heusner WW, et al. Pathogenic weight-control behaviors of young competitive swimmers. *Physician Sportsmed.* 1987;5:75–76.
10. Hamilton LH, Brocks-Gunn J, Warren MP. Sociocultural influences on eating disorders in professional female ballet dancers. *Int J Eat Disord.* 1985;4:465–477.
11. Rosen LW, Hough DO. Pathogenic weight-control behaviors of female college gymnasts. *Physician Sportsmed.* 1988;9:141–144.
12. Smith NJ. Excessive weight loss and food aversion in athletes simulating anorexia nervosa. *Pediatrics.* 1980;1:109–113.
13. Sykora C, Grilo CM, Wilfly DE, Brownell KD. Eating, weight, and dieting disturbances in male and female lightweight and heavyweight rowers. *Int J Eat Disord.* 1993;2:203–211.
14. Wilmore JH. Eating and weight disorders in female athletes. *Int J Sport Nutr.* 1991;1:104–117.
15. American Psychiatric Association. *Diagnostic and Statistical Manual of Mental Disorders 3rd ed.* Washington, DC: American Psychiatric Association; 1987:65–69.
16. Szmuckler GI, Eisler I, Gillies C, Hayward ME. The implications of anorexia nervosa in a ballet school. *J Psychiatr Res.* 1985;19:177–181.
17. Thompson RA, Trattner-Sherman R. *Helping Athletes with Eating Disorders.* Champaign, IL: Human Kinetics; 1993.
18. Bassoe HH. Anorexia/bulimia nervosa: The development of anorexia nervosa and of mental symptoms. Treatment and the outcome of the disease. *Acta Psychiatr Scand;* 1990;82:7–13.
19. American Psychiatric Association. *Diagnostic and Statistical Manual of Mental Disorders.* 4th ed. Washington, DC: American Psychiatric Association; 1994:1–2.
20. Sundgot-Borgen J, Larsen S. Nutrient intake and eating behavior of female elite athletes suffering from anorexia nervosa, anorexia athletica and bulimia nervosa. *Int J Sport Nutr.* 1993;3:431–442.
21. Pugliese MT, Lifshitz F, Grad G, Fort P, Marks-Katz M. Fear of obesity. A cause of short stature and delayed puberty. *N Engl J Med.* 1983;309:513–518.
22. Warren BJ, Stanton AL, Blessing DL. Disordered eating patterns in competitive female athletes. *Int J Eat Disord.* 1990;5:565–569.
23. Sundgot-Borgen J. Risk and trigger factors for the development of eating disorders in female elite athletes. *Med Sci Sports Exerc.* 1994;4:414–419.
24. Andersen AE. Diagnosis and treatment of males with eating disorders. In: Andersen AE, ed. *Males with Eating Disorders.* New York: Brunner/Mazel; 1990:133–162.
25. Rucinski A. Relationship of body image and dietary intake of competitive ice skaters. *J Am Diet Assoc.* 1989;89:98–100.
26. Steen SN, Brownell KD. Current patterns of weight loss and regain in wrestlers: Has the tradition changed? *Med Sci Sports Exerc.* 1990;22:762–768.

27. Blouin AG, Goldfield GS. Body image and steroid use in male bodybuilders. *Int J Eat Disord.* 1995;2:159–165.

28. Andersen AE. Eating disorders in males: a special case. In: Brownell KD, Rodin J, Wilmore JH, eds. *Eating, Body Weight and Performance in Athletes. Disorders of Modern Society.* Philadelphia: Lea & Febiger; 1992;172–188.

29. Brownell KD, Rodin J, Wilmore JH. Prevalence of eating disorders in athletes. In: Brownell KD, Rodin J, Wilmore JH, eds. *Eating, Body Weight and Performance in Athletes. Disorders of Modern Society.* Philadelphia: Lea & Febiger; 1992;128–143.

30. Hamilton LH, Brocks-Gunn J, Warren MP, Hamilton WG. The role of selectivity in the pathogenesis of eating problems in ballet dancers. *Med Sci Sports Exerc.* 1988;20:560–565.

31. Rosen LW, McKeag DB, Hough DO. Pathogenic weight-control behaviors in female athletes. *Physician Sportsmed.* 1986;14:79–86.

32. Sundgot-Borgen J, Corbin CB. Eating disorders among female athletes. *Physician Sportsmed.* 1987;15(2):89–95.

33. Garfinkel PE, Garner DM, Goldbloom, DS. Eating disorders: implications for the 1990s. *Can J Psychiatry.* 1987;32:624–631.

34. Katz JL. Some reflections on the nature of the eating disorders. *Int J Eat Disord.* 1985;4:617–626.

35. Garner DM, Olmsted MP, Polivy J. *Manual of Eating Disorder Inventory.* Odessa: Psychological Assessment Resources; 1984.

36. Clifton EJ. Eating disorders in female athletes: identification and management. *Kentucky AHPERD J.* 1991;1:30–32.

37. Sacks MH. Psychiatry and sports. *Ann Sports Med.* 1990;5:47–52.

38. Epling WF, Pierce WD. Activity based anorexia nervosa. *Int J Eat Disord.* 1988;7:475–485.

39. Epling WF, Pierce WD, Stefan L. A theory of activity based anorexia. *Int J Eat Disord.* 1983;3:27–46.

40. Costill DL. Carbohydrate for exercise: dietary demands for optimal performance. *Int J Sports Med.* 1988;9:1–18.

41. Katz JL. Eating disorders in women and exercise. In: Shangold and Mirken, eds. *Physiology and Sports Medicine.* Philadelphia: Davis Company; 1988;248–263.

42. Brownell KD, Steen SN, Wilmore JH. Weight regulation practices in athletes: analysis of metabolic and health effects. *Med Sci Sports Exerc.* 1987;6:546–556.

43. Wilson T, Eldredge KL. Pathology and development of eating disorders: implications for athletes. In: Brownell

KD, Rodin J, Wilmore JH, eds. *Eating, Body Weight and Performance in Athletes. Disorders of Modern Society.* Philadelphia: Lea & Febiger; 1992:115–127.

44. Yates A. *Compulsive Exercise and Eating Disorders.* New York: Brunner/Mazel; 1991.

45. Williamson DA, Netemeyer RG, Jackman LP, Andersen DA, Funsch CL, Rabalis JY. Structural equation modeling of risks for the development of eating disorder symptoms in female athletes. *Int J Eat Disord.* 1995;4:387–393.

46. Wolf EMB, Wirth JC, Lohman TG. Nutritional practices of coaches in the Big Ten. *Physician Sportsmed.* 1975;2:112–124.

47. Parr RB, Porter MA, Hodgson SC. Nutrient knowledge and practice of coaches, trainers, and athletes. *Physician Sportsmed.* 1984;3:127–138.

48. Hsu LKG. *Eating Disorders.* New York: Guilford Press; 1990.

49. Johnson C, Connor SM. *The Etiology and Treatment of Bulimia Nervosa.* New York: Basic Books; 1987.

50. Mitchell JE. *Bulimia Nervosa.* Minneapolis, MN: University of Minnesota Press; 1990.

51. Erp-Bart AMJ, Fredrix LWHM, Binkhorst RA, et al. Energy intake and energy expenditure in top female gymnasts. In: Brinkhorst, et al (eds). *Children and Exercise XI.* Champaign, IL: University Park Press; 1985:218–223.

52. Welch PK, Zager KA, Endres J. Nutrition education, body composition and dietary intake for female college athletes. *Physician Sportsmed.* 1987;15:63–74.

53. Fogelholm M. Effects of bodyweight reduction on sports performance. *Sports Med.* 1994;4:249–267.

54. Ingjer F, Sundgot-Borgen J. Influence of body weight reduction on maximal oxygen uptake in female elite athletes. *Scand J Med Sci Sports.* 1991;1:141–146.

55. Klinzing JE, Karpowicz W. The effect of rapid weight loss and rehydration on a wrestling performance test. *J Sports Med Phys Fitness.* 1986;26:149–156.

56. Fogelholm GM, Koskinen R, Laakso J. Gradual and rapid weight loss: effects on nutrition and performance in male athletes. *Med Sci Sports Exerc.* 1993;25:371–377.

57. Mansfield MJ, Emans SJ. Growth in female gymnasts: should training decrease during puberty? *Pediatrics.* 1993;122:237–240.

58. Theintz MJ, Howald H, Weiss U. Evidence of a reduction of growth potential in adolescent female gymnasts. *J Pediat.* 1993;122:306–313.

59. Clark N. How to help the athlete with bulimia: practical tips and case study. *Int J Sport Nutr.* 1993;3:450–460.

60. Eisenman PA, Johnson SC, Benson JE. *Coaches' Guide to Nutrition and Weight Control.* 2nd ed. Champaign, IL: Leisure Press; 1990.

CHAPTER 12

Female Athletes and Bone

David L. Nichols and Charlotte F. Sanborn

Despite new therapies and heightened awareness, the consequences of poor bone health have continued to increase in recent years. Osteoporosis now affects almost one out of every two women at some point in their lives. Medical costs are close to $10 billion per year, and approximately 50,000 deaths each year can be attributed to osteoporosis.[1] Osteoporosis has classically been defined as a pathologic condition associated with an increased loss of bone mass, resulting in a greater risk for fractures. The level of bone mass that is necessary to qualify as osteoporotic is still debated. However, the World Health Organization (WHO) has recently defined osteoporosis as a bone mass measurement more than 2.5 standard deviations below the young adult mean.[2] Based on these criteria, the number of U.S. women at risk for fracture is estimated to be 26 million.[3]

Prevention of osteoporosis can be accomplished by maximizing peak bone density and maintaining that bone density. Exercise appears to have positive effects in this regard. Weight-bearing exercise can result in greater bone mass for the active person as compared to an inactive person.[4–10] The positive impact on bone health is seen whether this activity comes in the form of an exercise program, such as walking, running, or weight training, or as part of participation in an athletic program.

Female varsity athletes, because of their training, exercise more, are generally stronger, and have greater lean body mass than the nonathletic female. As a result, they generally have higher bone densities than nonathletic women.[7,11–17] However, female athletes also have a higher incidence of amenorrhea (≤ 3 menses/year) than do nonathletes.[18] A number of studies conducted over the last several years have reported that amenorrheic athletes have lower bone mineral density than those with regular menstrual cycles,[19–21] placing them at an increased risk for osteoporosis both now and in the future.

This chapter will focus on the factors associated with bone health in athletic women and what role these factors may play in either increasing or decreasing bone mineral density (BMD). A brief overview of bone physiology and its role in osteoporosis as well as information on the measurement of bone mineral density is given first.

BONE PHYSIOLOGY

Bone tissue not only provides a support structure for the body but is also the major reserve of calcium and phosphorus.[22] Two main types of bone tissue are known—cortical and trabecular. Cortical or compact bone forms the dense outer wall of bone. Cortical bone comprises almost 80% of the total skeleton whereas trabecular bone makes up the remaining 20%.[22] Trabecular bone, also known as cancellous or spongy bone, can be found at the ends of long bones, within the central core of the shaft, and as the primary component of vertebrae. It is a lacy network of interconnecting rods or plates of bone. Trabecular bone has a much higher surface-to-volume ratio than cortical bone, making it much more metabolically active.[22,23] Cortical bone may be more responsive to weight-bearing or mechanical stress whereas trabecular bone seems to be influenced more by hormonal or metabolic factors.[24] For the three most common sites of osteoporotic fracture, the spine, hip (femoral neck), and wrist (distal radius), trabecular bone composes approximately 50%, 25%, and 80% of each site, respectively.

Changes in bone are the result of the continual process of bone resorption and bone formation known as bone remodeling. There are three types of bone cells that are responsible for the process of remodeling—osteoblasts, osteoclasts, and osteocytes.[22,23] Osteoclasts function in bone resorption by eroding old bone and osteoblasts then form new bone. Osteocytes may mediate the entire process although their exact function is unknown.[22] The remodeling process takes from 14 to 18 weeks to complete. However, the process is usually shortest and occurs with greater frequency in trabecular bone.[22,23] Remodeling is involved in the growth of bone, changes in bone density, and the regulation of calcium levels in the body.

The process of remodeling occurs throughout the life span. Once peak bone mass has been achieved, bone formation generally equals bone resorption (that is, the density of the bone remains unchanged). Peak bone density (or peak bone mass), for most purposes, is defined as the highest amount of bone mass attained during life. The age at which peak bone density is achieved still remains unclear.[25] Peak bone mass has been reported to occur when a person is in his or her 20s or 30s,[26] but other research has suggested it occurs as early as age 18.[27–29] There is the possibility that after growth ceases, resorption slightly exceeds formation, resulting in the decline in bone mass seen with aging. However, as with many things, the age-related decline may be the result of changes in other factors such as exercise or calcium nutrition. Nevertheless, because the rate of the age-related decline in bone

density is apparently the same regardless of the initial BMD, a person may be able to remain above the critical fracture threshold for osteoporosis by maximizing peak bone density. The key influences of peak bone density, other than genetics, are hormonal status, exercise, and calcium.

The accelerated bone loss associated with menopause, and also seen in amenorrheic younger women, clearly establishes the importance of estrogen in maintaining bone mass.[19,20,30–33] The absence of estrogen apparently results in greater resorption of bone by osteoclasts while the rate of bone formation remains unchanged, resulting in decreases in bone mass. Estrogen may also have a direct effect on bone, as estrogen receptors in osteoblasts have been discovered.[34]

The effects of mechanical strain on bone remodeling are not totally understood. However, it appears that when strain is increased, such as with exercise, osteoblast activity is stimulated while osteoclast activity remains at normal levels.[35,36] The result of the greater osteoblast activity would be an increase in bone mineral density. Conversely, during periods of weightlessness or extended bed rest, osteoblast activity decreases and osteoclast activity again remains constant, resulting in decreases in bone density.[37,38]

Calcium is a major component of bone, and more than 99% of the body's calcium is stored in the bone.[39] Calcium is vital to the proper functioning of many physiologic processes, including muscle and heart contractions; therefore, serum calcium levels are tightly regulated. When calcium is unavailable in the blood and is needed elsewhere in the body, it is removed from the bone by osteoclasts.[22,39] When calcium levels are restored, osteoblasts replace calcium in the bone. However, if serum calcium remains low for extended periods, as a result of low dietary calcium or poor absorption, too little bone formation and too much resorption take place, weakening the bones and making them susceptible to fractures.[39] Thus, adequate calcium intake is essential for good bone health. However, monitoring of serum calcium levels or urinary calcium excretion does not appear to be useful in assessing changes in bone turnover or bone density.[40]

Thus, changes in bone mineral density occur as the result of the alteration of the physiologic process of bone remodeling. Osteoporosis develops when bone resorption greatly exceeds formation, causing decreases in BMD. The principal cause of osteoporosis in women is the loss of ovarian function after menopause. However, ovarian dysfunction can also occur in younger women, sometimes as the result of participation in athletics, placing them at risk for osteoporosis as well.

MEASUREMENT OF BONE MINERAL DENSITY

The primary means of assessing changes in bone as a result of exercise or other interventions is to measure bone mineral content (also known as bone mass). Measurements of bone mineral content are generally expressed as the amount of bone mineral (primarily hydroxyapatite) per unit of area, which gives bone mineral density (grams of bone mineral content per square centimeter of bone; g/cm^2). Accurate measurement of bone mineral density is important in any study attempting to determine the factors associated with changes in bone density. During the past 20 years, rapid advances have been made in techniques used for measuring bone mineral density.[25] These advances have resulted in increased precision, less radiation exposure, and the ability to measure fracture-prone sites.[25,41] These methods include quantitative computed tomography (QCT), single and dual photon absorptiometry (SPA, DPA), and single and dual energy X-ray absorptiometry (SXA, DXA). All of these methods are based on the principle of the absorption, or attenuation, by bone, of a collimated radiation beam. The higher the attenuation, the greater the bone mass. Single and dual photon absorptiometry use a radionuclide as the source, whereas QCT, SXA, and DXA use X-rays.[41]

BMD is most often measured in the spine, hip (femoral neck), and wrist, because these are the most common sites for fracture in osteoporosis.

The accuracy of predicting bone density (and fracture risk) at one site based on measurement of BMD at another site is low (50% or less). In addition, amenorrheic athletes have been shown to have normal density in the wrist but significantly low BMD in the spine.[21] Thus, measurement from all three sites is preferable, but minimally from the spine and hip, because consequences of fracture are the highest at these two sites.

Dual energy X-ray absorptiometry is now the most widely used method for determining bone density.[41] This technique uses X-rays emitted at two different energy levels to allow for the distinction of bone tissue from the surrounding soft tissue. With DXA, radiation exposure is very low (less than 5 mrem/scan), measurements of bone mineral density are both more precise and more accurate, and scanning time is considerably less than with any other method.[25,41] With DXA, the patient is recumbent on a scanning table while transmissions from the energy source located beneath the scanning table are recorded with a computer.

A more recent variation on DXA is the peripheral DXA (pDXA). The advantage of pDXA is that it is small and relatively lightweight and can thus be transported much more readily. Therefore, it has the potential to become widely used as a way of measuring bone density outside of the clinical or research setting. Unfortunately, pDXA is limited to measurements of the forearm or calcaneus.

Biochemical markers of bone metabolism are also sometimes used to monitor therapy or progression of bone disease. Although these markers generally show poor correlations with actual measures of bone density ($r = 0.3$ or less), they can be useful for assessing relative rates of bone formation or resorption. The advantage of biochemical markers is that they can detect alterations in bone formation or resorption in a matter of weeks whereas detecting changes in bone mineral density may take several months.[40] Serum markers of bone formation include osteocalcin and bone alkaline phosphatase. These appear to be the most sensitive markers of formation.[42] Bone resorption markers are typically measured in urine samples, with the most widely used being N-telopeptide, C-telopeptide, and deoxypyridinoline. The telopeptides are thought to be more sensitive than deoxypyridinoline.[43] Although biochemical markers appear worthwhile for detecting changes in bone turnover in research studies, the clinical usefulness of any of these markers in monitoring individual patients has been questioned because of their wide day-to-day variability and their lack of any significant association with changes in BMD.[44–47]

RESEARCH ON FEMALE ATHLETES AND BONE MINERAL DENSITY

Participation in athletics has the potential for increasing bone mineral density. Indeed a number of studies, both cross-sectional and longitudinal, have found positive effects on bone health from the training associated with sports participation.[7,11–17] Some of those studies are illustrated in Figures 12–1 and 12–2. However, there is not yet sufficient evidence to suggest that one type of athletic activity produces a better osteogenic effect than another athletic activity. It does appear that those sports that involve a high degree of impact (gymnastics or volleyball) are more beneficial to bone than those sports without impact loading (swimming or cycling).[11,16,48]

Fehling and colleagues[11] compared BMD in female collegiate athletes involved in impact loading sports (volleyball and gymnastics) to those involved in an active loading sport (swimming) and to controls. Gymnasts and volleyball players had 10% to 20% higher BMD at all sites measured as compared to either swimmers or control subjects. The BMD of the swimmers was not different than the control subjects'.

Risser and his colleagues[16] reported similar results; they studied bone mineral density in 29 female collegiate athletes participating in volleyball, swimming, and basketball. They were compared with 13 control subjects. Volleyball players' lumbar spine BMD was 24% higher than that of swimmers and 11% higher than that of control subjects. Both volleyball and basketball players had greater BMD in the calcaneus than swimmers and control subjects.

Site-specific responses in BMD to training have also been reported.[11,15] That is, bone density is higher at sites specifically loaded by a sport as compared to BMD at the same site in athletes competing in a different sport. Arm BMD in gymnasts has been found to be higher than arm BMD in volleyball players, possibly as a result of the impact loading of gymnastics on the arms.[11]

Increases in the BMD of athletes have been seen over the course of a competitive season.[6] Gymnasts and sedentary control subjects had BMD assessments of the lumbar spine (L2–L4) and femoral neck using DXA both before and after a 27-week gymnastics season. Initial BMD was 8% higher in the gymnasts at both sites, but gymnasts still had an increase of 1.3% in BMD at both the lumbar spine and femoral neck after 27 weeks of training. There were no increases for control subjects. Similar results have been reported in recreational runners[10] and weight lifters[5,10,49] who have shown 1% to 2% gains in bone density after training.

Although the mechanical loading associated with athletic training can be beneficial to bone, potential skeletal health problems may exist for the female athlete. As a result of the pressure to excel at her sport, or to achieve the leanest body, the female athlete is often driven to extreme measures for both training and weight loss. Consequently, there is a higher prevalence of amenorrhea and eating disorders in the female athlete as compared to the general population.[50–52] The term "disordered eating" is now typically used, because of the wide variety of eating problems noted among female athletes.[53] Either amenorrhea or disordered eating can lead to decreased bone density and an increased risk for osteoporosis. The presence and association of all three disorders—amenorrhea, disordered eating, and osteoporosis—have recently been referred to as the female athlete triad.[53]

Unfortunately, the exact cause of amenorrhea in female athletes has not been fully determined,

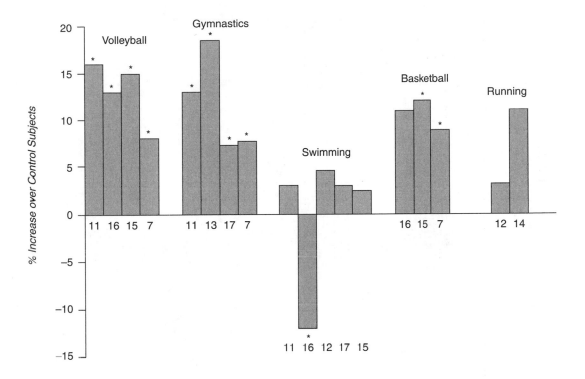

Figure 12–1 Studies Examining Lumbar Bone Mineral Density (BMD) in Athletic Teams and Sedentary Controls. *Indicates the value is significantly different than that of control subjects (P < .05). The number under each bar refers to the corresponding reference number at the end of this chapter.

and it is probable that athletic amenorrhea has a number of possible contributing factors. The two most current theories are a negative energy balance, which may lead to hypothalamic dysfunction, or excess cortisol levels that inhibit release of gonadotropins.[54] Regardless of the cause, the lack of estrogen rapidly decreases bone density, and if the amenorrhea persists long enough, some of the bone mass lost may not be regained.[21,55]

The majority of studies examining amenorrheic athletes have reported 10% to 25% lower BMD at the lumbar spine in the athlete as compared to eumenorrheic control subjects.[20,21,55–62] However, although studies consistently report lower BMD in amenorrheic athletes at the more trabecular site of the lumbar spine, lower BMD has not always been found in the more cortical,

peripheral sites.[57,62] More recent studies, though, have reported significantly lower BMD at a number of different skeletal sites in amenorrheic athletes.[60,63] An illustration of several studies that investigated BMD in amenorrheic athletes is presented in Figure 12–3.

Lindberg et al[39] compared lumbar spine and radial bone density in amenorrheic, oligomenorrheic, and eumenorrheic runners (mean age = 30.4 years) along with sedentary controls and postmenopausal women (mean age = 62.9 years). BMD of both trabecular (lumbar) and cortical (radial) bone was significantly lower in the amenorrheic runners when compared to the eumenorrheic runners and control subjects. Trabecular BMD in the amenorrheic runners was even lower than that found in the postmenopausal women.

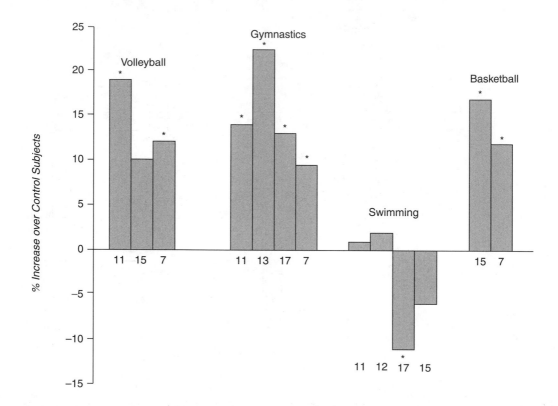

Figure 12–2 Studies examining Femoral Neck Bone Mineral Density (BMD) in Athletic Teams and Sedentary Controls. *Indicates the value is significantly different than that of control subjects (P < .05). The number under each bar refers to the corresponding reference number at the end of this chapter.

Drinkwater et al[20] also studied BMD in a group of amenorrheic and eumenorrheic runners. Amenorrheic runners had significantly less BMD in the lumbar spine when compared to the eumenorrheic group. In a follow-up study,[55] it was reported that seven athletes who regained their menses increased lumbar BMD by 6%. However, their values were still significantly less than those of eumenorrheic athletes. The two athletes who remained amenorrheic exhibited further decreases in BMD. Similar findings have been reported in dancers who increased BMD 14% over a 2-year period after regaining their menses, but still had values significantly below those of normal control subjects.[21]

There is limited evidence that suggests that certain forms of athletic activity may be of sufficient intensity to counteract the bone loss often associated with amenorrhea.[64] Gymnasts were reported to have 10% to 18% higher bone density at the femoral neck and lumbar spine than runners despite similar prevalence of amenorrhea. In addition, the gymnasts had 10% higher femoral neck bone density when compared to eumenorrheic control subjects.[64] One important point is that the gymnasts were significantly younger than the runners in this study. It is unknown what effects continued amenorrhea might have on the BMD of the gymnasts, because amenorrheic athletes in other studies have

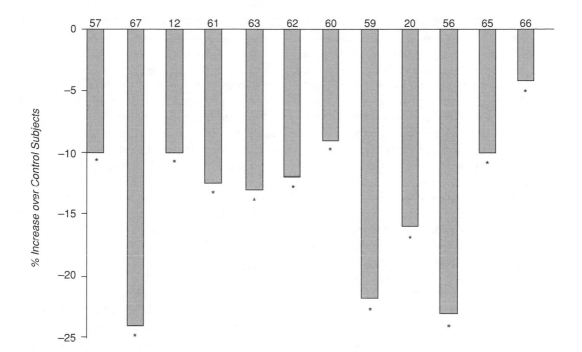

Figure 12–3 Studies Examining Lumbar Bone Mineral Density (BMD) in Athletes with Amenorrhea. *Indicates the value is significantly different than that of control subjects (P < .05). The number above each bar refers to the corresponding reference number at the end of the chapter. The last two studies on the right are those involving athletes with stress fractures.

shown continued declines in BMD as long as the amenorrhea is still present.[55]

Stress fractures appear to be more common not only in women with low bone mass,[65] but in amenorrheic women as well.[63] Although studies have shown higher incidences of amenorrhea in stress fracture groups, the groups with fracture did not always have lower bone mass.[66] Therefore, it is unknown if the increased rate of stress fractures in amenorrheic women is a result of the concomitant decrease in bone mass or is somehow related to the etiology of amenorrhea. The risk of stress fracture for the amenorrheic athlete is thus greater, not only because of strain placed on the bones as a result of training, but by the amenorrhea as well. An illustration of some studies examining stress fractures in female athletes is given in Figure 12–3.

Case Study

A 20-year-old, female, collegiate, cross-country runner is referred for assessment. She is approximately 15% underweight. She reports having had no menstrual cycles for the past 6 months, but has experienced no previous bouts of amenorrhea. She has been training competitively for 10 years.

A thorough dietary and menstrual history must be obtained to discount the possibility of any patterns of disordered eating or other menstrual irregularities. A careful determination of the athlete's energy intake and expenditure should also be made. This should at least include estimating caloric intake based on a 3- or 7-day dietary record, estimating basal metabolic rate, using an appropriate method such as The Harris-

Benedict equation, and estimating daily energy expenditure by determining both the volume and intensity of training, along with time spent doing other moderate to vigorous activities (climbing stairs, walking back and forth to class, etc). Weight-loss patterns over the previous 2 or 3 years should also be established as much as possible. This will allow ascertainment of the athlete's energy balance. It can thus be determined if a negative caloric balance might be contributing to the recent bout of amenorrhea. For a more thorough review of nutritional evaluation, please refer to the work by Johnson.[67]

Assessment of follicle-stimulating hormone (FSH) in women with amenorrhea is recommended.[68] Determination of serum levels of estrogen and progesterone might also be worthwhile, but this is advisable only if serial blood samples can be obtained to give an accurate estimate of overall levels of the two hormones. If blood samples are taken, cortisol levels could also be measured if it is not cost-prohibitive. An accurate evaluation of these hormones could aid in determining the possible factors associated with the loss of menstrual function. For a more complete review of clinical evaluation of amenorrhea, please see the work by Marshall.[68]

A measurement of bone mineral density should be made if it is easily accessible and within cost constraints. It should not be considered a necessity at this point. However, if the amenorrhea persists, or if the athlete had reported frequent problems with menstrual irregularities in the past, or has a pattern of disordered eating, then a BMD measurement would be highly advisable.

After a thorough initial assessment, the athlete can be counseled on ways to regain her menses. This may include a reduction in intensity or volume of training, a 2% to 3% increase in weight, an increase in total caloric intake, and an increase in calcium intake, particularly if BMD was low. If these measures do not work, or if the athlete is unwilling to make the necessary changes to regain her menses, some form of estrogen replacement therapy should be considered in an effort to counteract the bone loss that is taking place. Follow-up measurements of bone density would be indicated if the use of replacement therapy is initiated, especially given that there are only limited prospective studies on the use of estrogen replacement therapy in amenorrheic athletes.[69] In addition, if a pattern of disordered eating is detected, the athlete should be referred to a qualified therapist for counseling as well as to a medical doctor for further clinical evaluation.

CONCLUSION

Generally speaking, participation in athletics provides many potential benefits, both physically and mentally, for the participant. Most athletes are leaner, stronger, and more cardiovascularly fit than their more sedentary counterparts, and bone density can be anywhere from 5% to 15% higher in the female athlete when compared to control subjects. Increases in BMD have also been seen over the course of an athletic season.[7] In addition, participation in exercise programs, such as running or weight training, outside the realm of athletic programs, can increase BMD from 1% to 2%,[4,5,10,49,70] although declines in BMD have been seen after detraining.[4,70]

It must be stressed, however, that many young women are driven to extreme measures to excel at their sport or achieve the ideal lean athletic image. These extreme measures can sometimes lead to what is now known as the female athlete triad, which not only reduces bone density, but compromises many other aspects of a woman's health as well. The "ideal" female athlete would be one who enjoys her sport and the many positive benefits associated with it, while also being aware of the potential negative health issues.

REFERENCES

1. Chrischilles EA, Shireman T, Wallace R. Costs and health effects of osteoporotic fractures. *Bone.* 1994;15:377–385.

2. Kanis JA, Melton LJ, Christiansen C, Johnston CC, Khaltaev N. The diagnosis of osteoporosis. *J Bone Miner Res.* 1994;9:1137–1141.

3. Melton LJ. How many women have osteoporosis now? *J Bone Miner Res.* 1995;10:175–177.

4. Dalsky GP, Stocke KS, Ehsani AA, Slatopolsky E, Lee WC, Birge SJ. Weight-bearing exercise training and lumbar bone mineral content in postmenopausal women. *Ann Intern Med.* 1988;108:824–828.

5. Lohman TG, Going S, Pamenter RW, et al. Effects of resistance training on regional and total bone mineral density in premenopausal women: A randomized prospective study. *J Bone Miner Res.* 1995;10:1015–1024.

6. Nichols DL, Sanborn CF, Bonnick SL, Ben-Ezra V, Gench B, DiMarco NM. The effects of gymnastics training on bone mineral density. *Med Sci Sports Exerc.* 1994;26:1220–1225.

7. Nichols DL, Sanborn CF, Gench B, DiMarco NM. Relationship of regional body composition to bone mineral density in college females. *Med Sci Sports Exerc.* 1995;27:178–182.

8. Pruitt LA, Jackson RD, Bartels RL. Weight-training effects on bone mineral density in early postmenopausal women. *J Bone Miner Res.* 1992;7:179–185.

9. Simkin A, Ayalon J, Leichter I. Increased trabecular bone density due to bone-loading exercises in postmenopausal osteoporotic women. *Calcif Tissue Int.* 1987;40:59–63.

10. Snow-Harter C, Bouxsein ML, Lewis BT, Carter DR, Marcus R. Effects of resistance and endurance exercise on bone mineral status of young women: A randomized exercise intervention trial. *J Bone Miner Res.* 1992;7:761–769.

11. Fehling PC, Alekel L, Clasey J, Rector A, Stillman RJ. A comparison of bone mineral densities among female athletes in impact loading and active loading sports. *Bone.* 1995;17:205–210.

12. Heinrich CH, Going SB, Pamenter RW, Perry CD, Boyden TW, Lohman TG. Bone mineral content of cyclically menstruating female resistance and endurance trained athletes. *Med Sci Sports Exerc.* 1990;22:558–563.

13. Kirchner EM, Lewis RD, O'Connor PJ. Effect of past gymnastics participation on adult bone mass. *J App Physiol.* 1996;80:226–232.

14. Kirk S, Sharp CF, Elbaum N, et al. Effect of long distance running on bone mass in women. *J Bone Min Res.* 1989;4:515–522.

15. Lee EJ, Long KA, Risser WL, Poindexter HBW, Gibbons WE, Goldzieher J. Variations in bone status of contralateral and regional sites in young athletic women. *Med Sci Sports Exerc.* 1995;27:1354–1361.

16. Risser WL, Lee EJ, LeBlanc A, Poindexter HBW, Risser JHM, Schneider V. Bone density in eumenorrheic female college athletes. *Med Sci Sports Exerc.* 1990;22:570–574.

17. Taaffe DR, Snow-Harter C, Connolly DA, Robinson TL, Brown MD, Marcus R. Differential effects of swimming versus weight-bearing activity on bone mineral status of eumenorrheic athletes. *J Bone Miner Res.* 1995;10:586–593.

18. Sanborn CF, Wagner WW. Athletic amenorrhea. In: Drinkwater BL, ed. *Female Endurance Athletes.* Champaign, IL: Human Kinetics; 1986:125–148.

19. Davies MC, Hall ML, Jacobs HS. Bone mineral loss in young women with amenorrhoea. *BMJ.* 1990;790–793.

20. Drinkwater BL, Nilson K, Chesnut CH III, Bremner WJ, Shainholtz S, Southworth MB. Bone mineral content of amenorrheic and eumenorrheic athletes. *N Engl J Med.* 1984;311:277–281.

21. Jonnavithula S, Warren MP, Fox RP, Lazaro MI. Bone density is compromised in amenorrheic women despite return of menses: A 2-year study. *Obstet Gynecol.* 1993;81:669–674.

22. Buckwalter JA, Glimcher MJ, Cooper RR, Recker R. Bone biology. Part I: structure, blood supply, cells, matrix, and mineralization. *J Bone Joint Surg.* 1995;77-A:1256–1275.

23. Marks SC, Popoff SN. Bone cell biology: The regulation of development, structure, and function in the skeleton. *Am J Anat.* 1988;183:1–44.

24. Mora S, Goodman WG, Loro ML, Roe TF, Sayre J, Gilsanz V. Age-related changes in cortical and cancellous vertebral bone density in girls: Assessment with quantitative CT. *Am J Roentgen.* 1994;405–409.

25. Sowers MR, Galuska DA. Epidemiology of bone mass in premenopausal women. *Epidemiol Rev.* 1993;15:374–398.

26. Rodin A, Murby B, Smith MA, et al. Premenopausal bone loss in the lumbar spine neck of femur: a study of 225 Caucasian women. *Bone.* 1990;11:1–5.

27. Bonjour J-P, Theintz G, Buchs B, Slosman D, Rizzoli R. Critical years and stages of puberty for spinal and femoral bone mass accumulation during adolescence. *J Clin Endocrinol Metab.* 1991;73:555–563.

28. Matkovic V, Jelic T, Wardlaw GM, et al. Timing of peak bone mass in caucasian females and its implication for the prevention of osteoporosis. Inference from a cross-sectional model. *J Clin Invest.* 1994;93:799–808.

29. Rosenthal DI, Mayo-Smith W, Hayes CW, et al. Age and bone mass in premenopausal women. *J Bone Miner Res*. 1989;4:533–538.

30. Christiansen C, Riis BJ, Rodbro P. Prediction of rapid bone loss in postmenopausal women. *Lancet*. 1987; 1105–1108.

31. Ettinger BF, Genant HK, Cann CE. Long-term estrogen replacement therapy prevents bone loss and fractures. *Ann Intern Med*. 1985;102:319–324.

32. Hedlund LR, Gallagher JC. The effect of age and menopause on bone mineral density of the proximal femur. *J Bone Miner Res*. 1989;4:639–646.

33. Pouilles JM, Tremollieres F, Ribot C. The effects of menopause on longitudinal bone loss from the spine. *Calcif Tissue Int*. 1993;52:340–343.

34. Eriksen E, Colvard D, Berg N, et al. Evidence of estrogen receptors in normal human osteoblast-like cells. *Science*. 1988;241:84–86.

35. Buckwalter JA, Glimcher MJ, Cooper RR, Recker R. Bone biology. Part II: formation, form, modeling, remodeling, and regulation of cell function. *J Bone Joint Surg*. 1995;77–A:1276–1289.

36. Lanyon LE. Using functional loading to influence bone mass and architecture: Objectives, mechanisms, and relationship with estrogen of the mechanically adaptive process in bone. *Bone*. 1996;18:37S–43S.

37. Donaldson CL, Hulley SB, Vogel JM, Hattner RS, Bayers JH, McMillan DE. Effect of prolonged bed rest on bone mineral. *Metabolism*. 1970;19:1071–1084.

38. Mack PB, Vogt FB. Roentgenographic bone density changes in astronauts during representative Apollo space flight. *Am J Roentgenol, Radium Ther Nuc Med*. 1971;113:621–633.

39. Kanis JA. Calcium nutrition and implications for osteoporosis. Part I. Children and healthy adults. *Eur J Clin Nutr*. 1994;48:757–767.

40. Akesson K. Biochemical markers of bone turnover. *Acta Orthop Scand*. 1995;66:376–386.

41. Genant HK, Engelke K, Fuerst T, et al. Noninvasive assessment of bone mineral and structure: state of the art. *J Bone Miner Res*. 1996;11:707–730.

42. Delmas PD. Clinical use of biochemical markers of bone remodeling in osteoporosis. *Bone*. 1992;13:S17–S21.

43. Eyre D. New biomarkers of bone resorption. *J Clin Endocrinol Metab*. 1992;74:470A–470C.

44. Bollen A, Martin MD, Leroux BG, Eyre DR. Circadian variation on urinary excretion of bone collagen cross-links. *J Bone Miner Res*. 1995;10:1844–1852.

45. Cosman F, Nieves J, Wilkinson C, Schnering D, Shen V, Lindsay R. Bone density change and biochemical indices of skeletal turnover. *Calcif Tissue Int*. 1996;58: 236–243.

46. Panteghini M, Pagani F. Biological variation in bone-derived biochemical markers in serum. *Scand J Clin Lab Invest*. 1995;55:609–616.

47. Schlemmer A, Hassager C, Jensen SB, Christiansen C. Marked diurnal variation in urinary excretion of pyridinium cross-links in premenopausal women. *J Clin Endocrinol Metab*. 1992;74:476–480.

48. Snow CM. Exercise and bone mass in young premenopausal women. *Bone*. 1996;18:51S–55S.

49. Friedlander AL, Genant HK, Sadowsky S, Byl NN, Gluer C. A two-year program of aerobics and weight training enhances bone mineral density of young women. *J Bone Miner Res*. 1995;10:574–585.

50. Feicht CB, Johnson TS, Martin BJ, Sparkes KE. Secondary amenorrhea in athletes. *Lancet*. 1978;2:1145–1146.

51. Loucks AB, Horvath SM. Athletic amenorrhea: a review. *Med Sci Sports Exerc*. 1985;17:56–72.

52. Rosen LW, Hough DO. Pathogenic weight control behaviors of female college gymnasts. *Physician Sports Med*. 1988;16:141–146.

53. Yeager KK, Agostini R, Nattiv A, Drinkwater BL. The female athlete triad: disordered eating, amenorrhea, osteoporosis. *Med Sci Sports Exerc*. 1993;25:775–777.

54. Loucks AB. Effects of exercise training on the menstrual cycle: existence and mechanisms. *Med Sci Sports Exerc*. 1990;22:275–280.

55. Drinkwater BL, Nilson K, Ott SM, Chesnut CH III. Bone mineral density after resumption of menses in amenorrheic athletes. *JAMA*. 1986;256:308–382.

56. Drinkwater BL, Bruemner B, Chesnut CH III. Menstrual history as a determinant of current bone density in young athletes. *J Am Med Wom Assoc*. 1990;263:545–548.

57. Hetland ML, Haarbo J, Christiansen C. Running induces menstrual disturbances but bone mass is unaffected, except in amenorrheic women. *Am J Med*. 1993;95:53–60.

58. Howat PM, Carbo ML, Wozniak P. The influence of diet, body fat, menstrual cycling, and activity upon the bone density of females. *J Am Diet Assoc*. 1989;89: 1305–1307.

59. Lindberg J, Fears W, Hunt M, Powell M, Boll D, Wade C. Exercise induced amenorrhea and bone density. *Ann Int Med*. 1984;101:647–648.

60. Rencken ML, Chesnut CH III, Drinkwater BL. Bone density at multiple skeletal sites in amenorrheic athletes. *JAMA*. 1996;276:238–240.

61. Rutherford OM. Spine and total body bone mineral density in amenorrheic endurance athletes. *J Appl Physiol*. 1993;74:2904–2908.

62. Snead DB, Weltman A, Weltman JY, et al. Reproductive hormones and bone mineral density in women runners. *J Appl Physiol*. 1992;72:2149–2156.

63. Myburgh KH, Bachrach LK, Lewis BT, Kent K, Marcus R. Low bone mineral density at axial and appendicular sites in amenorrheic athletes. *Med Sci Sports Exerc.* 1993;25:1197–1202.

64. Robinson TL, Snow-Harter C, Taaffe DR, Gillis DE, Shaw J, Marcus R. Gymnasts exhibit higher bone mass than runners despite similar prevalence of amenorrhea and oligomenorrhea. *J Bone Miner Res.* 1995;10:26–35.

65. Myburgh KH, Hutchins J, Fataar AB, Hough SF, Noakes TD. Low bone density is an etiologic factor for stress fracture in athletes. *Ann Intern Med.* 1991; 113:754–759.

66. Carbon R, Sambrook PN, Deakin V, et al. Bone density of elite female athletes with stress fractures. *Med J Aust.* 1990;153:373–376.

67. Johnson MD. Disordered eating. In: Agostini RA, ed. *Medical and Orthopedic Issues of Active and Athletic Women.* Philadelphia: Hanley & Belfus; 1994:141–151.

68. Marshall LA. Clinical evaluation of amenorrhea. In: Agostini RA, ed. *Medical and Orthopedic Issues of Active and Athletic Women.* Philadelphia: Hanley & Belfus; 1994:154–163.

69. Cumming DC. Exercise-associated amenorrhea, low bone density, and estrogen replacement therapy. *Arch Intern Med.* 1996;156:2193–2195.

70. Vuori I, Heinonen A, Sievanen H, Kannus P, Pasanen M, Oja P. Effects of unilateral strength training and detraining on bone mineral density and content in young women: A study of mechanical loading and deloading on human bones. *Calcif Tissue Int.* 1994;55:59–67.

CHAPTER 13

Nutrition for the School-Age Child Athlete

Suzanne Nelson Steen

Participation in athletics often begins at an early age and has become an important part of growing up for many children. In addition to providing children with opportunities for personal enjoyment, social interaction, and skill development, athletic participation can be used to introduce children and their families to sound nutritional practices that may provide an important lifelong health benefit.[1–4]

Children have the right to enjoy physical activity and to strive for success. This can be compromised, however if they are misinformed about how much and what foods to eat and drink for activity. The purpose of this chapter is to provide guidelines to help ensure that young athletes are guaranteed appropriate nutrition for exercise, compatible with optimal needs for growth and development. Before turning to a discussion of sports nutrition for the school-age child, please take a moment to review the Young Athlete's Bill of Rights (Exhibit 13–1).[5]

EVALUATION OF GROWTH

Achieving normal growth and development is a key concern in school-age children. To this end, all children should have their weight, height, weight for height, and standard height for age evaluated and assessed by a qualified health professional using National Center for Health Statistics (NCHS) growth charts (see Figures 13–1 through 13–4).[6]

Routine plotting of weight and height on growth charts is essential to identify growth patterns that are indicative of acute or chronic malnutrition (stunting, failure to thrive) or overnutrition (obesity). Growth retardation, obesity, iron-deficiency anemia, dental disease, and poor academic performance indicate that many children may be at nutritional risk.[7,8]

Because height and weight taken once do not lend themselves to interpretation of growth status, measurements should be recorded at regular intervals to accurately reflect the growth patterns of the child.[9] Usually, normal childhood growth occurs between the 5th and 95th percentile. During the first 2 years of age, some fluctuation in height and weight within the 5th and 95th percentile is expected as both infants and children demonstrate individual spurts in growth. However, children generally maintain their height and weight between the same percentiles (that is, 50th–75th percentile, also referred to as growth channel) during the preschool and early childhood years.

Although individual children differ in their rates of growth, they should follow the same channels. When either height or weight deviates from the child's usual growth percentile, the etiology of the change should be investigated.

A more precise evaluation of growth is necessary when height and weight fall in markedly different percentiles (for example, height 25th percentile, weight 75th percentile) because the height and weight of a child should be in propor-

217

Exhibit 13–1 Young Athlete's Bill of Rights

1. The right to have the opportunity to participate in sports regardless of ability level.
2. The right to participate at a level commensurate with the child's developmental level.
3. The right to have qualified adult leadership.
4. The right to participate in a safe and healthy environment.
5. The right of each child to share leadership and decision making.
6. The right to play as a child and not as an adult.
7. The right to proper preparation for participation in sports.
8. The right to equal opportunity to strive for success.
9. The right to be treated with dignity by all involved.
10. The right to have fun through sports.

Source: Reprinted with permission from *American Journal of Diseases of Children*, Vol. 142, p. 143, © 1988, American Medical Association.

tion to one another. Assessment of weight in relation to height enables assessment of current nutrition status and growth that is specific to the child's body size. At a single point in time, weight for height is a more sensitive index of appropriate growth than weight for age, because appropriateness of body weight is dependent on total body size, not on age.

In contrast to the weight for height assessment, height for age comparison is an index of previous nutrition and growth status. A reduction in height velocity is slower to develop in the presence of undernutrition than a decrease in weight velocity. Therefore, it is an index of *chronic* malnutrition.

Age- and sex-specific standards have been developed to separate the genetic contribution of parental stature from other factors that affect a child's linear growth, such as malnutrition or disease. A child's actual height can be adjusted with a factor derived from the average of each parent's height. This method is recommended for evaluating children whose height for age is lower than the 5th percentile.[10,11]

The actual increments in height and weight during the school-age years are small compared with those of infancy and adolescence. Weight increases an average of 2 to 3 kg each year until the child is 9 or 10 years old. Then, rate of weight increases, which is an initial sign of approaching puberty. Height increments average 5 to 6 cm per year from age 2 until the pubertal acceleration.[9]

At puberty, children undergo hormonal changes that mark the beginning of adolescence. Nutritional needs before and during this period of rapid growth increase significantly. In addition to growth charts, the Tanner stages of sexual development (Sexual Maturity Ratings) can be used to monitor maturing athletes (Exhibit 13–2).[12]

This numerical system has been established for describing children in terms of how their bodies are changing and developing sexually. By using the Tanner staging system, the athletic capabilities of children can be estimated so that boys and girls are trained properly and appropriately nourished. Regular monitoring of growth allows trends to be identified early and when necessary appropriate intervention given to ensure that long-term growth is not compromised.

Weight and Body Composition

Studies have shown that extra weight can be detrimental to performance, particularly when body mass must be moved through space, either horizontally or vertically, in athletics such as running and jumping.[13] Consequently, many ask what weight, or range of weights, is ideal for an athlete to achieve optimal performance. Unfortunately, there is no easy answer, particularly for the growing young athlete.

Although appropriate weight loss may result in an improvement in athletic performance, there is a point beyond which further weight loss leads to a deterioration in performance and may jeopardize the health of the athlete as well.[13] For the

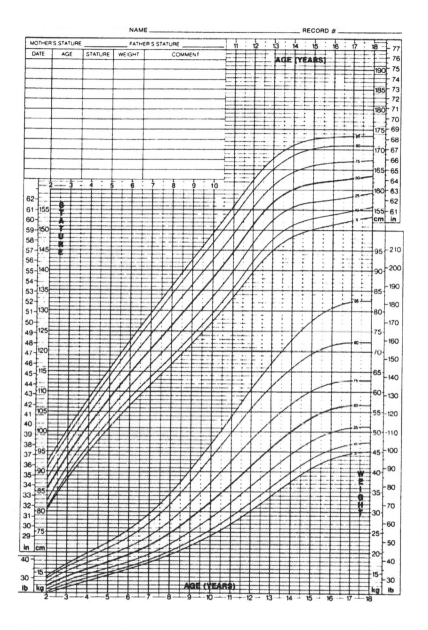

Figure 13–1 Girls: 2 to 18 Years Physical Growth NCHS Percentiles. *Source:* Adapted from Hamill PVV, Drizd TA, Johnson CL, Reed RB, Roche AF, Moore WM, Physical Growth: National Center for Health Statistics Percentiles, *American Journal of Clinical Nutrition*, Vol. 32, pp. 607–629, © 1979. Data from the National Center for Health Statistics (NCHS), Hyattsville, MD. Reprinted with permission of Ross Laboratories, Columbus, OH, from *NCHS Growth Charts*, © 1982 Ross Laboratories.

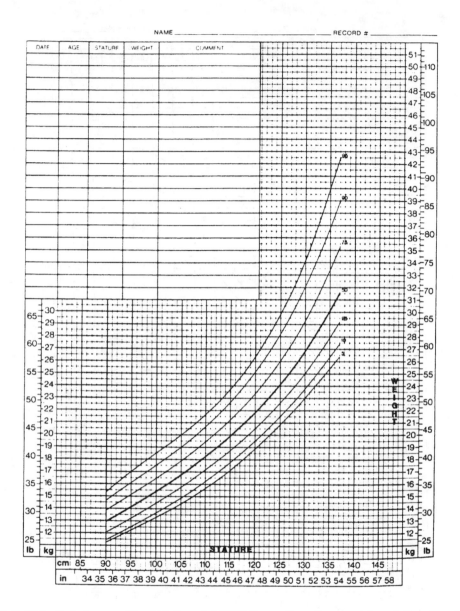

Figure 13–2 Girls: Prepubescent Physical Growth NCHS Percentiles. *Source:* Adapted from Hamill PVV, Drizd TA, Johnson CL, Reed RB, Roche AF, Moore WM, Physical Growth: National Center for Health Statistics Percentiles, *American Journal of Clinical Nutrition*, Vol. 32, pp. 607–629, © 1979. Data from the National Center for Health Statistics (NCHS), Hyattsville, MD. Reprinted with permission of Ross Laboratories, Columbus, OH, from *NCHS Growth Charts*, © 1982 Ross Laboratories.

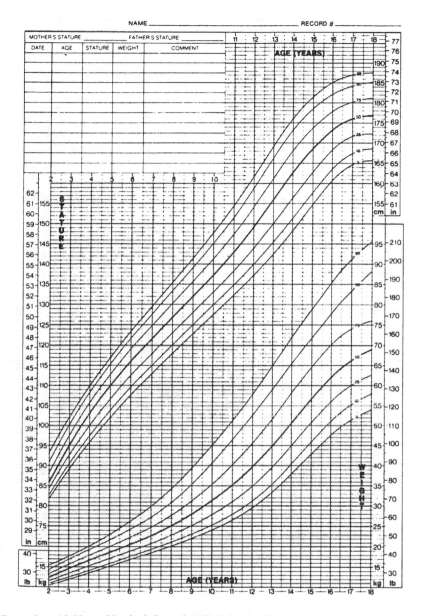

Figure 13–3 Boys: 2 to 18 Years Physical Growth NCHS Percentiles. *Source:* Adapted from Hamill PVV, Drizd TA, Johnson CL, Reed RB, Roche AF, Moore WM, Physical Growth: National Center for Health Statistics Percentiles, *American Journal of Clinical Nutrition*, Vol. 32, pp. 607–629, © 1979. Data from the National Center for Health Statistics (NCHS), Hyattsville, MD. Reprinted with permission of Ross Laboratories, Columbus, OH, from *NCHS Growth Charts*, © 1982 Ross Laboratories.

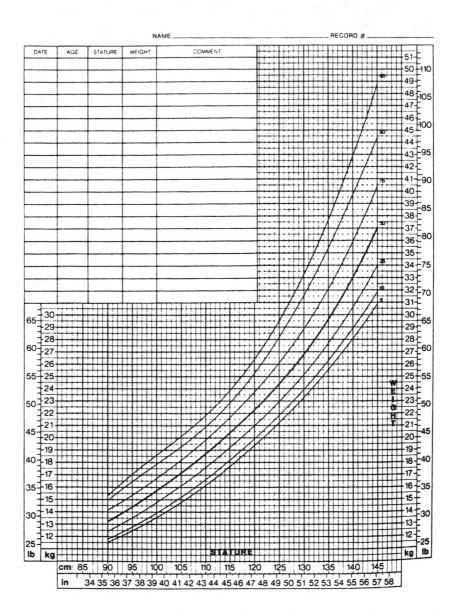

Figure 13–4 Boys: Prepubescent Physical Growth NCHS Percentiles. *Source:* Adapted from Hamill PVV, Drizd TA, Johnson CL, Reed RB, Roche AF, Moore WM, Physical Growth: National Center for Health Statistics Percentiles, *American Journal of Clinical Nutrition,* Vol. 32, pp. 607–629, © 1979. Data from the National Center for Health Statistics (NCHS), Hyattsville, MD. Reprinted with permission of Ross Laboratories, Columbus, OH, from *NCHS Growth Charts,* © 1982 Ross Laboratories.

Exhibit 13–2 Tanner Stages of Development

Stage		Boys	Girls
1		Prepubescent	Prepubescent
		First appearance of pubic hair	First appearance of pubic hair
2		Growth of genitalia	Development of genitalia
	Peak growth spurt in girls	Increased activity of sweat glands	Increased activity of sweat glands
		Pubic hair extends to scrotum	Pubic hair thicker, coarser, curly
3		Growth and pigmentation of genitalia	Breasts enlarge; pigmentation continues
		Changes in voice	Genitals well developed
	Peak growth spurt in boys	Beginning of acne	Beginning of acne
		Pubic hair thickens, facial hair begins	Pubic hair abundant, armpit hair begins
4		Growth and pigmentation of genitalia	Breasts enlarge and mature
		Voice deepens	Genitals assume adult structure
		Acne (may be severe)	Acne (may be severe)
			Menarche begins
		Increased distribution of hair	Increased pubic hair distribution
5		Genitals fully mature	Breasts fully mature
		Acne may persist and increase	Increased severity of acne (if present)

Source: Data from J.M. Tanner, *Growth at Adolescence*, 2nd ed., © 1962, Blackwell Scientific Publications.

young athlete, the effects of weight loss on growth rate, nutritional status, hormone levels, and bone mineral content are of special concern in addition to the psychological stress that may result in an eating problem.

It is now widely recognized that weight per se is not an appropriate marker of performance capabilities, and that the existing weight of the athlete should not be used as an index to establish goal weights.[13] Instead, body composition of the athlete needs to be evaluated, in which an estimation of the amount of lean and fat tissue is calculated.

Body Composition Assessment

Although body composition assessment has important implications for health, fitness, and performance,[14] evaluation of children is complicated by several factors that affect the conceptual basis for estimating fat and lean tissue.[14–16] First, children have higher body water content and lower bone mineral content[14–16] and therefore have a lower body density than adults. Equations developed for prepubescent children that use conversion constants derived from adult samples are not appropriate for children because they may overestimate body fatness by 3% to 6% and underestimate lean body weight.[15,16]

Another limitation is that the chemical composition of the fat-free mass changes as the child passes through puberty.[14–16] Slaughter and colleagues[16] found that significant changes in the relation of skinfolds to density occur from prepubescence to puberty and from puberty to postpubescence. As a result, estimates of body fatness by skinfolds, body widths, and circumferences may reflect alterations in the composition of the fat-free body components, which include water, mineral, and protein, rather than alterations in actual fat content.

To overcome these limitations, estimates of body fat in children must take a multicomponent approach to assessing body composition rather than the traditional two-compartment model of fat and fat-free densities.[14–16] Lohman[17] has proposed equations for estimating percent body fat from body density on the basis of age and gender. These equations were derived by substituting estimated fat-free body densities by age and sex (along with the assumed fat density of 0.90 g/mL) into the Siri equation (a prediction equation used for calculating percentage body fat). These equations are listed in Table 13–1.

Skinfold equations that use a multicomponent approach to assess body composition and account for the chemical immaturity of children have been developed by Slaughter and colleagues.[16] The Tanner Scale of pubertal development was used to assess the maturational level of the children.[12] These equations (Exhibit 13–3) are recommended for predicting percent body fat in children 8 to 18 years old.

Another approach is to simply track changes in skinfold thickness instead of calculating percent-

age body fat. The sum of specific skinfolds (for example, triceps plus calf) may be used. Lohman[15] has proposed that all children, whether athletes or not, should be given the opportunity to follow changes in their body composition throughout childhood and adolescence. In conjunction with a sound nutrition program, children can learn to appreciate the relationship between body composition and health risks and benefits, as well as physical performance.[15] This approach can also assist teachers and coaches to intervene early with children who start to develop either excess adiposity or extreme leanness. With skinfold assessment on a biyearly basis, screening for a potential problem can occur so that treatment can be initiated in a timely manner in an effort to prevent obesity or an eating disorder.

Inappropriate Use of Weight

From a practical standpoint, body composition measures can be used by a qualified health professional to monitor changes in fat and lean tissue during training. Although helpful in evaluating the fitness and performance of mature athletes, body composition measures should never be used in the prepubescent athlete to manipulate body fat for sports participation or to set stringent weight loss guidelines. Doing so may adversely affect normal growth and development. This point needs to be made clear to coaches, parents, and athletes.

Because of the potential consequences of extreme weight loss, the issue of determining an appropriate weight for health is important to address. Body composition tables that show percent body-fat values for male and female athletes are not suitable to use for children because the majority of measurements were taken on athletes 19 years and older. There are currently no standards of comparison for young athletes that are specific for sport and gender. No tables are available that provide an "optimal or ideal weight" for performance (if one does in fact exist) among children or older athletes.

However, as defined earlier, body composition measures from skinfolds in combination

Table 13–1 Body-Fat Equations

Age (years)	Males	Females
7–8	% fat = 5.38 Db − 4.97	% fat = 5.43 Db − 5.03
9–10	% fat = 5.30 Db − 4.89	% fat = 5.35 Db − 4.95
11–12	% fat = 5.23 Db − 4.81	% fat = 5.25 Db − 4.84
13–14	% fat = 5.07 Db − 4.64	% fat = 5.12 Db − 4.69
15–16	% fat = 5.03 Db − 4.59	% fat = 5.07 Db − 4.64

Note: Db = body density (determined by underwater weighing)

Source: Adapted with permission from T.G. Lohman, Assessment of Body Composition in Children, *Pediatric Exercise Science*, Vol. 1, pp. 19–30, © 1989.

with growth charts and sound clinical judgment can be used to determine a range of weights for a particular young athlete based on optimal health. Lohman[15,17] has suggested that once body fat is determined, Figures 13–5 and 13–6 can be used to assess health risks and to determine an optimal range of weights.

These figures were derived from the equations presented by Slaughter et al.[16] It should be noted that the equations are more exact than the charts, because of the small change in the relationship of skinfolds to percent fat by age. Recognizing both individual variability and methodologic error, if a child falls above the optimal range, it is reasonable for the health professional to recommend that the child's body weight be slowly titrated down toward the upper end of this range. This can be accomplished by a modest reduction in calories combined with healthy eating and gradual increases in physical activity. Conversely, a young athlete who falls within the very low range can be encouraged to increase weight toward the optimal range for health. An example of how to determine a healthy weight range is shown in Exhibit 13–4.

NUTRITION REQUIREMENTS

School-age children tend to be repetitious in their food choices, and the foods they include in their diets remain relatively constant from month to month.[18] The caloric and nutrient content of the diet should be evaluated, and excess consumption of high-calorie, low-nutrient density foods, unusual foods, and consistently omitted food categories should be noted.

Methods of Dietary Assessment

A 24-hour recall, food frequency, food record, or a combination of these methods can be used to obtain dietary information (Exhibit 13–5).

Most children recall food items fairly reliably, but quantities less accurately. Therefore, the methodology chosen should be adjusted to consider the physical and emotional differences between children and older athletes. Establishing a good rapport with the child is of primary importance to facilitate future recommendations.

It is also important to interview the parent(s) about their impressions of the child's diet. Ideally, the child and parent(s) should be interviewed separately. Otherwise, children may report what they think the parent wants them to be eating instead of the actual intake. Comparing and combining information from both parent and child will provide a complete picture of the child's habits and rationale for consumption of certain foods.

Meal Patterns

Meal patterns can be identified by asking the child when, where, and with whom he or she typically eats. For example, does the child eat breakfast? Does the child have lunch at school or at home? What is the frequency of snacking?

Exhibit 13–3 Skinfold Equations

Skinfold Equations

For predicting % body fat in children and youth (8–18 years)

For sum of triceps and subscapular less than 35 mm use:

White male:

Prepubescent	% fat = 1.21 (T + S) – 0.008 (T + S)^2 – 1.7
Pubescent	% fat = 1.21 (T + S) – 0.008 (T + S)^2 – 3.4
Postpubescent	% fat = 1.21 (T + S) – 0.008 (T + S)^2 – 5.5

Black male:

Prepubescent	% fat = 1.21 (T + S) – 0.008 (T + S)^2 – 3.2
Pubescent	% fat = 1.21 (T + S) – 0.008 (T + S)^2 – 5.2
Postpubescent	% fat = 1.21 (T + S) – 0.008 (T + S)^2 – 6.8
All females:	% fat = 1.33 (T + S) – 0.013 (T + S)^2 – 2.5

For sum of triceps and subscapular greater than 35 mm use:

All males:	% fat = 0.783 (T + S) + 1.6
All females:	% fat = 0.546 (T + S) + 9.7

For triceps and calf:

Males	% fat = 0.735 (T + C) + 1.0
Females	% fat = 0.610 (T + C) + 5.1

Skinfold Measurement Locations

- Triceps (upper arm): Vertical fold raised midway between right olecranon and acromion processes on posterior of brachium.
- Subscapula (back): Skinfold picked up 1 cm below inferior angle of right scapula inclined downward laterally in natural cleavage.
- Medial calf: Vertical skinfold is raised on medial side of right calf just above level of maximal calf girth.
- Abdominal (stomach): Horizontal fold 3 cm lateral and 1 cm inferior to midpoint of umbilicus.

Note: C = calf; S = subscapular; T = triceps.

Source: Reprinted from Skinfold Equations for Estimation of Body Fatness in Children and Youth, Vol. 60, No. 5, 1988, by M. H. Slaughter et al., by permission of the Wayne State University Press. Copyright © 1988, Wayne State University Press.

Are dinners spent with family or eaten alone? What times of day does the child eat meals in relation to practice? Are fluids consumed during and after practice?

Many children skip breakfast.[18] Some studies suggest that children who eat breakfast have a better attitude, school record, and problem-solving ability compared to children who do not eat breakfast.[19,20] In addition, breakfast helps to replenish glycogen stores depleted during an overnight fast, to ensure that the child has adequate energy stores for afternoon training. It is important to encourage children to find foods they like to eat for breakfast. These do not need to be traditional foods. Food composition, not social tradition, is the best strategy. Breakfast should provide between a quarter and a third of the nutrients for the day.

The child's lunch may be provided by the school or brought from home. Because food choices are often influenced by the child's friends, it is important to ask the child whom he or she typically eats lunch with and why he or she chooses certain foods. Studies have shown that the school lunch is usually more nutritious than a lunch brought from home.[21] This is be-

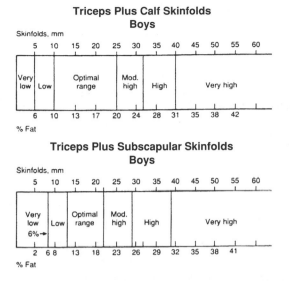

Figure 13–5 Percent-Fat Charts for Boys. *Source:* Reprinted with permission from T.G. Lohman, 1987, *Measuring Body Fat Using Skinfolds* (Champaign, IL: Human Kinetics), 84.

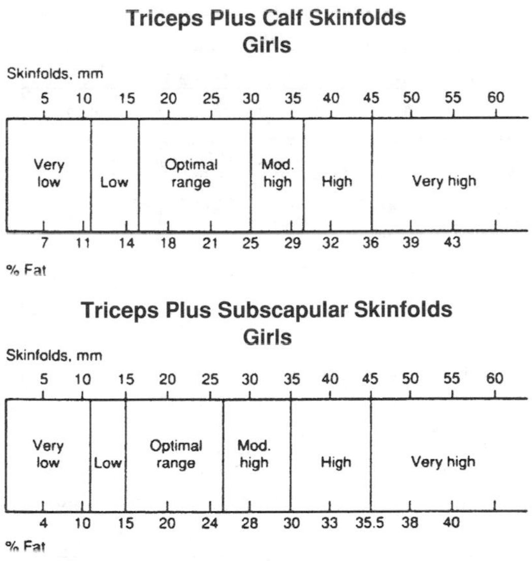

Figure 13–6 Percent-Fat Charts for Girls. *Source:* Reprinted with permission from T.G. Lohman, 1987, *Measuring Body Fat Using Skinfolds* (Champaign, IL: Human Kinetics), 84.

cause box lunches typically contain less variety, and include only favorite foods.[21] In addition, they are limited to foods that travel well and do not require heating or refrigeration. Even if a nutritious lunch is packed at home, the parent does not necessarily know what portion is eaten, traded, or thrown away.

Snacks may significantly contribute to the child's nutrient intake and eating style.[18] The quality of snacks eaten may determine whether nutrient requirements are being met. Therefore, the frequency of snacking and type of snacks are important considerations. For example, does the child typically snack during the morning or afternoon? What are the child's favorite snacks? Are they prepared at home or purchased from a vending machine?

Calorie Needs

Calorie requirements should be estimated based on current dietary intake, rate of growth, age, and physical activity. Energy needs for the school-age child are modest compared to the adolescent period of rapid growth and high nutritional demands.[2,3,18,22,23]

There may be large variability in energy intakes of healthy growing children of the same age and sex. For example, a 7-year-old boy and a 10.5-year-old girl approaching puberty have significantly different factors determining their energy needs even though they have the same recommended dietary allowance (RDA).[24] The RDA can be used to estimate caloric needs for normal growth and development per kilogram of body weight as shown in Table 13–2.

If reported energy intake seems low, several factors to consider are whether the child has adequate time to eat, is a finicky eater, is trying to lose weight, or has an underlying medical problem. The nutritionist needs to be cognizant of the significant numbers of children who live in poverty and frequently do not have access to sufficient calories and nutrients.[25,26] Social changes such as unemployment, the increasing number of dual-income families, and one-parent families have an impact on the food availability and food selection of children.[26]

Exhibit 13–4 Determining a Healthy Weight Range

Example:
  Male: Height: 59.5 in.   Weight: 124 lb
  Skinfolds: Triceps: 36 mm   Calf: 20 mm

Step 1: Determine % body fat (use appropriate formula from Exhibit 13–3
     % body fat = 0.735 (triceps and calf) + 1.0

$$= 0.735\ (56) + 1.0 = 42.2\ (0.422)$$

Step 2: Determine how much weight is fat
     Fat weight = actual weight × % body fat

$$= 124 \times 0.422 = 52.3\ \text{lb of fat}$$

Step 3: Determine fat-free weight
     Fat-free weight = actual weight − fat weight

$$= 124 - 52.3 = 71.7\ \text{lb}$$

Step 4: Calculate optimum healthy range of weight between 10% and 20% body fat
     Healthy weight at 10% = fat-free weight ÷ .9 = 71.7 ÷ .9 = 79 lb
     Healthy weight at 20% = fat-free weight ÷ .8 = 71.7 ÷ .8 = 89.6 lb

Healthy range of weight is 79 to 89.6 lb

To estimate how many calories the child may be expending during activity, specific questions should be asked about the training schedule: First of all, in what sport(s) is the child involved? Does he or she participate in competitions, and at what level? What have his or her accomplishments been so far? How often does the child train, and for how long? The intensity of activity can be estimated by asking him or her to describe a typical training session or more precisely, have the child keep an exercise diary that documents time spent doing various activities. Caloric expenditures for various activities that are specific for children are available and are presented in Table 13–3.

These data can be used as a guide to calculate calories expended per kilogram of body weight. It is important to recognize that children are more inefficient with their movements and thus potentially require more calories per unit of body weight. For example, compared with adults, children (age 6–8 years old) require 20% to 30% more oxygen per unit of body weight to run at a particular speed.[27–29] In older children, the difference is less.

Dietary Recommendations

What is the most appropriate diet for the child athlete? Adequate energy and nutrients should be obtained from a diet that emphasizes complex carbohydrates, moderate amounts of protein, and low-fat foods to support growth and physical activity.[23] This can be achieved by planning intake to include a variety of foods from each of the major food groups as illustrated by the food pyramid.[30] The key messages of variety, balance, and moderation in food choices should be promoted. Especially for the child, the pyramid serves as a visual guide for choosing foods and helping to plan healthful meals.

As shown in Figure 13–7, each section of the pyramid represents a food category and gives a range for the number of recommended servings to be consumed daily. Each day, the young athlete should consume at least 2 to 3 servings from the milk group, 2 to 3 servings from the meat and protein group, 4 servings from the vegetable group, 3 servings from the fruit group, and 9 servings from the bread and grain group. Foods containing the majority of calories from fat or

Exhibit 13–5 Food Frequency Form for Children

How Often Do You Eat the Different Foods Listed Below?

Food	Every Day (Always)	3-4 Times/Week (Often)	Every 2 or 3 Weeks (Sometimes)	Don't Eat (Never)
Dairy Products				
Milk, whole				
Milk, 2%				
Nonfat				
Cottage cheese				
Cream cheese				
Other cheeses				
Yogurt				
Ice cream				
Sherbet				
Puddings				
Margarine				
Butter				
Other: _____				
Meats				
Beef, hamburger				
Poultry				
Pork, ham				
Bacon, sausage				
Cold cuts, hot dogs				
Other: _____				
Fish				
Canned tuna				
Breaded fish				
Fresh or frozen fish				
Eggs				
Peanut Butter				
Grain Products				
Bread, white				
Bread, whole wheat				
Rolls, biscuits				
Muffins				
Pancakes, waffles				
Bagels				
Pasta, spaghetti				
Pasta, macaroni/cheese				
Rice				
Crackers				
Other: _____				
Cereals				
Sugar coated				

continues

Exhibit 13–5 continued

Food	Every Day (Always)	3-4 Times/Week (Often)	Every 2 or 3 Weeks (Sometimes)	Don't Eat (Never)
High fiber (bran)				
Natural (granola)				
Plain (Cheerios)				
Fortified				
Other: _____				
Fruits				
Oranges, orange juice				
Tomatoes, tomato juice				
Grapefruit, grapefruit juice				
Strawberries				
Cranberry juice				
Apples, apple juice				
Grapes, grape juice				
Fruit drink				
Peaches				
Bananas				
Other: _____				
Vegetables				
Peppers				
Potatoes				
Lettuce				
Broccoli				
Spinach				
Carrots				
Corn				
Squash				
Peas				
Green beans				
Beets				
Other: _____				
Snacks and Sweets				
Chips (potato, corn)				
Pretzels				
Popcorn				
French fries				
Cookies				
Cake, pie				
Pastries, doughnuts				
Candy				
Sugar, honey, jelly				
Soda, regular				
Soda, diet				
Cocoa				
Other: _____				

What Are Your Five Favorite Foods?

1. _____   2. _____   3. _____   4. _____   5. _____

Table 13–2 Estimated Average Calories and Protein Needs per Kilogram Body Weight for Children and Adolescents

Age (years)	Calories/kg	Protein (gm/kg)
4–6	90	1.2
7–10	70	1.0
11–14 (m)	55	1.0
11–14 (f)	47	1.0
15–18 (m)	45	0.9
15–18 (f)	40	0.8

Note: Values are based on *Recommended Dietary Allowances*. 10th ed. The RDA energy recommendations are derived from longitudinal intake data and represent average energy intake consistent with good health and appropriate growth in healthy persons. Protein recommendations are determined from the measurement of minimum protein intakes necessary to maintain nitrogen balance in practically all growing, healthy persons plus a safety factor to account for individual variation.

Source: Data from *Recommended Dietary Allowances,* 10th ed., © 1989, National Academy of Science.

Table 13–3 Caloric Equivalents of Child's Activities in kcal per 10 Minutes of Activity

Activity	Body Weight (kg)									
	20	25	30	35	40	45	50	55	60	65
Basketball	34	43	51	60	68	77	85	94	102	110
Calisthenics	13	17	20	23	26	30	33	36	40	43
Cycling										
10 km/hr	15	17	20	23	26	29	33	36	39	42
15 km/hr	22	27	32	36	41	46	50	55	60	65
Figure skating	40	50	60	70	80	90	100	110	120	130
Ice hockey (on-ice time)	52	65	78	91	104	117	130	143	156	168
Running										
8 km/hr	37	45	52	60	66	72	78	84	90	95
10 km/hr	48	55	64	73	79	85	92	100	107	113
Soccer (game)	36	45	54	63	72	81	90	99	108	117
Swimming 30 m/min										
breast	19	24	29	34	38	43	48	53	58	62
front crawl	25	31	37	43	49	56	62	68	74	80
back	17	21	25	30	34	38	42	47	51	55
Tennis	22	28	33	39	44	50	55	61	66	72
Walking										
4 km/hr	17	19	21	23	26	28	30	32	34	36
6 km/hr	24	26	28	30	32	34	37	40	43	48

Source: Adapted with permission from O. Bar-Or. *Pediatric Sports Medicine for the Practitioner,* © 1983, Springer-Verlag.

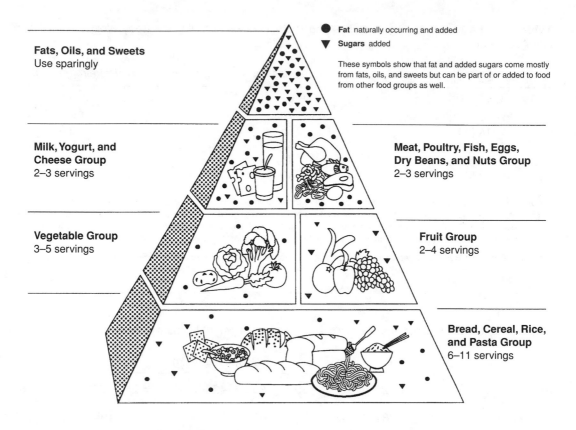

How Many Servings of Each Food Group Does the Active Child Need Each Day?

Food Group	No. of Servings
Bread	9
Vegetable	4
Fruit	3
Milk	2–3
Meat	2–3

Caloric level is about 2200. The exercising child may need an additional 500 to 1000 calories each day, depending on the frequency, intensity, and duration of physical activity.

Figure 13–7 The Food Guide Pyramid for the Growing Child Athlete. *Source:* Food guide pyramid reprinted from U.S. Department of Agriculture. Text below pyramid © 1995, The American Dietetic Association, *Play Hard, Eat Right*, used by permission.

sugars at the top of the pyramid are not eliminated, but should be consumed occasionally as an addition to, and not in place of, other nutrient-dense foods.

In general, providing servings within these recommended ranges will supply the necessary nutrients and calories (2200 calories) most active children require. However, depending on the frequency, intensity, and duration of physical activity, the exercising child may need an additional 500 to 1000 calories each day. Children should be encouraged to distribute calories throughout the day at regular mealtimes and snacks. This will ensure the presence of readily available sources of energy to support growth and training activity.

Young athletes can meet their vitamin and mineral needs while following diets that include the foods and servings recommended in the food guide pyramid.[23] If it is determined that the child's intake is low for certain micronutrients, strategies to increase consumption from food should be discussed with the parent.[1] Because the young child relies for the most part on the foods that are brought into the house, an evaluation of foods that are purchased by the parents or caretakers is informative. A food shopping frequency form can be used to help elucidate which foods are purchased on a regular basis and which are typically omitted (Exhibit 13–6).

In addition to purchasing more healthful foods, favorite foods can be made more nutritionally dense or acceptable substitutions can be made with similar foods. There are many different food choices available that will supply adequate amounts of vitamins and minerals for even the choosiest of eaters. Variety in the family menu will underscore the importance of eating different foods to provide the range of nutrients necessary for growth and development. Ideally, this variety is most easily achieved in regularly scheduled meals at home plus nutritious snacks. To be effective in getting the child to actually eat the recommended foods, it is important to suggest changes that are compatible with the eating style of the child.

Based upon the information obtained from the initial questions on dietary patterns and nutritional adequacy, sports nutrition issues that are pertinent for this age group can be considered, which include thermoregulation and fluid needs, pre- and postevent meals, weight control practices, and food supplements.

THE SPECIAL FLUID NEEDS OF CHILDREN

All athletes need to maintain adequate hydration to replace losses during exercise. However, compared with adults and even adolescents, pre-adolescent children must be especially careful to drink enough during exercise for several reasons. Although children's physiologic responses to exercise are generally similar to those of adults, there are several age- and maturation-related differences in their response.[31,32] As shown in Table 13–4, children respond to the combined stresses of exercise and climatic heat differently than do adults. Children tolerate temperature extremes less efficiently than adults.[31,33] They have a lower sweating rate (absolute and per single gland) that potentially decreases capacity to evaporate heat loss.[34,35] In addition, a child experiences a greater heat production in exercise and has less ability to transfer this heat from the muscles to the skin.

Relative surface area is greater for a child compared to an adult. For example, for an 8-year-old child the ratio of surface area to mass is 360–380 cm^2/kg compared to 240–260 cm^2/kg for an adult of medium size.[31] This results in excessive heat gain in extreme heat and heat loss in the cold. Children also have a lower cardiac output at given metabolic level that potentially decreases capacity for heat convection from core to periphery during strenuous exercise.[31]

The previous morphologic and functional characteristics do not interfere with the ability of the child exercising to adequately dissipate heat in a neutral or mildly warm climate.[31] However, children are at a disadvantage when exposed to extreme heat or cold. The greater the temperature gradient between the air and the skin, the greater the affect on the child.

Acclimatization to exercising in the heat is more gradual in children than in adolescents or adults.[36] A child may require five to six sessions to achieve the same degree of acclimatization acquired by an adult in two to three sessions in the same environment. From a practical standpoint, the intensity and duration of exercise

Exhibit 13–6 Food Shopping Frequency Form for Parents

	Frequency of Purchase				
Food Item	Always	Often	Sometimes	Rarely	Never
Dairy Products					
Milk, whole					
Milk, 2%					
Nonfat					
Cottage cheese					
Cream cheese					
Other cheeses					
Yogurt					
Ice cream					
Sherbet					
Puddings					
Margarine					
Butter					
Other: _____					
Meats					
Beef, hamburger					
Poultry					
Pork, ham					
Bacon, sausage					
Cold cuts, hot dogs					
Other: _____					
Fish					
Canned tuna					
Breaded fish					
Fresh, frozen fish					
Eggs					
Peanut Butter					
Grain Products					
Bread, white					
Bread, whole wheat					
Rolls, biscuits					
Muffins					
Pancakes, waffles					
Bagels					
Pasta, spaghetti					
Pasta, macaroni/cheese					
Rice					
Crackers					
Other: _____					
Cereals					
Sugar coated					
High fiber (bran)					

continues

Exhibit 13–6 continued

Food Item	Frequency of Purchase				
	Always	*Often*	*Sometimes*	*Rarely*	*Never*
Natural (granola)					
Plain (Cheerios)					
Fortified					
Other: _____					
Fruits					
Oranges, orange juice					
Tomatoes, tomato juice					
Grapefruit, grapefruit juice					
Strawberries					
Cranberry juice					
Apples, apple juice					
Grapes, grape juice					
Fruit drink					
Peaches					
Bananas					
Other: _____					
Vegetables					
Peppers					
Potatoes					
Lettuce					
Broccoli					
Spinach					
Carrots					
Corn					
Squash					
Peas					
Green beans					
Beets					
Other: _____					
Snacks and Sweets					
Chips, potato, corn					
Pretzels					
Popcorn					
French fries					
Cookies					
Cake, pie					
Pastries, doughnuts					
Candy					
Sugar, honey, jelly					
Soda, regular					
Soda, diet					
Cocoa					
Other: _____					

Table 13–4 Physiologic Responses of Children to Exercise in the Heat: Comparison with Adults

Characteristic	Typical for Children, vs Adults
Metabolism heat of locomotion	Higher
Sweating rate per m² skin	Lower
Sweating rate per gland	Much lower
Sweating threshold	Higher
Population density of HASG	Higher
Cardiac output/L O₂ uptake	Lower
Blood flow to skin	Higher
Sweat NaCl content	Lower
Sweat lactate and H+	Higher
Exercise tolerance time	Shorter
Acclimatization to heat	Slower
Core temperature increase with dehydration	Faster

Note: HASG = heat-activated sweat glands

Source: Courtesy of Gatorade Sports Science Institute, Chicago, Illinois.

should be restrained during the first 4 to 5 days of beginning an exercise program, particularly in the heat. Over a period of 1.5 weeks, activity can be slowly increased.[31] The major physiologic changes that occur during heat acclimatization include a reduction in heart rate and body temperature, an increase in sweat rate, and a decreased concentration of salt in the sweat.[31,37]

Dehydration and Heat Disorders

Because children sweat less, have a lower cardiac output, do not tolerate temperature extremes, and acclimate to heat more slowly than young adults,[31,35] they are at increased risk for dehydration. As little as a 2% decrease in body weight from fluid loss can lead to a significant decrease in muscular strength and stamina.[38] For example, this translates into a 1.2-lb loss for a 60-lb athlete.

As shown in Table 13–5 the progressive effects of dehydration are serious. As a person becomes dehydrated, heart rate increases, blood flow to the skin decreases, and body temperature can increase steadily to dangerous levels.[39] Coaches need to be familiar with the symptoms

Table 13–5 Effects of Dehydration

% Body Weight Lost	Symptoms
0.5	Thirst
2	Stronger thirst, discomfort, appetite loss
3	Dry mouth, reduced urine
4	Increased effort, flushed skin, impatience, apathy
5	Difficulty concentrating
6	Impaired temperature regulation
8	Dizziness, labored breathing, confusion
10	Spasticity, imbalance, swollen tongue, delirium
11	Kidney failure, circulatory insufficiency

Source: Adapted with permission from J.E. Greenleaf and W.J. Fink, Fluid Intake and Athletic Performance, in *Nutrition and Athletic Performance*, W. Haskell, ed., © 1982, Bull Publishing.

of heat distress and procedures for obtaining and providing immediate treatment (Exhibit 13–7).

As shown in Table 13–6, there are certain groups of children who are at a particularly high risk of heat illness due to certain diseases and medical conditions.[37,40] One common underlying factor among the conditions listed alphabetically (not by severity) is that they may induce hypohydration, either through excessive fluid loss or insufficient intake. Excessive fluid loss may be observed in the following conditions: bulimia, congenital heart disease, diabetes mellitus, diabetes insipidus, gastroenteritis, fever, obesity, and vomiting. Insufficient fluid intake may occur in persons with anorexia nervosa, cystic fibrosis, mental retardation, and renal failure.

Children who are obese are at a disadvantage when exercising in the heat. As shown by Haymes et al,[35] rectal temperature and heart rate increased more quickly in boys who were mildly obese (31.2% body fat) compared to controls who were leaner during 70 minutes of intermittent exercise and rest. According to Bar-Or[40] possible reasons for the deficient thermoregulation in children who are obese include the following: 1) A relatively small amount of heat is needed to increase the temperature of a given mass of fat. 2) Hypohydration denotes a relatively higher percentage of water loss in persons who are obese, because fat has a lower water content than most other tissues. 3) When children who are obese exercise at the same intensity, compared to children who are not obese,

Exhibit 13–7 Symptoms and Treatment of Heat Disorders

Symptoms	Disorder	Treatment
Thirst Nausea Chills Clammy skin Throbbing heart Muscle pain, spasms	Heat cramps	4–8 oz of cold water every 10–15 minutes. Move athlete to shade and remove any excess clothing.
Reduced sweating Dizziness Headache Shortness of breath Weak, rapid pulse Lack of saliva Extreme fatigue	Heat exhaustion	Stop exercise, move athlete to cool place. Take off wet clothes, place icebag on head. Have athlete drink 16 oz (2 cups) of water for every pound of weight lost.
Lack of sweat, urine Dry, hot skin Swollen tongue Hallucinations Rapid pulse Unsteady gait Fainting Low blood pressure Loss of consciousness Shock	Heat stroke	Call for emergency medical treatment. Place ice bags on back of head. Remove wet clothing. If athlete is conscious, help take a cold shower. If in shock, elevate feet.

Source: Adapted with permission from J.E. Greenleaf and W.J. Fink, Fluid Intake and Athletic Performance, in *Nutrition and Athletic Performance*, W. Haskell, ed., © 1982, Bull Publishing.

Table 13–6 Diseases and Conditions That Predispose the Exercising Child to Heat-Related Illness

Disease or Condition	Insufficient Drinking	Excessive Sweating	Insufficient Sweating	Potential Hypohydration	Insufficient Heat Convection to Skin	Other
				Possible Mechanisms		
Anorexia nervosa	X			X	X	Thermoregulatory insufficiency
Bulimia	X			X	X	
Congenital (cyanotic) heart disease		X		X		Excessive salt loss
Cystic fibrosis	X	X		X		Diuresis
Diabetes (mellitus and insipidus)	X			X		
Diarrhea and vomiting				X	X	
Fever		X		X	X	Thermoregulatory insufficiency
No acclimatization			X			
Low aerobic fitness			X			
Mental deficiency	X			X		
Obesity		X				Low specific heat, high heat production
Undernutrition	X		X	X		Thermoregulatory insufficiency

Courtesy of Gatorade Sports Science Institute, Chicago, Illinois.

their relative effort is greater (and increase of core temperature is higher) due to a low maximal aerobic capacity.

The type of clothing worn during exercise affects the body's ability to cool itself. Heavy clothing can be a contributing factor to heat stress. Therefore, children who participate in certain sports may be at an increased risk for dehydration and heat illness. For example, football and hockey players wear protective gear, which reduces the ability of the body to cool itself. Mathews and associates[41] evaluated young men who exercised on a treadmill while wearing a football uniform, or a pair of shorts, no shirt, and a backpack that weighed the same as the uniform. They showed that athletes with the football uniforms had increased heat production as indicated by an increase in rectal temperature. This is because the uniforms allowed for only 30% to 40% evaporation to occur, whereas the shorts and backpack allowed for 70% evaporation to occur.

Swimmers may not recognize that they are losing body water through sweat in the pool. They can also become dehydrated by sitting around the pool in a hot, humid environment between exercise sessions. Figure skaters may not realize the importance of fluid replacement because they are in a cool environment. In addition, the typical attire of gloves, tights, and body suits, and/or sweats reduces the ability of the body to cool itself.

Athletes in sports that have weight categories for competition, such as wrestling or lightweight rowing, may purposefully restrict fluid and/or food intake in an effort to lose weight, potentiating the risk of dehydration.[42-44] Athletes in sports where appearance and leanness are critically evaluated by judges and audience such as gymnastics, ballet, and figure skating may also be at increased risk for dehydration if fluid and/or food deprivation are used to control weight.[44-46]

To prevent dehydration and reduce the risk of heat injury, the timing of practice can be adjusted depending on weather conditions. Workouts should be scheduled for the coolest time of the day (before 10 am, after 6 pm), especially in warm, humid weather conditions. Extreme heat and humidity are valid reasons to cancel practice or competition (Table 13–7).

Prevention of Heat Illness: Fluid Requirements

Heat stroke ranks second to head injury among reported causes of death in secondary school athletes. Heat illness can be prevented through education and establishing healthy fluid intake habits at an early age. Because a substantial level of dehydration can be reached before the body ever feels "thirsty," special emphasis should be placed on ensuring adequate fluid intake in children before, during, and after physical activity. Guidelines for fluid replacement are shown in Figure 13–8.

Children, like adults, do not usually drink enough when offered fluids during exercise in the heat.[32,33,37] However, one important difference is that for any given level of hypohydration, children's core temperatures increase faster than those of adults.[33] During prolonged exercise, children and adolescents may not recognize the symptoms of heat strain and push themselves to the point of heat-related illness.[31,33,40] From a practical standpoint, this suggests that it is important to prevent, or significantly reduce, "voluntary dehydration" in children. This can be accomplished by providing children with a personalized bottle and encouraging them to drink at regular, frequent intervals—and beyond thirst. For example, Bar-Or suggests that children younger than 10 years old should drink until they do not feel thirsty, and then drink an additional half a glass of liquid.[40] Supervision of fluid intake is essential, particularly for children, because they do not instinctively drink enough fluid to replace water losses.[32,33,37]

Fluid losses can be monitored by weighing the athlete before and after exercise. Serial weighing can identify the athlete who is becoming chronically dehydrated during repetitive training. Another practical strategy would be to weigh the athlete during several training sessions and then predict how much fluid the athlete needs for sub-

Table 13–7 Restraints on Activities at Different Levels of Heat Stress

WBGT		
°C	°F	Restraints on Activities
< 24	< 75	All activities allowed, but be alert for prodromes of heat-related illness in prolonged events
24.0–25.9	76.0–78.6	Longer rest periods in the shade Enforce drinking every 15 minutes
26–28	79–84	Stop activity of unacclimatized and other persons with high risk Limit activities of all others (disallow long-distance races, cut down further duration of other activities)
> 29	> 84	Cancel all athletic activities

Note: WBGT = wet bulb globe temperature. This is an index of climatic heat stress that can be measured on the field by the use of a psychrometer. This apparatus, available commercially, is composed of three thermometers. One ("wet bulb") has a wet wick around it, to monitor humidity. Another is inside a hollow black ball ("globe"), to monitor radiation. The third is a simple thermometer ("temperature"), to measure air temperature. The heat stress index is calculated as

WBGT = 0.7 WB temp + 0.2 G temp + 0.1 temp

It is noteworthy that 70% of the stress is due to humidity, 20% to radiation, and only 10% to air temperature.

Source: Used with permission of the American Academy of Pediatrics, *Sports Medicine: Health Care for Young Athletes*, 2nd ed., American Academy of Pediatrics, 1991.

sequent workouts. Fluid losses should be replaced during and after exercise. Children should be allowed to take "fluid breaks" to promote adequate hydration. In addition, fluids should be readily available and never be withheld as a disciplinary measure.

Choosing the Right Fluids

Although plain water is the most economical source of fluid to hydrate the body, children may be more likely to drink sufficient amounts if they are given flavored fluids. To enhance a child's willingness to drink, beverages consumed during exercise should be palatable and stimulate thirst.[40] In a recent study,[47] to examine the effect of drink flavor and composition on voluntary drink and hydration, 9- to 12-year-old boys performed three 3-hour exercise sessions (four 20-minute cycling bouts at 50% maximal O_2 uptake followed by 25 minutes' rest) in a warm climate. One of the following three beverages was assigned to each session in a Latin-square sequence: unflavored water (W), grape-flavored

water (FW), and grape-flavored water plus 6% carbohydrate and 18 mmol/l NaCl (CNa). Drinking was ad libitum. The results were striking—the children stayed better hydrated when they drank sports drinks (38 oz) compared to drinking plain (20 oz) or flavored water (30 oz). The authors concluded that although flavoring of water reduces children's voluntary dehydration, further addition of 6% carbohydrates and 18 mmol/l NaCl prevents it altogether.

Diluted fruit juice (diluted at least twofold—2 cups of water for every 1 cup of juice) is another option for fluid replacement during activity. However, diluted juice may not eliminate thirst compared to a sport drink. More research is needed to identify whether diluted fruit juice is an optimal choice for fluid replacement during exercise. Undiluted juice or carbonated soda should never be used during activity because they typically contain too much carbohydrate (10% to 12%) and may cause gastric discomfort and delay gastric emptying. Caffeinated beverages (iced tea, certain soft drinks) should also be avoided because they promote diuresis. Particu-

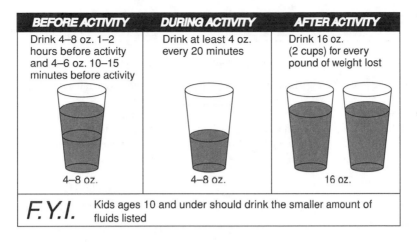

BEFORE ACTIVITY	DURING ACTIVITY	AFTER ACTIVITY
Drink 4–8 oz. 1–2 hours before activity and 4–6 oz. 10–15 minutes before activity	Drink at least 4 oz. every 20 minutes	Drink 16 oz. (2 cups) for every pound of weight lost
4–8 oz.	4–8 oz.	16 oz.

F.Y.I. Kids ages 10 and under should drink the smaller amount of fluids listed

Figure 13–8 Gatorade Fluid Guidelines for Players. Courtesy of Gatorade Sports Science Institute, Chicago, Illinois.

larly for children, the potential side effects of consuming caffeine—agitation, nausea, muscle tremors, palpitations, and headaches—are not conducive to optimal performance.

Meyer and colleagues[32] have demonstrated that sweat $[Na+]$ and $[Cl-]$ tended to increase with maturation whereas sweat $[K+]$ was lower in young adults compared with prepubescent females and males. Because children have a lower sweating rate than young adults, total Na+ and Cl– losses per kilogram body weight from sweat were higher in young adults compared with those of the prepubescent and pubescent groups. However, no maturational differences were found in K+ losses. The authors speculate that a protective mechanism may exist in children against excessive salt loss, which accompanies their lower sweating rate. It is not clear whether the lower NaCl content in children's sweat justifies the use of more dilute beverages for children than adults; more research is needed.[32,40]

PRE- AND POSTEVENT MEAL

The pre-event meal serves two main purposes—first, to prevent athletes from feeling hungry before or during activity, and second, to help supply fuel to the muscles during training and competition. Still, most of the energy needed for any sports event is provided by whatever the child has eaten during the prior week. The most optimal plan is to offer foods that the child finds pleasing 2 to 3 hours before exercise. The food should be high in carbohydrate, contain low to moderate amounts of protein, and be low fat.[1,22] In addition, consumption of at least 240 mL fluid (water or juice) should be encouraged.

High-fat and high-protein foods should be avoided because they take longer to digest than carbohydrate foods and, if eaten for the pre-event meal, can contribute to indigestion and nausea. Children should also avoid eating simple carbohydrates such as sugar, candy, honey, or soft drinks before exercise. They do not provide "quick energy," and some athletes are more sensitive than others to changes in blood glucose levels when simple sugars are eaten. Instead, complex carbohydrates, which are found in breads, cereals, pasta, rice, and other starchy foods, should be included in the pre-event meal. These foods are digested relatively quickly, so that the child's stomach is empty and blood sugar level is stable before practice or competition.

The child can make choices depending upon food availability and preferences based upon the guidelines shown in Exhibit 13–8.

Exhibit 13–8 Guidelines for Eating Before an Event

1 to 2 Hours Before	2 to 3 Hours Before	3 or More Hours Before
Fruit or vegetable juice, sport drink	Fruit or vegetable juice, sport drink	Fruit or vegetable juice, sport drink
Fresh fruit (low fiber)	Fresh fruit	Fresh fruit
	Breads, bagels with jam	Breads, bagels
	English muffins with jam	English muffins
		Peanut butter, lean meat, low-fat cheese
		Low-fat yogurt
		Baked potato
		Cereal with low-fat (1%) milk
		Pasta with tomato sauce

Ideally, the previous guidelines should be considered regarding pre-event meal for the child. However, some children prefer not to eat because they feel nervous or excited. Under these circumstances, the child should never be pressured to eat; instead liquids such as sport drinks or juice should be encouraged.

After exercise, fluids should be offered to promote hydration and complex carbohydrates encouraged to replenish glucose stores. Some parents may inappropriately use food as a bribe to encourage a winning performance. Parents should be advised that special treats should not be used to reward a child that does well and withheld if he does not do well. Whether the child competed successfully or not should have no bearing upon postexercise intake.

WEIGHT-CONTROL PRACTICES

Sometimes, healthy nutrition practices are disregarded in the pursuit of athletic prowess. The emphasis may be on what will make the child a better athlete, rather than what will make him or her a happy, healthy child. This may be in part because parents and coaches are not well-informed about a child's stage of maturation, nutritional needs, emotions, and/or physical ability.

Unfortunately, some parents and coaches have misconceptions about how much the pre-

pubescent child should eat. Some encourage their children to eat excessively, with the erroneous belief that this will build strength and endurance at a faster rate. To the contrary, indiscriminate consumption, in which food intake exceeds the child's caloric requirement, may be the start of a lifelong struggle with being overweight.

At the other extreme are parents and coaches who promote a diet restricted in calories and nutrients, that may compromise the health of the child.[1] Given the current focus on lowering cholesterol and fat, some parents inappropriately narrow the child's food choices (excluding red meat, dairy products) in an attempt to control weight or to minimize the future risk of heart disease. Prepubescent children should receive 30% of total calories from fat, because lower levels of fat intake may not adequately support growth and development.[48] Parents can encourage long-term healthful habits without compromising growth by offering foods with moderate amounts of unsaturated fats and reducing (not eliminating) foods that are high in saturated fats.

Exercise demands by parents or coaches to reduce body weight by running laps, calisthenics, or extra practice time can be excessive. Especially during hot temperatures, fatigue, heat exhaustion, and illness can be the result. If the child does need to lose fat weight, a medically supervised weight control plan that focuses on weight monitoring, caloric stabilization, and increased activity is recommended.[1,4,22]

The Special Case of "Making Weight"

Scholastic wrestlers must meet a certain weight classification to compete. It is a common practice throughout the competitive season for wrestlers to restrict food and fluid intake to compete at one to three weight classes below their normal weight.[43,44,49] Wrestlers typically believe that this practice, known as "making weight," gives them a competitive edge over smaller opponents. Wrestlers, coaches, and parents may not realize the negative physiologic impact this practice may have on their bodies.

Studies have shown that making weight decreases blood and plasma volumes, reduces cardiac function during submaximal work (for example, higher heart rate, smaller stroke volume, and reduced cardiac output), impairs thermoregulation, decreases renal blood flow and renal filtration, and increases electrolyte losses.[5,38] The calorie and micronutrient content of wrestlers' diets during training are typically inadequate.[42]

From a performance standpoint, making weight can lead to liver and muscle glycogen depletion, dehydration, reduced muscular strength, and decreased performance work time.[5,38] Because wrestlers rarely regain all of their lost fluid weight after the official weigh-in, they may be competing under suboptimal physiologic conditions. Other athletes at risk for extreme weight loss methods are gymnasts, figure skaters, and dancers—participants in activities where a certain physique is promoted to achieve the "ideal" thin appearance.

In an effort to preclude the use of erratic weight loss practices by some young athletes, it is imperative to establish healthy weight-control guidelines with the prepubescent child. Through nutrition education, coaches, parents, and athletes can be apprised about the consequences of rapid and extreme weight reduction by fluid and food restriction and healthy alter-

natives for achieving a suitable competitive weight.[4,22]

Although the majority of parents are appropriately supportive and considerate of the young child's needs, some are not as well-informed about weight control. It is imperative to develop effective strategies to counter demanding parents who may be exploiting their child for their own satisfaction or personal gain. Nutritional requirements for growth and development must be placed before athletic considerations.

FOOD SUPPLEMENTS

Research is lacking on the use of dietary supplements and other performance-enhancing aids by child athletes. However, many older athletes consume substances, including vitamin and mineral supplements, in an effort to improve performance. Unfortunately, many self-proclaimed "experts" and clever marketing strategies by companies are eager to convince athletes that their products will improve athletic performance by increasing muscle mass, preventing fat gain, enhancing strength, or supplying energy, to name just a few. These "experts" may insist that the athletes' fatigue and muscle soreness are due to a special vitamin or mineral deficiency. In fact, when there is a nutritional reason for fatigue, it is usually insufficient calories, insufficient carbohydrates, or dehydration.

Although vitamin and mineral supplementation may improve the nutritional status of persons consuming marginal amounts of nutrients from food, and may improve performance in persons with deficiencies, no scientific evidence supports the general use of supplements to improve athletic performance.[50,51] Certainly, for the child who consistently is unable to incorporate certain foods into the diet or is chronically restricting intake, a one-a-day multivitamin and multimineral (100% of the RDA) is prudent to ensure adequate intake of micronutrients. However, there is no place in the diet of a healthy child for megadoses of vitamins, minerals, or other performance-enhancing substances.[23] Unsupervised, indiscriminate use of vitamin, mineral, and other substances raises safety concerns.[52]

Well-meaning, but misinformed parents and coaches may advise children to take supplements in an effort to promote early athletic development and improve performance and as "health insurance."[1] However, eventual maturity and athletic prowess do not necessarily depend upon how early a child reaches adolescence, and in any event, the process will not be facilitated by dietary supplements. Providing children with supplements can give them a false sense of security and may encourage faulty eating habits. They may assume that their morning dose of supplements provides them with all of the nutrients that they need, so that they can eat candy and soda instead of cereal and fruit juice.

Another disadvantage of supplement use is that child athletes may erroneously associate improvements in performance with whatever supplements they may be taking. They may be less likely to attribute progress to training, hard work, and a balanced diet. This type of false reinforcement may also encourage children to try other types of supplements and substances (including possibly steroids) and lead to a snowball effect with undesired consequences.

To move away from this reliance on "supplement insurance," young athletes need to feel confident about eating ordinary foods. Parents, coaches, and health professionals must emphasize how regular foods promote muscle growth and optimal performance. From a practical standpoint, this is yet another important reason to encourage young athletes to keep records of what they eat, when and how hard they train, and

how their performance improves. These records can be used to illustrate the importance of good dietary and training habits as the cause of improvement rather than leaving the child to erroneously associate athletic accomplishments with a pill.[1]

Hopefully, if children understand why extra vitamins and minerals are not necessary, they will learn to refrain from using them at an early age and continue to do so during adolescence, when peer pressure is amplified. For the young athlete, the key to health and performance cannot be found in any one food or supplement, but in a proper combination of foods that provides many different nutrients that the body requires. Variety and moderation is the best strategy to achieve balance.

CONCLUSION

When working with the prepubescent athlete, the challenge for health professionals is to provide the child, coach, and parents with appropriate nutrition information to promote training and performance after meeting needs for growth and development. Meal patterns, and caloric and nutritional adequacy of the diet should be evaluated followed by questions and recommendations about sports-related issues and practices. In addition to promoting a healthy dietary intake, explanation of basic nutrition concepts as they are related to exercise is important to help establish good habits at an early age, and to dispel any misconceptions that the child has already heard or will most likely be exposed to as an adolescent.

REFERENCES

1. Jennings DS, Steen SN. *Play Hard, Eat Right: A Parents' Guide to Sports Nutrition for Children*. Minnetonka, MN: Chronimed Publishing; 1995.

2. Steen SN. Nutrition and the young athlete: special considerations. *Sports Med.* 1994;17(3):152–162.

3. Steen SN. Nutrition for the competitive athlete. In: Rickert VI, ed. *Adolescent Nutrition.* New York: Chapman & Hall; 1996.

4. Coleman E, Steen SN. *The Ultimate Sports Nutrition Book.* Palo Alto, CA: Bull Publishing Co; 1996.

5. American Medical Association. Committee on the medical aspects of sports: wrestling and weight control. *JAMA.* 1967;201:541.

6. Hamill PVV, Drizd TA, Johnson CL, Reed RB, Roche AF, Moore WM. Physical growth: National Center for Health Statistics Percentiles. *Am J Clin Nutr.* 1979; 32:607–629.

7. Splett P, Story M. Child nutrition objective for the decade. *J Am Diet Assoc.* 1991;91:665–668.

8. Meyers A. Undernutrition, hunger, and learning in children. *Nutr News.* 1989;52:1.

9. Chumlea WC. Growth and development. In: Queen PM, Lang CE, eds. *Handbook of Pediatric Nutrition.* Gaithersburg, MD: Aspen Publishers; 1993:3–25.

10. Garn SM, Rohmann CG. Interaction of nutrition and genetics in the timing of growth and development. *Pediatr Clin North Am.* 1966;13:353.

11. Himes JH, Roche AF, Thissen D, Moore WM. Parent-specific adjustments for evaluation of recumbent length and stature of children. *Pediatrics.* 1985;75:304.

12. Tanner JM. *Growth at Adolescence.* 2nd ed. Oxford, England: Blackwell Scientific Publications; 1962.

13. Wilmore JH. Body weight standards and athletic performance. In: Brownell KD, Rodin J, Wilmore JH, eds. *Eating, Body Weight, and Performance in Athletes: Disorders of Modern Society.* Philadelphia: Lea & Febiger; 1992:315–329.

14. Boileau RA, Lohman TG, Slaughter MH, Horswill CA, Stillman RJ. Problems associated with determining body composition in maturing youngsters. In: Brown EW, Banta CF, eds. *Competitive Sports for Children and Youth: An Overview of Research and Issues.* Champaign, IL: Human Kinetics; 1988.

15. Lohman TG. *Advances in Body Composition Assessment.* Champaign, IL: Human Kinetics; 1992.

16. Slaughter MH, Lohman TG, Boileau CA, et al. Skinfold equations for estimation of body fatness in children and youth. *Hum Biol.* 1988;60:709–723.

17. Lohman TG. Assessment of body composition in children. *Pediatr Exerc Sci.* 1989;1:19–30.

18. Lucas B. Normal nutrition from infancy through adolescence. In: Queen PM, Lang CE, eds. *Handbook of Pediatric Nutrition.* Gaithersburg, MD: Aspen Publishers; 1993:145–170.

19. Pollitt E, Leibel RL, Greenfield D. Brief fasting, stress, and cognition in children. *Am J Clin Nutr.* 1981; 34:1526.

20. Simeon DT, Grantham-McGregor S. Effects of missing breakfast on the cognitive functions of school children of differing nutritional status. *Am J Clin Nutr.* 1989;49:646.

21. Ho CS, Gould RA, Jensen LN. Evaluation of the nutrient content of school, sack and vending lunch of junior high school students. *Sch Food Serv Res Rev.* 1991;15:85–90.

22. Steen SN. *Sports Nutrition for Young Athletes.* San Marcos, CA: Nutrition Dimension, Inc; 1994.

23. American Dietetic Association. Timely statement on the nutrition guidance for child athletes in organized sports. *J Am Diet Assoc.* 1996;96(6):610–612.

24. National Research Council. *Recommended Dietary Allowances.* 10th ed. Washington, DC: National Academy Press; 1989.

25. Community Childhood Hunger Identification Project. *A Survey of Childhood Hunger in the United States. Executive Summary.* Washington, DC: Food Research Action Center; 1991.

26. The Kellogg Children's Nutrition Survey. *Executive Summary.* Battle Creek, MI: Kellogg Co; 1991.

27. Astrand PO. *Experimental Studies of Physical Working Capacity in Relation to Sex and Age.* Copenhagen, Denmark: Munskgaard; 1952.

28. Krahenbuhl GS, Pangrasi R. Characteristics associated with running performance in young boys. *Med Sci Sports Exerc.* 1983;15:488.

29. Daniels J. Differences and changes in VO$_2$ among runners 10-18 years of age. *Med Sci Sports Exerc.* 1978;10:200–212.

30. U.S. Department of Agriculture and U.S. Department of Health and Human Services. *Food Guide Pyramid: A Guide to Daily Food Choices.* 1993.

31. Bar-Or O. Climate and the exercising child—a review. *Int J Sports Med.* 1980;1:53–65.

32. Meyer F, Bar-Or O, MacDougall D, Heigenhauser GJF. Sweat electrolyte loss during exercise in the heat: effects of gender and maturation. *Med Sci Sports Exerc.* 1992;24(7):776–781.

33. Bar-Or O, Dotan R, Inbar O, Rothstein A, Zonder H. Voluntary hypohydration in 10- to 12-year-old boys. *J Appl Physiol.* 1980;48:104.

34. Drinkwater BL, Kupprat IC, Denton JE, Crist JL, Horvath SM. Response of pubertal girls and college women to work in the heat. *J Appl Physiol.* 1997; 43:1046–1053.

35. Haymes EM, McCormick RJ, Buskirk ER. Heat tolerance of exercising lean and obese prepubertal boys. *J Appl Physiol.* 1975;39:457.

36. Wagner JA, Robinson S, Tzankoff SP, Marino RP. Heat tolerance and acclimatization to work in the heat in relation to age. *J Appl Physiol.* 1972;33:616–622.

37. Bar-Or O, Blimkie CJR, Hay JA, MacDougal JD, Ward DS, Wilson WM. Voluntary dehydration and heat tolerance in cystic fibrosis. *Lancet.* 1992;339:696–699.

38. American College of Sports Medicine. Position stand on weight loss in wrestlers. *Med Sci Sports Exerc.* 1976;8:xi.

39. American College of Sports Medicine. Position stand on exercise and fluid replacement. *Med Sci Sports Exerc.* 1996;28:i–vi.

40. Bar-Or O. Children's responses to exercise in hot climates: implications for performance and health. *Gatorade Sports Sci Exch.* 1994;7(49).

41. Mathews DK, Fox EL, Tamzo D. Physiological responses during exercise and recovery in a football uniform. *J Appl Physiol*. 1969;26:611–615.

42. Steen SN, McKinney S. Nutritional assessment of college wrestlers. *Phys Sports Med*. 1986;14(11):100–116.

43. Steen SN, Brownell KD. Patterns of weight loss and regain in wrestlers: has the tradition changed? *Med Sci Sports Exerc*. 1990;22(6):762–768.

44. Brownell KD, Steen SN. Weight cycling in athletes: implications for behavior, health and physiology. In: Brownell, KD, Rodin J, Wilmore JH, eds. *Eating, Body Weight, and Performance in Athletes: Disorders of Modern Society*. Philadelphia: Lea & Febiger; 1992:159–171.

45. Garner G, Rosen L. Eating disorders among athletes: research and recommendations. *J Appl Sport Sci Res*. 1991;5(2):100–107.

46. Sherman RA, Thompson RT. *Helping Athletes with Eating Disorders*. Champaign, IL: Human Kinetics; 1993.

47. Boguslaw W, Bar-Or O. Effect of drink flavor and NaCl on voluntary drinking and hydration in boys exercising in the heat. *J Appl Physiol*. 1996;80(4):1112–1117.

48. Committee on Nutrition, American Academy of Pediatrics. Statement on children, dietary fat and cholesterol. *Pediatrics*. 1992;90:469.

49. Steen SN, Oppliger RA, Brownell KD. Metabolic implications of repeated weight loss and regain in high school wrestlers. *JAMA*. 1988;260:47–50.

50. Singh A, Moses FM, Deuster PA. Chronic multivitamin-mineral supplementation does not enhance physical performance. *Med Sci Sports Exerc*. 1992;24:726–732.

51. Haymes EM. Vitamin and mineral supplementation in athletes. *Int J Sport Nutr*. 1991;1:146–149.

52. American Dietetic Association. Position stand on enrichment and fortification of foods and dietary supplements. *J Am Diet Assoc*. 1994;94(6):661–662.

CHAPTER 14

Eating while Traveling

Jacqueline R. Berning

Competing away from home presents a number of challenges for athletes. Jet lag, unfamiliar playing fields, changes in sleep and training are just a few of the obstacles traveling athletes encounter. No matter where athletes are competing, it is important that they choose the proper fuel for optimal performance. Too often, traveling athletes will skip meals, eat insufficient amounts of carbohydrates, and compete dehydrated. Athletes who consume diets that are chronically deficient in carbohydrates and fluid can experience a progressive depletion of glycogen stores, which may cause a decrease in endurance, precision, and speed.[1]

SURVEY FINDINGS

Surveys of elite national swimmers revealed that, like typical Americans, they consumed more fat than carbohydrates in their diets.[2,3] Furthermore, when given a nutrition knowledge test, they did well on basic nutrition knowledge (knowing the food groups) but poorly when it came to choosing foods that were high in a specific nutrient. For example, when asked to name a nutritious carbohydrate, 63% chose an apple, but 38% chose French fries. When asked which food is a good source of protein, 63% chose the correct answer of chicken, but 37% chose oatmeal. Overall, 62% of the swimmers picked the correct answers; 38%, however, were unable to select the proper balance of foods necessary

for the energy demands of their sport. If athletes cannot make proper food choices, they cannot be expected to select a proper diet that is required for peak performance.

In other surveys of competitive swimmers ages 13 to 20 years, several misconceptions were reported.[4] For example, more than half of them believed that everyone should take supplements, that vitamin E improves performance, that supplementing with B vitamins gives you a boost of energy, and that milk consumption the day of competition impairs performance. A study of male track, baseball, and football teams found that only 28% could define glycogen loading, 69% did not know which foods were a good source of carbohydrates, and 54% did not know the major functions of vitamins.[5] A nutrition knowledge questionnaire completed by adolescent gymnasts showed that more than 50% of the girls could not define a complex carbohydrate and did not know that carbohydrates were an important source of energy for exercise.[6] Instead, 75% of the girls erroneously believed that protein was the best source of energy. Volleyball players had difficulty with questions about food sources of quality protein, vitamin C, good sources of energy, carbohydrate loading, and caloric requirements for training.[7] However, they were knowledgeable about the importance of eating a variety of foods, vitamin supplementation, and the differences between plant and animal fats. Massad and colleagues found that when high school athletes were more knowledgeable about nutrition information they were less likely to use supplements.[8]

Not only athletes have a lack of nutrition knowledge or improper eating habits. It has been found that 29% of those 18 to 22 years old skip breakfast, with that number approaching 50% for the high school age group. Nearly a quarter regularly miss lunch and 86% of these young people eat in fast food restaurants each week. An average family of four eats together fewer than five times per week. With this type of dietary intake and lack of nutrition knowledge, it is easy for athletes to make improper food choices while training at home and while traveling.

MAKING WISE FOOD CHOICES

A suggested distribution of calories for most competitive athletes is 10% to 15% protein, 25% to 30% fat, and 50% to 60% carbohydrates.[1] Endurance athletes (triathletes, cyclists, and marathon runners), however, should be consuming 60% to close to 70% of their total calories from carbohydrates because one of the limiting factors in prolonged human performance is glycogen depletion.[9] Athletes who consume diets chronically deficient in carbohydrates can experience a progressive depletion of glycogen stores.[9] This may cause a decrement in endurance, precision, and speed.

Recently, several diet plans have been promoted to athletes that are based on lowering carbohydrate consumption and increasing protein intake. The promoters of these diets have aligned themselves with well-known athletes or teams as endorsements. The scientific basis for a low-carbohydrate, high-protein diet is not supported by scientific research. As a matter of fact, consuming protein at the expense of carbohydrate has been associated with the development of cardiovascular disease and may decrease the ability of athletes to perform aerobic endurance exercise as well as anaerobic exercises, as shown in the following research studies. Sherman et al[10] found that consuming carbohydrates an hour before exercise can actually improve performance. In another study,[11] they

found that carbohydrate feeding 3 to 4 hours before exercise can also enhance performance by filling muscle and liver glycogen stores. Other researchers like Coyle et al[12,13] found that feeding carbohydrates to athletes during exercise lasting an hour or longer aided performance by providing glucose for the exercising muscles to use when they are running low on glycogen. And, taking in carbohydrates immediately after exercise can increase glycogen synthesis after the exercise.[14] Athletes who consume inadequate amounts of carbohydrates may be setting themselves up for less than optimal performances.

Because athletes have a high requirement for carbohydrates but often have a difficult time making wise food choices, eating while away from home becomes even more difficult for athletes who travel to away games and competitions.

PRACTICAL APPLICATIONS

The food guide pyramid for athletes (Figure 14–1) offers an easy method for selecting a nutritionally balanced diet. Foods are classified according to their nutrient content. By eating a variety of foods from each group every day, the athlete will obtain the needed nutrients for a nutritionally sound diet. During periods of heavy training, athletes should increase their consumption from the bread, fruit, and vegetable group. This will increase their carbohydrate intake and help minimize the gradual decline of muscle glycogen and the feelings of fatigue that occur with heavy training.

Another way to ensure that athletes make wise food choices on the road is to determine where they will eat before mealtime. For example, at a suitable restaurant, the athletes should ask for a pasta meal within their budget. Usually, the manager or chef can accommodate them, especially if this request is made on a regular basis when an athlete is in town. Pasta meals, burritos with beans and rice, cold cereal with low-fat milk, baked potatoes, and fruits and vegetables

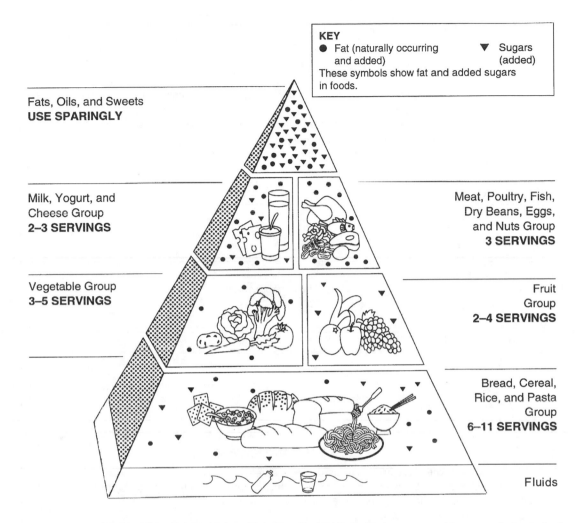

KEY
● Fat (naturally occurring and added)   ▼ Sugars (added)
These symbols show fat and added sugars in foods.

Fats, Oils, and Sweets
USE SPARINGLY

Milk, Yogurt, and
Cheese Group
2–3 SERVINGS

Meat, Poultry, Fish,
Dry Beans, Eggs,
and Nuts Group
3 SERVINGS

Vegetable Group
3–5 SERVINGS

Fruit
Group
2–4 SERVINGS

Bread, Cereal,
Rice, and Pasta
Group
6–11 SERVINGS

Fluids

Use the Food Guide Pyramid to help you select the foods you need for top performance. Start with plenty of bread, cereals, rice, and pasta; vegetables; and fruits. Add two to three servings from the milk group and two to three servings from the meat group.

Each of these food groups provides some, but not all, of the nutrients you need. No one food group is more important than another—for top performance you need them all! Go easy on fats, oils, and sweets, the foods in the small tip of the pyramid.

Figure 14–1 Food Guide Pyramid for Athletes—A Plan for Daily Training Food Choices. *Source:* Food guide pyramid reprinted from U.S. Department of Agriculture. Text below pyramid reprinted with permission from L. Houtkooper and University of Arizona Board of Regents, Tucson, Arizona.

can usually be found in restaurants and provide the easiest and cheapest sources of carbohydrates.

If a hotel offers food service, the coach or trainer should contact the catering manager and

request high-carbohydrate meals within their budget. Exhibit 14–1 gives guidelines for choosing meals while traveling.

As long as the team or school is paying for the meals, the type and quality of food can be cho-

Exhibit 14–1 Guidelines for Choosing Meals while Traveling

BREAKFAST HINTS

- Try pancakes, waffles, French toast, bagels, muffins, cereal, fruit, or juices for a high-carbohydrate breakfast.
- Juice, dried fruit, fresh fruit, pretzels, and bagels are good snacks to pack when away from home.
- Breakfast is the easiest meal in which to consume carbohydrate-rich foods.
- Avoid meals that contain high-fat choices such as bacon or sausage.

Suggested breakfast menus:

Orange juice, 1 cup
Pancakes with syrup (3)
1 banana sliced on pancakes   547 calories, 90% carbohydrate

Apple juice, 6 ounces
Raisin Bran, large bowl
Low-fat milk, 1 cup
Banana   498 calories, 95% carbohydrate

Bran muffin, large
Hot cocoa
Raisins or fresh fruit   310 calories, 69% carbohydrate

Plain English muffin
Strawberry jam, 2 Tbsp.
Scrambled egg
Orange juice, 1 cup
Low-fat yogurt, 1 cup

LUNCH HINTS

- Emphasize the bread in sandwiches rather than the fillings.
- Avoid hamburgers with toppings, fried fish, fried chicken, and French fries at fast food restaurants.
- Try baked potatoes, salads with fat-free dressing, plain hamburgers, chili, or plain burritos and tacos at fast food restaurants because they have less fat.
- Choose fruit juices or low-fat milk rather than soft drinks.

Suggested lunch menus:

Large turkey sandwich on two
   slices of bread
Low-fat fruited yogurt, 1 cup
Orange juice, 1 cup   1017 calories, 60% carbohydrate

Plain baked potato
Chili, 1 cup
Chocolate milkshake   916 calories, 62% carbohydrate

Vegetable soup, 1 cup
Baked chicken, 1 breast
Bread, 1 slice
Applesauce, 1 cup
Low-fat fruited yogurt, 1 cup   737 calories, 71% carbohydrate

continues

Exhibit 14–1 continued

DINNER HINTS

- When traveling, find a restaurant that offers pasta, baked potatoes, rice, breads, vegetables, and salads.
- Order thick-crust pizza and double the amount of vegetable toppings like green peppers, mushrooms, onions, tomatoes, instead of pepperoni and sausage.
- Try restaurants that offer Italian foods such as spaghetti, lasagna, breads, and salads.
- Vegetable soups accompanied by crackers, bread, and muffins can add to a low-fat, carbohydrate-rich meal.

Suggested dinner menus:

Minestrone soup, 1 cup
Spaghetti, 2 cups
Marinara sauce, 2/3 cup
Parmesan cheese, 1 Tbsp
Bread sticks, 2
Low-fat milk, 1 cup   977 calories, 68% carbohydrates

Turkey, 4 oz
Stuffing, 1/2 cup
Mashed potatoes, 1 cup
Peas, 1 cup
Roll
Low-fat milk, 1 cup   960 calories, 55% carbohydrate

Lean roast beef, 3 oz
Rice, 1 1/2 cups
Corn, 1 cup
Rolls, 2
Low-fat milk, 1 1/2 cups   1320 calories, 60% carbohydrates

---

sen. Athletes should be able to ask for special foods and get a reasonable price. The hotel or restaurant wants their business. Athletes can also be taught how to order from the menu for better nutrition. For example, ordering a la carte might be more expensive, but it can offer greater variety and increase the carbohydrate content of a diet. Requesting substitutions like a baked potato instead of French fries, whole wheat bread for white bread, jelly instead of fat-loaded pats of butter, and skim milk or fruit juice instead of calorie-dense soda, and asking for salad dressing on the side to help control the amount of fat in a diet are ways athletes can make small changes when eating out that will make a significant difference in their nutritional status. All-you-can-eat buffets should be approached with caution. Some athletes regard buffet dining as a personal

challenge, with the goal to get more than their money's worth by filling up their plate until it is overflowing. Athletes should be taught how to survey the entire buffet line and how to decide what foods are high in carbohydrate and low in fat and stick to those foods. Athletes who "fill up" on nutritious foods first will get all the fuel and nutrients they need to compete and stay healthy. Exhibit 14–2 lists key words to look for when reading a menu.

If athletes or athletic departments cannot afford all three meals at a restaurant, then they should choose breakfast for a team meal. With selections like cereal (hot or cold), bagels, English muffins, pancakes, toast, fruit and fruit juices, breakfast can be inexpensive and an easy way to get carbohydrate-rich foods. If their budget does not allow restaurant meals or if they are

1. Fat content must be watched when selecting menu items. If you see one of the following words describing a food, try to make another selection: **fried, crispy, breaded, scampi style, creamed, buttery, au gratin, gravy**.
2. Adjectives that represent lower-fat foods are the following: **marinara, steamed, boiled, broiled, tomato sauce, in its own juice, poached, charbroiled**.
3. Restaurant choices

   Depending on the restaurant you go to, the following are some tips when selecting foods:

   • **Mexican**—Choose pot beans instead of refried beans and chicken or bean burritos and tostadas. Ask for baked soft corn tortillas instead of deep fat fried shells or flour tortillas. Use salsa instead of sour cream and guacamole. Watch the chip intake.
   • **Italian**—Pasta with marinara sauce is good, but watch the cream sauces. Pizza, plain or with vegetables, is a good choice. Salads with dressing on the side and bread with butter on the side are good choices. Low-fat Italian ices and low-fat frozen yogurt are better than rich dessert choices.
   • **Chinese**—Stir fry and steamed dishes, such as chicken and vegetables with rice, are good choices. Minimize your intake of deep fried items such as egg rolls, wontons, and sweet and sour pork.
   • **Burger places**—Salad bars are great, but use a low-fat or nonfat dressing. Look for grilled burgers, hold the mayonnaise, and go light on the cheese. Watch your French fry intake (select a baked potato with a topping on the side if you can), and drink juice or low-fat milk instead of the milkshake.
   • **Breakfast cafes**—Always ask for margarine on the side when ordering pancakes, toast, bagels, and waffles. Select fruit, fruit juices, and whole grain cereals, breads, and muffins. Watch your caffeine intake.

on only a day trip, a nearby grocery store offers a great variety of foods. Many grocery stores have a delicatessen or a soup and salad bar, and athletes can always pick up fresh fruits, vegetables, fruit juices, low-fat milk, and dairy products as well as breads, bagels, muffins, and low-fat luncheon meats. Not only are grocery stores easy and fast, they can also be a cheaper source of meals than restaurants. Athletes can choose foods from all five food groups and come away with nutritious food choices that can enhance their performance.

Another way to urge athletes to make more nutritious food choices is to bring or pack a cooler with nutritious snacks for the road trip. Usually, athletes who travel by bus or van tend to consume candy, soda pop, and potato chips. To cut down on these types of foods, pack a cooler with high-carbohydrate foods. Exhibit 14–3 lists examples of nutritious, high-carbohydrate snacks for athletes traveling.

SMART FOOD CHOICES AT FAST FOOD RESTAURANTS

It's 7:00 PM and the team has just finished competing. They shower, dress, and pile into the team bus or van. It's now 8:15 PM They are hungry, on a limited budget, and have a 2-hour drive home. Where do they eat? Like many traveling teams and athletes, they stop at a fast food restaurant. Although fast foods can be high in fat and low in calcium and in vitamins A and C, an athlete can make wise food selections by using the chart shown in Exhibit 14–4.

By making a few wise food choices at fast food restaurants, athletes can change a calorie-dense meal into a nutrient-dense meal. Try teaching the following tips to athletes next time they step up to the counter at their favorite fast food chain:

• Have them think about what they've already eaten and what they will eat later in

Exhibit 14–3 Packing the Cooler

- Fluids—water, sports drinks, fruit juices
- Turkey sandwiches
- Fresh and dried fruit
- Low- or nonfat yogurt
- Vegetables
- Part-skim string cheese
- Energy bars
- Low-fat, ready-to-eat cereal
- Bagels, breads, and rolls
- Rice cakes
- Breadsticks
- Pretzels
- Graham crackers
- Animal crackers
- Fig bars, Nutrigrain bars
- Ginger snaps and vanilla wafers

the day. For example, if they had a deluxe meal combo for lunch, they might decide to cut back and have a lighter dinner.

- Have them try to include low-fat dairy products and at least two vegetables or fruits with each meal.
- Try limiting the amount of salad dressing (or use fat-free dressing), mayonnaise, and other special sauces.
- Try some of the new lower-fat items at their favorite fast food chain (like the grilled McChicken sandwich).
- Suggest they share French fries, a large sandwich, a baked potato, or dessert with another teammate. Or take half home for another meal.

INTERNATIONAL TRAVEL

Although making wise food choices while traveling is no easy task, trying to find familiar and nutritious foods during international travel and competition is extremely difficult. Most athletes who travel internationally have problems finding enough food as well as finding foods that are familiar and have been prepared in a way that doesn't present any potential food safety hazard.

Problems and Solutions

Athletes who travel to other countries have a 50-50 chance of contracting traveler's diarrhea, a sometimes serious, always annoying, bacterial infection of the digestive tract. The risk is high because, for one thing, other countries' cleanliness standards for food and water are often lower than those of the United States and Canada. Another reason for the high incidence is that every region's microbes are different, and although persons are immune to those in their own neighborhoods, traveling athletes have not had the chance to develop immunity to the pathogens in the places they are competing.

To protect against disease-causing organisms not found at home, traveling athletes should drink only bottled water, even if just brushing their teeth. They should drink only boiled, bottled, canned, or carbonated beverages without ice cubes. This way they are sure nothing has been added to the drink. Many athletes make the mistake of using ice in their beverages when traveling abroad. The ice is usually made from the local water supply and will be contaminated with local pathogens that traveling athletes have no immunity to. Athletes need to be careful not to swallow any water if they are swimming or showering; however, swimming pools that are well chlorinated are probably safe.

HOW CAN ATHLETES AVOID TRAVELER'S DIARRHEA?

Because contaminated food and water can cause traveler's diarrhea, athletes need to be careful of what they eat or drink. They should choose restaurants that are well-known or recommended by reliable people like hotel managers, and coaches and athletes who have traveled in the area before. The U.S. Embassy is also a reliable place to get information about the restaurants and water conditions. Also, whenever possible, athletes should avoid food sold on the streetcorners or in open air markets. They should be careful at buffets, especially outdoors, and make sure that when foods are

When eating a meal at a fast food restaurant, don't make it a dietary disaster. A typical fast food meal is high in fat and low in carbohydrates, calcium, vitamin A, and vitamin C. It is difficult to choose a high-carbohydrate meal at a fast food restaurant; however, the food choices below have a higher carbohydrate content and nutrient density. Satisfy athletes' hunger and nutrition needs by using the following suggestions:

McDonald's

Breakfast
- Cheerios, Wheaties, fat-free muffins (apple and blueberry), hotcakes (no sausage), English muffins, and apple, orange, or grapefruit juice.

Lunch and Dinner
- Grilled chicken sandwich, plain hamburger or cheeseburger, side salad with light vinaigrette or reduced-calorie French dressing. Juice or milk to drink, or vanilla, chocolate, or strawberry milkshake or low-fat frozen yogurt cone.

Subway

Lunch and Dinner
- Turkey breast sub or roast beef sub on whole wheat bread; watch the mayonnaise; side salad with low-calorie or regular dressing but use half the amount.

Hardees

Breakfast
- Pancakes without the sausage and bacon. Watch the amount of butter and syrup. Oat bran muffin with orange juice would be another good choice.

Lunch and Dinner
- Regular cheeseburger and hamburgers are relatively low in fat and would make good choices. The following are other low-fat, high-carbohydrate choices: roast beef sandwich, ham and cheese sandwich, turkey club, grilled chicken breast sandwich, garden salad with low-calorie dressing, mashed potatoes with gravy (it's fat-free). Top off the meal with a twist ice cream cone.

Taco Bell

Lunch and Dinner
- Any of the Border light items have half the fat of the regular items. If these are not available, then try the bean burrito, regular taco, soft taco, chicken fajita, pinto and cheese, or the rice side order. Low-fat milk is also available. Avoid items that have extra cheese, added sour cream, or guacamole—they are high in fat.

Arby's

Breakfast
- There are not many good choices here. Try the blueberry muffin with orange juice, the plain biscuit, or the cinnamon nut danish.

Lunch and Dinner
- Good choices include the regular roast beef sandwich, grilled chicken deluxe, grilled chicken barbeque, and turkey sub. Most of the light menu is very good, especially light roast turkey deluxe, the light roast chicken deluxe, or the light roast beef deluxe. Pick a baked potato to go with the sandwich instead of the fries, but watch the toppings that you add. Add a garden salad and you have a complete meal. If you don't want the salad, then pick their vegetable soup or the chicken noodle soup.

Wendy's

Lunch and Dinner
- Wendy's single hamburger and grilled chicken sandwich are the best choices from the regular sandwiches. If you want the bacon cheeseburger, then pick the junior version because it is smaller and has less fat. Even though you will not be full, try filling up on the salads or baked potatoes, but watch the toppings and dressings. Ask for the plain baked potato and then get the toppings on the side so you can control how much you add. The salad bar is an excellent choice but again watch the amount of chicken salad and potato salad you add. Wendy's also carries low-fat dressings. If you choose regular dressing, use half the amount you usually do. Their

continues

Exhibit 14–4 continued

Frosties contain 2 g of fat for the small size; if you made good food choices that are low in fat and high in nutrition, then you can reward yourself with a small Frostie.

Pizza Hut
Lunch and Dinner
- Order a thicker crust pizza, like the hand-tossed or pan pizza because they are higher in carbohydrates. Also try to order more vegetables on your pizza, like green peppers and onions, and try to avoid adding extra cheese, pepperoni, and sausage. Your best bets are the veggie lovers' pizza, the supreme or super supreme pizza, or the pepperoni pizza. Try adding a salad to your meal, but not one that is dripping in salad dressing. Choose the low-fat dressing or use half the amount that you usually need. Bread sticks are lower in fat; use them as an appetizer. There are other items on the menu that are not pizza and tend to be lower in fat. The ham and cheese sandwich and the spaghetti can have a salad added to them to make them filling and low in fat.

Burger King
Breakfast
- Burger King is not the best stop for breakfast items. If you must eat here, then try the blueberry muffins and the orange juice.

Lunch and Dinner
- Once again, if you find yourself in any of these fast food hamburger places, the plainer the item, the less fat. Good choices are the cheeseburger and the hamburger. If you feel like something different, order the Whopper Jr. It has less fat than the full-sized hamburger with the same name. Try the BK Broiler chicken sandwich. The worst choices are Double Whopper with cheese, bacon double cheeseburger, and the fried chicken sandwich. Add a garden salad with low-calorie dressing or use a half serving of the regular dressing. Try to avoid the French fries. If you're still hungry, eat another plain hamburger or cheeseburger.

KFC
Lunch and Dinner
- If you want the fried chicken, one way to not get as much fat is to pull off the skin and fried coating. You still get some of the flavor, but two-thirds less fat. Although the skinless chicken sounds like it should have less fat, it doesn't—they still fry the skinless chicken. The Chicken Little sandwich is not bad, with only 5 g of fat; add some mashed potatoes with gravy (it's fat free); however, the fries, coleslaw, and potato salad have at least 10 g of fat for one serving. Try the corn-on-the-cob or a garden salad with low-calorie dressing or use a half serving of regular dressing. Another tasty low-fat option is to choose the KFC rotisserie chicken. Adding corn-on-the-cob, mashed potatoes and gravy, and a salad will give you a satisfying meal as well as one that is high in carbohydrates and nutritionally balanced.

served that the hot foods are served hot and the cold foods cold.

Athletes also need to be careful about the amount and type of food eaten while traveling. Athletes should try to keep their eating habits as close to normal as possible. If they are not usually big fruit eaters, they shouldn't overconsume fruit while traveling. Eating too much of any food, even if it is a type of food an athlete eats all the time, increases his or her chances of having diarrhea. Also, people in many countries have their last meal of the day late into the evening. Having athletes wait late to eat after competition may adversely affect the next day's performance. The athlete should try to stick to the same time of eating as he or she did when training at home.

What Type Of Foods Should An Athlete Eat?

Cooked foods are the best choice because the cooking process kills most organisms that can cause diarrhea. Well-cooked vegetables and meats are good choices. Milk and milk products can be risky because they require pasteurization and complete refrigeration. Milk products may be safe at first-class hotels, but if they have not been properly refrigerated or have been sitting on a buffet line without ice for a long time, it is best to pass on them. Also, fruits that can be peeled, like oranges, grapefruit, and bananas, are safer because the part you eat is naturally protected by the skin. It is recommended that you peel the fruit yourself. Packing nonperishable foods from home helps on those days when the food that is being served is suspect. Exhibit 14–5 lists foods that travel well and are nonperishable.

What Should Athletes Do if They Have Traveler's Diarrhea?

If athletes develop diarrhea, they should stop eating solid foods until the gas, cramps, and stomach pains go away. Athletes should drink large amounts of a sport drink or fluid-replacement drink with bottled water, if these drinks are available. Otherwise, the BRAT diet should be followed, that is *B* for bananas; *R* for rice, *A* for applesauce, and *T* for toast. Those foods are usually available no matter what country athletes are traveling in, and they help restore muscle and liver glycogen. Carbonated beverages should be kept to a minimum. Athletes should not take medication that might stop the diarrhea. Their bodies are trying to get rid of the microbe that is causing the diarrhea, and taking medication may

prevent their bodies from getting rid of the microbe. If the diarrhea persists for more than 48 hours, the athlete should see a doctor.

GUIDELINES FOR EATING AT ALL-DAY EVENTS

Some athletic events such as swim meets, track meets, wrestling tournaments, volleyball tournaments, and tennis tournaments can last all day, and competition may continue for several days. When athletes participate in a sport that lasts all day, they need to replenish carbohydrate stores and make sure they are well-hydrated for peak performance. It is also important that athletes eat after competition to make sure that they will have enough energy in the muscles for the next day's competition.

The same diet principle used to plan the meal before competition can also apply to foods eaten at an all-day competition. If a swimmer races at 10:00 AM and again in 2 hours, foods that are high in protein and fat will more than likely be in the swimmer's stomach, causing some type of gastrointestinal (GI) distress as he or she gets ready to race. The following guidelines have been recommended to help athletes make wise food choices at athletic events that last all day.

If an athlete has an hour or less between events or heats, he or she should stick with car-

Exhibit 14–5 Nonperishable Foods to Pack for International Travel

Assorted cold cereals (individual packs)	Fig Newtons
Packets of instant oatmeal	Pretzels
Carnation Instant Breakfast	Healthy cookies like Snackwell's
Fruit Roll-Ups	Canned tuna
A variety of fruit bars like Nutrigrain bars	Canned baked beans
Jars of peanut butter	Dried fruit that is packaged (raisins, apples, bananas, apricots, cranberries)
Canned or tetra pak fruit juices	
Bread sticks	Microwaved popcorn—select those that have less than 30% of the calories from fat
A variety of healthy crackers	
Graham crackers	Canned fruits
Vanilla wafers	Canned puddings

bohydrate foods that are in liquid form, such as juices and sports drinks. If athletes want something solid, they should try fruits like oranges, peaches, pears, and bananas. These foods are mostly carbohydrates and water, and they will be digested quickly and, therefore, will not cause as much of a problem with stomach cramping or GI distress. Another key point to making food choices with a limited time between competition is to limit the amount of food an athlete eats. The more he or she consumes of anything, the longer it will take to digest, especially when the athlete is nervous.

If an athlete has 2 to 3 hours between events or heats, he or she should add more solid carbohydrates like bagels, hot or cold cereal, and English muffins along with some type of fruit like bananas, apples, oranges, and peaches. The athlete also needs to make sure that he or she is still drinking fluids, like a sport drink for rehydration and restoration of muscle glycogen.

If an athlete has 4 hours or more between events or heats, he or she may have a meal, but the meal should be composed primarily of carbohydrates. For example, a turkey sandwich on two slices of whole grain bread, low-fat yogurt with fruit, and a sport drink or spaghetti with meat sauce, bread, and sport drink are all appropriate. If athletes have a certain meal pattern before competition that they think is a winning combination, then they should try and stick to it. They shouldn't try new combinations of foods or different foods during an important race or competition. If athletes are complaining of GI distress or stomach cramping, then they should try different foods during training or a lesser competition to see if the foods are agreeable to them. Athletes who make food choices at concession stands need to be taught how to make the best choices. Most concession stands are filled with high-fat, high-caloric foods that are not designed to maximize an athlete's performance. It is always wiser for athletes to pack a cooler from home with winning combinations than to rely on a concession stand. Exhibit 14–3 has a list of nutrient-dense, carbohydrate-rich foods that are easy to pack in a cooler.

PUTTING IT ALL TOGETHER

Because athletes have a high requirement for carbohydrates and also have a difficult time making wise food choices, they need to learn the following strategies on how to eat better while traveling to and from competitions. First, it is important to learn that the food guide pyramid can be used as a guide in making food decisions. Second, identify where athletes are going to eat; paying close attention to the type and amount of high-carbohydrate foods selected from restaurant menus will help them maximize their athletic potential. Last but not least, parents, coaches, and athletes must be good role models. What good does it do to talk about the importance of good nutrition for athletic performance when the parent or coach is on the sideline or pool deck overconsuming coffee and doughnuts? Athletes look up to coaches, trainers, and other athletes. To change athletes' eating habits, we must educate them so that they have the knowledge to make wise food choices, provide opportunities for them to practice making good food choices and, most important, set a good example.

CLINICAL CASE STUDY

Freddy, a 6′8″, 225 lb, 19-year-old male was a right-handed pitcher and was drafted as the number one draft choice for a major league baseball team. He was sent to an AA ball club in the minor league system in the Southeast and was put into the pitching rotation. Freddy was excited to belong to a major league ball team. He enjoyed the freedom he had in deciding his nonbaseball lifestyle. His eating and sleeping habits were determined by what he deemed necessary to make it in this league. The first month that he joined the ball team, he found out that the lifestyle of a ball player in the minors is a late one. After the game and shower it would be 11:00 PM and he would be hungry and go out to eat. He would get to bed around 1 or 2 AM, depending on what he did after eating with his teammates. He would sleep until noon and sometimes he would get up and get some food, but most of the time he would get up and read the paper and get to the ball field around 2 PM for batting practice. Sometimes, he would eat something from the concession stand or from the club house and then either watch the game or pitch, depending on the rotation. His first road trip was 12 days. The first day consisted of 9 hours in a bus to southern Georgia. He arrived at the bus after only 3 hours of sleep the night before and had not had any food. He slept most of the way and upon arrival at the ball field he was told he would be pitching that night. It was summer and the temperature of the playing field that night was over 100 degrees with high humidity. Freddy pitched three innings and had a seizure on the mound and collapsed. He was taken to the hospital where he was revived, and physicians determined that he was dehydrated, malnourished, and exhausted. After being told at the hospital to drink more fluids, get more rest, and consume nutritionally balanced meals, Freddy decided to consult a dietitian.

Nutritionist's Assessment

Although Freddy perceived his lifestyle and dietary habits to be adequate to perform in a minor league ball club, a computerized dietary analysis indicated that he was eating well above the recommended amount of dietary fat and was consuming too much alcohol. His consumption of carbohydrates was 40% of his total calories, and he had not eaten any fruits or vegetables in the month that he had been with the team. He drank milk rarely and only when he would stop by a convenience store to grab something to eat. He was consuming some water at the ball field when it was not his turn to pitch but did not drink water while pitching or with his meals, nor did he drink water at home. His food intake consisted primarily of fast foods. Occasionally, he would go to a sit-down restaurant but not by himself. He usually ordered some type of burger or other type of fast food. He skipped breakfast because he was too tired to get up and eat, but he tried to eat something at the ball field before the game.

Plan

1. *Increase fluid consumption.* To ensure adequate consumption of fluid, Freddy was taught to monitor his weight before and after practices and games. For every pound he lost during his workout or game he had to drink 2 cups of fluid. He also was told that for complete hydration, the color of his urine should be the color of a pale lemonade and if not, he was to drink whether he was thirsty or not. Freddy purchased some sports drinks and kept them in his apartment to drink in the afternoons and late evenings.

2. *Increase carbohydrate consumption.* To ensure adequate repletion of glycogen stores on a daily basis, consumption of high-carbohydrate foods was encouraged for each meal and for snacks at the ballpark. Freddy purchased some cereal, bread, frozen waffles, pancakes, and fruits like bananas and apples to consume when he woke up in the mid-morning after a game. For lunch, he stopped at a fast food restaurant on the way to the ball field; however, he chose a chicken sandwich, side salad, and either juice or milk to drink. After the game, Freddy either ate out after being taught how to order high-carbohydrate meals at restaurants, or he ate at home. High-carbohydrate menus and recipes were developed for Freddy during the counseling sessions.

3. *Increase fruit and vegetable consumption.* Freddy actually likes fruits and vegetables. He purchased a juicer and pots and pans and found that he could fix vegetables in a number of ways and enjoy their flavor and taste. The difficult part was consuming them while traveling. During the counseling session, strategies were developed for consumption of fruits and vegetables while traveling by either taking them in a cooler or purchasing some when he got into town.

By the time Freddy met with the dietitian, he had realized what he had done. He no longer goes out every night after the games. He made a schedule and tries very hard to stick to it. He now knows the importance of consuming a balanced diet that emphasizes carbohydrates and fluids. What happened to him scared him, and he thought that he might never be able to pitch again. He is currently still pitching and actually is doing very well. He has become a very outspoken player on the importance of nutrition in human performance. He was called up to the majors to try out as a big league pitcher; however, he did not make the team. Two years after having the seizure on the mound, he was named outstanding pitcher of the minor league system.

REFERENCES

1. Steen SN. Timely statement of the American Dietetic Association: nutrition guidance for adolescent athletes in organized sports. *J Am Diet Assoc.* 1996; 6: 611–612.

2. Berning JR, Troup JP, VanHandel PJ, Daniels J, Daniels N. The nutritional habits of young adolescent swimmers. *Int J Sport Nutr.* 1991;1:240–248.

3. VanHandel PJ, Cells KA, Bradley PW, Troup JP. Nutritional status of elite swimmers. *J Swim Res.* 1984;1:27–31.

4. Campbell ML, McFadyen KL. Nutritional knowledge, beliefs and dietary practices of competitive swimmers. *Can Home Econom J.* 1984;34:47.

5. Shoaf LR, McClellan PD, Birskovich KA. Nutrition knowledge, interests and information sources of male athletes. *J Nutr Educ.* 1986;18:243.

6. Loosli AR, Benson J, Gillien DM, Bourdet K. Nutrition habits and knowledge in competitive adolescent female gymnasts. *Physician Sportsmed.* 1986;14:118.

7. Perron M, Endres J. Knowledge, attitudes, and dietary practices of female athletes. *J Am Diet Assoc.* 1985;85:573.

8. Massad SJ, Shier NW, Koceja DM, Ellis NT. High school athletes and nutritional supplements: a study of knowledge and use. *Int J Sport Nutr.* 1995;5(3):232–245.

9. Costill DL, Sherman WM, Fink WJ. The role of dietary carbohydrate in muscle glycogen resynthesis after strenuous running. *Am J Clin Nutr.* 1981;34:1831–1836.

10. Sherman WM, Peden MC, Wright DA. Carbohydrate feedings 1 hour before exercise improves cycling performance. *Am J Clin Nutr.* 1991;54:866–870.

11. Sherman WM, Brodowica G, Wright DA, Allen WK, Simonsen J, Dernbach A. Effects of 4 hour preexercise carbohydrate feedings on cycling performance. *Med Sci Sports Exerc.* 1989;21:598–604.

12. Coyle EF, Habber JM, Hurley BF, Martin WH, Ehsani AA, Holloszy JO. Carbohydrate feeding during prolonged strenuous exercise can delay fatigue. *J Appl Physiol.* 1983;55:230–235.

13. Coyle EF, Coggan AR, Hemmert MK, Ivy JL. Muscle glycogen utilization during prolonged strenuous exercise when fed carbohydrate. *J Appl Physiol.* 1986; 61:165–172.

14. Zawadski KM, Yaspelkis BB, Ivy JL. Carbohydrate-protein complex increases the rate of muscle glycogen storage after exercise. *J Appl Physiol.* 1992;72(5):1854–1859.

Caloric Expenditure for Various Physical Activities

Source: Reprinted from *Nutrition for Fitness and Sport*, ed 2 (pp A44–A53) by MH Williams with permission of Wm C Brown Publishers, © 1995.

Body Weight

Kilograms	45	48	50	52	55	57	59	61	64	66	68	70	73	75	77	80	82	84	86	89	91	93	95	98	100
Pounds	100	105	110	115	120	125	130	135	140	145	150	155	160	165	170	175	180	185	190	195	200	205	210	215	220
Sedentary Activities																									
Lying quietly	.99	1.0	1.1	1.1	1.2	1.3	1.3	1.4	1.4	1.5	1.5	1.5	1.6	1.6	1.7	1.7	1.8	1.8	1.9	1.9	2.0	2.0	2.1	2.1	2.2
Sitting and writing, card playing, etc	1.2	1.3	1.4	1.5	1.5	1.6	1.7	1.7	1.8	1.8	1.9	2.0	2.0	2.1	2.2	2.2	2.3	2.4	2.4	2.5	2.5	2.6	2.7	2.7	2.8
Standing with light work, cleaning, etc	2.7	2.9	3.0	3.1	3.3	3.4	3.5	3.7	3.8	3.9	4.1	4.2	4.4	4.5	4.6	4.8	4.9	5.0	5.2	5.3	5.4	5.6	5.7	5.9	6.0
Physical Activities																									
Archery	3.1	3.3	3.5	3.6	3.8	4.0	4.1	4.3	4.5	4.6	4.8	4.9	5.1	5.3	5.4	5.6	5.7	5.9	6.0	6.2	6.4	6.5	6.7	6.9	7.0
Badminton																									
Recreational singles	3.6	3.8	4.0	4.2	4.4	4.6	4.7	4.9	5.1	5.3	5.4	5.6	5.8	6.0	6.2	6.4	6.6	6.7	6.9	7.1	7.3	7.4	7.6	7.8	8.0
Social doubles	2.7	2.9	3.0	3.1	3.3	3.4	3.5	3.7	3.8	3.9	4.1	4.2	4.4	4.5	4.6	4.8	4.9	5.0	5.2	5.3	5.4	5.6	5.7	5.9	6.0
Competitive	5.9	6.1	6.4	6.7	7.0	7.3	7.6	7.9	8.2	8.5	8.8	9.1	9.4	9.7	10.0	10.3	10.6	10.9	11.2	11.5	11.8	12.1	12.4	12.7	13.0
Baseball																									
Player	3.1	3.3	3.4	3.6	3.8	4.0	4.1	4.3	4.4	4.5	4.7	4.8	5.0	5.2	5.3	5.5	5.6	5.8	5.9	6.1	6.3	6.4	6.6	6.8	6.9
Pitcher	3.9	4.1	4.3	4.5	4.7	4.9	5.1	5.3	5.5	5.7	5.9	6.0	6.3	6.5	6.7	6.9	7.1	7.3	7.4	7.7	7.9	8.0	8.2	8.5	8.6
Basketball																									
Half court	3.0	3.1	3.3	3.5	3.6	3.8	3.9	4.1	4.2	4.4	4.5	4.7	4.8	5.0	5.1	5.3	5.4	5.6	5.7	5.9	6.0	6.2	6.4	6.5	6.7
Recreational	4.9	5.2	5.5	5.7	6.0	6.2	6.5	6.7	7.0	7.2	7.5	7.7	8.0	8.2	8.5	8.7	9.0	9.2	9.5	9.7	10.0	10.2	10.5	10.7	11.0
Vigorous competition	6.5	6.8	7.2	7.5	7.8	8.2	8.5	8.8	9.2	9.5	9.9	10.2	10.5	10.9	11.2	11.5	11.9	12.2	12.5	12.9	13.2	13.5	13.8	14.2	14.5
Bicycling, level (mph) (min/mile)																									
5 12:00	1.9	2.0	2.1	2.2	2.3	2.4	2.5	2.6	2.7	2.8	2.9	3.0	3.1	3.2	3.3	3.4	3.5	3.6	3.7	3.8	3.9	4.0	4.1	4.2	4.3
10 6:00	4.2	4.4	4.6	4.8	5.1	5.3	5.5	5.7	5.9	6.1	6.4	6.6	6.8	7.0	7.2	7.4	7.6	7.9	8.1	8.3	8.5	8.7	8.9	9.1	9.4
15 4:00	7.3	7.6	8.0	8.4	8.7	9.1	9.5	9.8	10.0	10.5	10.9	11.3	11.6	12.0	12.4	12.7	13.1	13.4	13.8	14.2	14.5	14.9	15.3	15.6	16.0
20 3:00	10.7	11.2	11.7	12.3	12.8	13.3	13.9	14.4	14.9	15.5	16.0	16.5	17.1	17.6	18.1	18.7	19.2	19.7	20.3	20.8	21.3	21.9	22.4	22.9	23.5
Bowling	2.7	2.8	3.0	3.1	3.3	3.4	3.5	3.7	3.8	3.9	4.1	4.2	4.4	4.5	4.6	4.8	4.9	5.0	5.2	5.3	5.5	5.6	5.7	5.9	6.0
Calisthenics																									
Light type	3.4	3.6	3.8	4.0	4.1	4.3	4.5	4.7	4.8	5.0	5.2	5.4	5.5	5.7	5.9	6.1	6.3	6.4	6.6	6.8	7.0	7.1	7.3	7.5	7.7
Timed vigorous	9.7	10.1	10.6	11.1	11.6	12.1	12.6	13.1	13.6	14.1	14.6	15.1	15.6	16.1	16.6	17.1	17.6	18.1	18.6	19.1	19.6	20.0	20.5	21.0	21.5
Canoeing (mph) (min/mile)																									
2.5 24	1.9	2.0	2.1	2.2	2.3	2.4	2.5	2.6	2.7	2.8	2.9	3.0	3.1	3.2	3.3	3.4	3.5	3.6	3.7	3.8	3.9	4.0	4.1	4.2	4.3
4.0 15	4.4	4.6	4.9	5.1	5.3	5.5	5.8	6.0	6.2	6.4	6.7	6.9	7.1	7.4	7.6	7.8	8.0	8.2	8.5	8.7	8.9	9.1	9.4	9.6	9.8
5.0 12	5.7	6.0	6.3	6.6	6.9	7.2	7.5	7.8	8.1	8.4	8.7	9.0	9.3	9.5	9.8	10.1	10.4	10.7	11.0	11.3	11.6	11.9	12.2	12.5	12.8

Body Weight

Kilograms	45	48	50	52	55	57	59	61	64	66	68	70	73	75	77	80	82	84	86	89	91	93	95	98	100
Pounds	100	105	110	115	120	125	130	135	140	145	150	155	160	165	170	175	180	185	190	195	200	205	210	215	220
Dancing																									
Moderately (waltz)	3.1	3.3	3.5	3.6	3.8	4.0	4.1	4.3	4.5	4.6	4.8	4.9	5.1	5.3	5.4	5.6	5.7	5.9	6.0	6.2	6.4	6.5	6.7	6.9	7.0
Active (square, disco)	4.5	4.7	5.0	5.2	5.4	5.6	5.9	6.1	6.3	6.6	6.8	7.0	7.3	7.5	7.7	7.9	8.2	8.4	8.6	8.9	9.1	9.3	9.5	9.8	10.0
Aerobic (vigorously)	6.0	6.3	6.7	7.0	7.3	7.6	7.9	8.2	8.5	8.8	9.1	9.4	9.7	10.0	10.3	10.6	10.9	11.2	11.5	11.8	12.1	12.4	12.7	13.0	13.3
Fencing																									
Moderately	3.3	3.5	3.6	3.8	4.0	4.1	4.3	4.5	4.6	4.8	5.0	5.2	5.3	5.5	5.7	5.8	6.0	6.2	6.3	6.5	6.7	6.8	7.0	7.1	7.3
Vigorously	6.6	7.0	7.3	7.7	8.0	8.3	8.7	9.0	9.4	9.7	10.0	10.4	10.7	11.0	11.4	11.7	12.1	12.4	12.7	13.1	13.4	13.8	14.1	14.4	14.8
Football																									
Moderate	3.3	3.5	3.6	3.8	4.0	4.1	4.3	4.5	4.6	4.8	5.0	5.2	5.3	5.5	5.7	5.8	6.0	6.2	6.3	6.5	6.7	6.8	7.0	7.1	7.3
Touch, vigorous	5.5	5.8	6.1	6.4	6.6	6.9	7.2	7.5	7.8	8.0	8.3	8.6	8.9	9.2	9.4	9.7	10.0	10.3	10.6	10.8	11.1	11.4	11.7	12.0	12.2
Golf																									
Twosome (carry clubs)	3.6	3.8	4.0	4.2	4.4	4.6	4.7	4.9	5.1	5.3	5.4	5.6	5.8	6.0	6.2	6.4	6.6	6.7	6.9	7.1	7.3	7.4	7.6	7.9	8.0
Foursome (carry clubs)	2.7	2.9	3.0	3.1	3.3	3.4	3.5	3.7	3.8	3.9	4.1	4.2	4.4	4.5	4.6	4.8	4.9	5.0	5.2	5.3	5.4	5.6	5.7	5.9	6.0
Power-cart	1.9	2.0	2.1	2.2	2.3	2.4	2.5	2.6	2.7	2.8	2.9	3.0	3.1	3.2	3.3	3.4	3.5	3.6	3.7	3.8	3.9	4.0	4.1	4.2	4.3
Handball																									
Moderate	6.5	6.8	7.2	7.5	7.8	8.2	8.5	8.8	9.2	9.5	9.9	10.2	10.5	10.9	11.2	11.5	11.9	12.2	12.5	12.9	13.2	13.5	13.8	14.2	14.5
Competitive	7.7	8.0	8.4	8.8	9.2	9.6	10.0	10.4	10.8	11.1	11.5	11.9	12.3	12.7	13.1	13.5	13.9	14.3	14.7	15.0	15.4	15.8	16.2	16.6	17.0
Hiking, pack (3 mph)	4.5	4.7	5.0	5.2	5.4	5.6	5.9	6.1	6.3	6.6	6.8	7.0	7.3	7.5	7.7	7.9	8.2	8.4	8.6	8.9	9.1	9.3	9.5	9.8	10.0
Hockey, field	5.0	6.3	6.7	7.0	7.3	7.6	7.9	8.2	8.5	8.8	9.1	9.4	9.7	10.0	10.3	10.6	10.9	11.2	11.5	11.8	12.1	12.4	12.7	13.0	13.3
Hockey, ice	6.6	7.0	7.3	7.7	8.0	8.3	8.7	9.0	9.4	9.7	10.0	10.4	10.7	11.0	11.4	11.7	12.1	12.4	12.7	13.1	13.4	13.8	14.1	14.4	14.8
Horseback riding																									
Walk	1.9	2.0	2.1	2.2	2.3	2.4	2.5	2.6	2.7	2.8	2.9	3.0	3.1	3.2	3.3	3.4	3.5	3.6	3.7	3.8	3.9	4.0	4.1	4.2	4.3
Sitting to trot	2.7	2.9	3.0	3.1	3.3	3.4	3.5	3.7	3.8	3.9	4.1	4.2	4.4	4.5	4.6	4.8	4.9	5.0	5.2	5.3	5.4	5.6	5.7	5.9	6.0
Posting to trot	4.2	4.4	4.6	4.8	5.1	5.3	5.5	5.7	5.9	6.1	6.4	6.6	6.8	7.0	7.2	7.4	7.6	7.9	8.1	8.3	8.5	8.7	8.9	9.1	9.4
Gallop	5.7	6.0	6.3	6.6	6.9	7.2	7.5	7.8	8.1	8.4	8.7	9.0	9.3	9.5	9.8	10.1	10.4	10.7	11.0	11.3	11.6	11.9	12.2	12.5	12.8
Horseshoes	2.5	2.6	2.8	2.9	3.0	3.1	3.3	3.4	3.5	3.7	3.8	3.9	4.0	4.2	4.3	4.4	4.5	4.7	4.8	4.9	5.2	5.2	5.3	5.4	5.6
Jogging (see Running)																									
Judo	8.5	8.9	9.3	9.8	10.2	10.6	11.0	11.5	11.9	12.3	12.8	13.2	13.6	14.1	14.5	14.9	15.4	15.8	16.2	16.6	17.1	17.5	17.9	18.4	18.8
Karate	8.5	8.9	9.3	9.8	10.2	10.6	11.0	11.5	11.9	12.3	12.8	13.2	13.6	14.1	14.5	14.9	15.4	15.8	16.2	16.6	17.1	17.5	17.9	18.4	18.8
Mountain climbing	6.5	6.8	7.2	7.5	7.8	8.2	8.5	8.8	9.2	9.5	9.8	10.2	10.5	10.8	11.2	11.5	11.8	12.1	12.5	12.8	13.1	13.5	13.8	14.1	14.5
Paddle ball	5.7	6.0	6.3	6.6	6.9	7.2	7.5	7.8	8.1	8.4	8.7	9.0	9.3	9.5	9.8	10.1	10.4	10.7	11.0	11.2	11.6	11.9	12.2	12.5	12.8
Pool (billiards)	1.5	1.6	1.6	1.7	1.8	1.9	1.9	2.0	2.1	2.2	2.2	2.3	2.4	2.5	2.6	2.6	2.7	2.8	2.9	2.9	3.0	3.1	3.2	3.2	3.3
Racquetball	6.5	6.8	7.1	7.5	7.8	8.1	8.4	8.8	9.1	9.4	9.8	10.1	10.4	10.7	11.1	11.4	11.7	12.0	12.4	12.7	13.0	13.4	13.7	14.0	14.4
Roller skating (9 mph)	4.2	4.4	4.6	4.8	5.1	5.3	5.5	5.7	5.9	6.1	6.4	6.6	6.8	7.0	7.2	7.4	7.6	7.9	8.1	8.3	8.5	8.7	8.9	9.1	9.4

Body Weight																									
Kilograms	45	48	50	52	55	57	59	61	64	66	68	70	73	75	77	80	82	84	86	89	91	93	95	98	100
Pounds	100	105	110	115	120	125	130	135	140	145	150	155	160	165	170	175	180	185	190	195	200	205	210	215	220

Running (steady state)

(mph)	(min/mile)																									
5.0	12:00	6.0	6.3	6.6	7.0	7.3	7.6	7.9	8.2	8.5	8.8	9.1	9.4	9.7	10.0	10.3	10.6	10.9	11.2	11.6	11.9	12.2	12.5	12.8	13.1	13.4
5.5	10:55	6.7	7.0	7.3	7.7	8.0	8.4	8.7	9.0	9.4	9.7	10.0	10.4	10.7	11.1	11.4	11.7	12.1	12.4	12.8	13.1	13.4	13.8	14.1	14.5	14.8
6.0	10:00	7.2	7.6	8.0	8.4	8.7	9.1	9.5	9.8	10.2	10.6	10.9	11.3	11.7	12.0	12.4	12.8	13.1	13.5	13.8	14.3	14.6	15.0	15.4	15.7	16.1
7.0	8:35	8.5	8.9	9.3	9.8	10.2	10.6	11.0	11.5	11.9	12.3	12.8	13.2	13.6	14.1	14.5	14.9	15.4	15.8	16.2	16.6	17.1	17.5	17.9	18.4	18.8
8.0	7:30	9.7	10.2	10.7	11.2	11.6	12.1	12.6	13.1	13.6	14.1	14.6	15.1	15.6	16.1	16.6	17.1	17.6	18.1	18.5	19.0	19.5	20.0	20.5	21.0	21.5
9.0	6:40	10.8	11.3	11.9	12.4	12.9	13.5	14.0	14.6	15.1	15.7	16.2	16.8	17.3	17.9	18.4	19.0	19.5	20.1	20.6	21.2	21.7	22.2	22.8	23.3	23.9
10.0	6:00	12.1	12.7	13.3	13.9	14.5	15.1	15.7	16.4	17.0	17.6	18.2	18.8	19.4	20.0	20.7	21.3	21.9	22.5	23.1	23.7	24.2	24.8	25.4	26.0	26.7
11.0	5:28	13.3	14.0	14.6	15.3	16.0	16.7	17.3	18.0	18.7	19.4	20.0	20.7	21.4	22.1	22.7	23.4	24.1	24.8	25.4	26.1	26.8	27.5	28.1	28.8	29.5
12.0	5:00	14.5	15.2	16.0	16.7	17.4	18.2	18.9	19.7	20.4	21.1	21.9	22.6	23.3	24.1	24.8	25.6	26.3	27.0	27.8	28.5	29.2	30.0	30.7	31.5	32.2

Sailing, small boat		2.7	2.9	3.0	3.1	3.3	3.4	3.5	3.7	3.8	3.9	4.1	4.2	4.4	4.5	4.6	4.8	4.9	5.0	5.2	5.3	5.4	5.6	5.7	5.9	6.0
Skating, ice (9 mph)		4.2	4.4	4.6	4.8	5.1	5.2	5.5	5.7	5.9	6.1	6.4	6.6	6.8	7.0	7.2	7.4	7.6	7.9	8.1	8.3	8.5	8.7	8.9	9.1	9.4

Skiing, cross country

(mph)	(min/mile)																									
2.5	24:00	5.0	5.2	5.5	5.7	6.0	6.2	6.5	6.7	7.0	7.2	7.5	7.8	8.0	8.3	8.5	8.8	9.0	9.3	9.5	9.8	10.0	10.3	10.6	10.8	11.1
4.0	15:00	6.5	6.8	7.2	7.5	7.8	8.2	8.5	8.8	9.2	9.5	9.9	10.2	10.5	10.9	11.2	11.5	11.9	12.2	12.5	12.9	13.2	13.5	13.8	14.2	14.5

Squash

Normal		6.7	7.0	7.3	7.7	8.0	8.4	8.7	9.1	9.5	9.8	10.1	10.5	10.8	11.2	11.5	11.8	12.2	12.5	12.9	13.2	13.5	13.9	14.2	14.6	14.9
Competition		7.7	8.0	8.4	8.8	9.2	9.6	10.0	10.4	10.8	11.1	11.5	11.9	12.3	12.7	13.1	13.5	13.9	14.3	14.7	15.0	15.4	15.8	16.2	16.6	17.0

Swimming (yards/min)

Backstroke

25		2.5	2.6	2.8	2.9	3.0	3.1	3.3	3.4	3.5	3.7	3.8	3.9	4.0	4.2	4.3	4.4	4.5	4.7	4.8	4.9	5.1	5.2	5.3	5.4	5.6
30		3.5	3.7	3.9	4.1	4.2	4.4	4.6	4.8	4.9	5.1	5.3	5.5	5.6	5.8	6.0	6.2	6.4	6.5	6.7	6.9	7.1	7.2	7.4	7.6	7.8
35		4.5	4.7	5.0	5.2	5.4	5.6	5.9	6.1	6.3	6.6	6.8	7.0	7.3	7.5	7.7	7.9	8.2	8.4	8.6	8.9	9.1	9.3	9.5	9.8	10.0
40		5.5	5.8	6.1	6.4	6.6	6.9	7.2	7.5	7.8	8.0	8.3	8.6	8.9	9.2	9.4	9.7	10.0	10.3	10.6	10.8	11.1	11.4	11.7	12.0	12.2

Breaststroke

20		3.1	3.3	3.5	3.6	3.8	4.0	4.1	4.3	4.5	4.6	4.8	4.9	5.1	5.3	5.4	5.6	5.7	5.9	6.0	6.2	6.4	6.5	6.7	6.9	7.0
30		4.7	5.0	5.2	5.4	5.7	5.9	6.2	6.4	6.7	6.9	7.1	7.4	7.6	7.9	8.1	8.3	8.6	8.8	9.1	9.3	9.5	9.8	10.0	10.3	10.5
40		6.3	6.7	7.0	7.3	7.6	8.0	8.3	8.6	8.9	9.3	9.6	9.9	10.2	10.5	10.9	11.2	11.5	11.9	12.2	12.5	12.8	13.1	13.5	13.8	14.1

Body Weight

Kilograms	45	48	50	52	55	57	59	61	64	66	68	70	73	75	77	80	82	84	86	89	91	93	95	98	100
Pounds	100	105	110	115	120	125	130	135	140	145	150	155	160	165	170	175	180	185	190	195	200	205	210	215	220
Front crawl																									
20	3.1	3.3	3.5	3.6	3.8	4.0	4.1	4.3	4.5	4.6	4.8	4.9	5.1	5.3	5.4	5.6	5.7	5.9	6.0	6.2	6.4	6.5	6.7	6.9	7.0
25	4.0	4.2	4.4	4.6	4.8	5.0	5.2	5.4	5.6	5.8	6.0	6.2	6.4	6.6	6.8	7.0	7.2	7.4	7.6	7.8	8.0	8.2	8.4	8.6	8.8
35	4.8	5.1	5.4	5.6	5.9	6.1	6.4	6.6	6.8	7.0	7.3	7.5	7.8	8.0	8.3	8.5	8.8	9.0	9.2	9.4	9.7	9.9	10.2	10.4	10.7
45	5.7	6.0	6.3	6.6	6.9	7.2	7.5	7.8	8.1	8.4	8.7	9.0	9.3	9.5	9.8	10.1	10.4	10.7	11.0	11.3	11.6	11.9	12.2	12.5	12.8
50	7.0	7.4	7.7	8.1	8.5	8.8	9.2	9.5	9.9	10.3	10.6	11.0	11.3	11.7	12.0	12.4	12.8	13.1	13.5	13.8	14.2	14.5	14.9	15.2	15.6
Table tennis	3.4	3.6	3.8	4.0	4.1	4.3	4.5	4.7	4.8	5.0	5.2	5.4	5.5	5.7	5.9	6.1	6.3	6.4	6.6	6.8	7.0	7.1	7.3	7.5	7.7
Tennis																									
Singles, recreational	5.0	5.2	5.5	5.7	6.0	6.2	6.5	6.7	7.0	7.2	7.5	7.8	8.0	8.3	8.5	8.8	9.0	9.3	9.5	9.8	10.0	10.3	10.6	10.8	11.1
Doubles, recreational	3.4	3.6	3.8	4.0	4.1	4.3	4.5	4.7	4.8	5.0	5.2	5.4	5.5	5.7	5.9	6.1	6.3	6.4	6.6	6.8	7.0	7.1	7.3	7.5	7.7
Competition	6.4	6.7	7.1	7.4	7.7	8.1	8.4	8.7	9.1	9.4	9.8	1C.1	10.4	10.8	11.1	11.4	11.8	12.1	12.4	12.8	13.1	13.4	13.7	14.1	14.4
Volleyball																									
Moderate, recreational	2.9	3.0	3.2	3.3	3.5	3.6	3.8	3.9	4.1	4.2	4.4	4.5	4.7	4.8	5.0	5.1	5.3	5.4	5.6	5.7	5.9	6.0	6.1	6.3	6.4
Vigorous, competition	6.5	6.8	7.1	7.5	7.8	8.1	8.4	8.8	9.1	9.4	9.8	1C.1	10.4	10.7	11.1	11.4	11.7	12.0	12.4	12.7	13.0	13.4	13.7	14.0	14.4
Walking (mph) (min/mile)																									
1.0 60:00	1.5	1.6	1.7	1.8	1.8	1.9	2.0	2.1	2.2	2.2	2.3	2.4	2.4	2.5	2.6	2.7	2.8	2.9	2.9	3.0	3.1	3.2	3.2	3.3	3.4
2.0 30:00	2.1	2.2	2.3	2.4	2.5	2.6	2.8	2.9	3.0	3.1	3.2	3.3	3.4	3.5	3.6	3.7	3.9	4.0	4.1	4.2	4.3	4.4	4.5	4.6	4.7
2.3 26:00	2.3	2.4	2.5	2.7	2.8	2.9	3.0	3.1	3.2	3.4	3.5	3.6	3.7	3.8	4.0	4.1	4.2	4.3	4.4	4.5	4.7	4.8	4.9	5.0	5.1
3.0 20:00	2.7	2.9	3.0	3.1	3.3	3.4	3.5	3.7	3.8	3.9	4.1	4.2	4.4	4.5	4.6	4.8	4.9	5.0	5.2	5.3	5.4	5.6	5.7	5.9	6.0
3.2 18:45	3.1	3.3	3.4	3.6	3.8	4.0	4.1	4.3	4.4	4.5	4.7	4.8	5.0	5.2	5.3	5.5	5.6	5.8	5.9	6.1	6.3	6.4	6.6	6.8	6.9
3.5 17:10	3.3	3.5	3.7	3.9	4.0	4.2	4.4	4.6	4.7	4.9	5.1	5.3	5.4	5.6	5.8	6.0	6.2	6.3	6.5	6.7	6.9	7.0	7.2	7.4	7.6
4.0 15:00	4.2	4.4	4.6	4.8	5.1	5.3	5.5	5.7	5.9	6.1	6.4	6.6	6.8	7.0	7.2	7.4	7.6	7.9	8.1	8.3	8.5	8.7	8.9	9.1	9.4
4.5 13:20	4.7	5.0	5.2	5.4	5.7	5.9	6.2	6.4	6.7	6.9	7.1	7.4	7.6	7.9	8.1	8.3	8.6	8.8	9.1	9.3	9.5	9.8	10.0	10.3	10.5
5.0 12:00	5.4	5.7	6.0	6.3	6.5	6.8	7.1	7.4	7.7	7.9	8.2	8.4	8.7	9.0	9.2	9.5	9.8	10.1	10.4	10.6	10.9	11.2	11.5	11.8	12.0
5.4 11:10	6.2	6.6	6.9	7.2	7.5	7.9	8.2	8.5	8.8	9.2	9.5	9.8	10.1	10.4	10.8	11.1	11.4	11.8	12.1	12.4	12.7	13.0	13.4	13.7	14.0
5.8 10:20	7.7	8.0	8.4	8.8	9.2	9.6	10.0	10.4	10.8	11.1	11.5	11.9	12.3	12.7	13.1	13.5	13.9	14.3	14.7	15.0	15.4	15.8	16.2	16.6	17.0
Water skiing	5.0	5.2	5.5	5.7	6.0	6.2	6.5	6.7	7.0	7.2	7.5	7.8	8.0	8.3	8.5	8.8	9.0	9.3	9.5	9.8	10.0	10.3	10.6	10.8	11.1
Weight training	5.2	5.4	5.7	6.0	6.2	6.5	6.8	7.0	7.3	7.6	7.8	8.1	8.3	8.6	8.9	9.1	9.4	9.7	9.9	10.2	10.5	10.7	11.0	11.2	11.5
Wrestling	8.5	8.9	9.3	9.8	10.2	10.6	11.0	11.5	11.9	12.3	12.8	13.2	13.6	14.1	14.5	14.9	15.4	15.8	16.2	16.6	17.1	17.5	17.9	18.4	18.8

Body Composition and VO$_{2\,max}$ Data for Male and Female Athletes of Varying Ages

Body Composition Values in Male and Female Athletes

Athletic Group or Sport	Sex	Age (yr)	Height (cm)	Weight (kg)	Relative Fat %	Reference
Baseball	male	20.8	182.7	83.8	14.2	Novak
	male	—	—	—	11.8	Forsyth
	male	26.0	185.4	87.5	16.2	Gurry
	male	27.3	185.8	86.4	12.6	Coleman
	male	27.4	183.1	88.0	12.6	Wilmore
Pitchers	male	26.7	188.1	80.8	14.7	Coleman
Infielders	male	27.4	183.1	83.2	12.0	Coleman
Outfielders	male	28.3	185.9	85.6	9.9	Coleman
Basketball	female	19.1	169.1	62.6	20.8	Sinning
	female	19.4	173.0	68.3	20.8	Vaccaro
	female	19.4	167.0	63.9	26.9	Conger
Centers	male	27.7	214.0	109.2	7.1	Parr
Forwards	male	25.3	200.6	96.9	9.0	Parr
Guards	male	25.2	188.0	83.6	10.6	Parr
Bicycling	male	—	180.3	67.1	8.8	Burke
	female	—	167.7	61.3	15.4	Burke
Canoeing/paddlers	male	23.7	182.0	79.6	12.4	Rusko
	male	20.1	179.9	76.3	10.4	Vaccaro
Dancing, ballet	female	15.0	161.1	48.4	16.4	Clarkson
General	female	21.2	162.7	51.2	20.5	Novak
Fencers	male	20.4	174.9	68.0	12.2	Vander
Football	male	19.3	186.8	93.1	13.7	Smith
	male	20.3	184.9	96.4	13.8	Novak
	male	—	—	—	13.9	Forsyth
Defensive backs	male	17–23	178.3	77.3	11.5	Wickkiser
	male	24.5	182.5	84.8	9.6	Wilmore
Offensive backs	male	17–23	179.7	79.8	12.4	Wickkiser
	male	24.7	183.8	90.7	9.4	Wilmore

Source: Reprinted from *Training for Sport and Activity: The Physiological Basis of the Conditioning Process*, ed 4, by JH Wilmore and DL Costill, with permission of Wm C. Brown Publishers, © 1993.

Body Composition Values in Male and Female Athletes

Athletic Group or Sport	Sex	Age (yr)	Height (cm)	Weight (kg)	Relative Fat %	Reference
Linebackers	male	17–23	180.1	87.2	13.4	Wickkiser
	male	24.2	188.6	102.2	14.0	Wilmore
Offensive linemen	male	17–23	186.0	99.2	19.1	Wickkiser
	male	24.7	193.0	112.6	15.6	Wilmore
Defensive linemen	male	17–23	186.6	97.8	18.5	Wickkiser
	male	25.7	192.4	117.1	18.2	Wilmore
Quarterbacks, kickers	male	24.1	185.0	90.1	14.4	Wilmore
Golf	female	33.3	168.9	61.8	24.0	Crews
Gymnastics	male	20.3	178.5	69.2	4.6	Novak
	female	14.0	—	—	17.0	Parizkova
	female	15.2	161.1	50.4	13.1	Moffatt
	female	19.4	163.0	57.9	23.8	Conger
	female	20.0	158.5	51.5	15.5	Sinning
	female	23.0	—	—	11.0	Parizkova
	female	23.0	—	—	9.6	Parizkova
Ice hockey	male	22.5	179.0	77.3	13.0	Rusko
	male	26.3	180.3	86.7	15.1	Wilmore
Jockeys	male	30.9	158.2	50.3	14.1	Wilmore
Orienteering	male	31.2	—	72.2	16.3	Knowlton
	female	29.0	—	58.1	18.7	Knowlton
Pentathlon	female	21.5	175.4	65.4	11.0	Krahenbuhl
Racquetball	male	25.0	181.7	80.3	8.1	Pipes
Lightweight	male	21.0	186.0	71.0	8.5	Hagerman
	female	23.0	173.0	68.0	14.0	Hagerman
Rowing	male	25.6	192.0	93.0	6.5	Secher
Rugby	male	28.1	181.6	86.3	9.1	Maud
Skating, speed	male	21.0	181.0	76.5	11.4	Rusko
Figure	male	21.3	166.9	59.6	9.1	Niinimaa
	female	16.5	158.8	48.6	12.5	Niinimaa
Skiing, alpine	male	25.9	176.6	74.8	7.4	Sprynarova
	male	16.5	173.1	65.5	11.0	Song
	male	21.0	178.0	78.0	9.9	Veicsteinas
	male	21.2	176.0	70.1	14.1	Rusko
	male	21.8	177.8	75.5	10.2	Haymes
	female	19.5	165.1	58.8	20.6	Haymes
Cross-country	male	21.2	176.0	66.6	12.5	Niinimaa
	male	22.7	176.2	73.2	7.9	Haymes
	male	25.6	174.0	69.3	10.2	Rusko
	female	20.2	163.4	55.9	15.7	Haymes
	female	24.3	163.0	59.1	21.8	Rusko
Nordic combination	male	21.7	181.7	70.4	8.9	Haymes
	male	22.9	176.0	70.4	11.2	Rusko
Ski jumping	male	22.2	174.0	69.9	14.3	Rusko

Body Composition Values in Male and Female Athletes

Athletic Group or Sport	Sex	Age (yr)	Height (cm)	Weight (kg)	Relative Fat %	Reference
Soccer	male	26.0	176.0	75.5	9.6	Raven
U.S. Junior	male	17.5	178.3	72.3	9.4	Kirkendall
U.S. Olympic	male	20.6	179.3	72.5	9.1	Kirkendall
U.S. Collegiate	male	20.0	175.3	72.4	10.9	Kirkendall
U.S. National	male	22.5	178.6	76.2	9.9	Kirkendall
M I S L	male	26.9	177.3	74.5	10.5	Kirkendall
Swimming	male	15.1	166.8	59.1	10.8	Vaccaro
	male	20.6	182.9	78.9	5.0	Novak
	male	21.8	182.3	79.1	8.5	Sprynarova
	female	19.4	168.0	63.8	26.3	Conger
Sprint	female	—	165.1	57.1	14.6	Wilmore
Middle distance	female	—	166.6	66.8	24.1	Wilmore
Distance	female	—	166.3	60.9	17.1	Wilmore
Synchronized swimming	female	20.1	166.2	55.8	24.0	Roby
Tennis	male	—	—	—	15.2	Forsyth
	male	42.0	179.6	77.1	16.3	Vodak
	female	39.0	163.3	55.7	20.3	Vodak
Track and field	male	21.3	180.6	71.6	3.7	Novak
	male	—	—	—	8.8	Forsyth
Runners	male	22.5	177.4	64.5	6.3	Sprynarova
distance	male	26.1	175.7	64.2	7.5	Costill
	male	26.2	177.0	66.2	8.4	Rusko
	male	26.2	177.1	63.1	4.7	Pollock
	male	40–49	180.7	71.6	11.2	Pollock
	male	47.2	176.5	70.7	13.2	Lewis
	male	55.3	174.5	63.4	18.0	Barnard
	male	50–59	174.7	67.2	10.9	Pollock
	male	60–69	175.7	67.1	11.3	Pollock
	male	70–75	175.6	66.8	13.6	Pollock
	female	19.9	161.3	52.9	19.2	Malina
	female	32.4	169.4	57.2	15.2	Wilmore
	female	37.8	165.1	54.1	15.5	Upton
	female	43.8	161.5	53.8	18.3	Vaccaro
Middle distance	male	20.1	178.1	71.9	6.9	Wilmore
	male	24.6	179.0	72.3	12.4	Rusko
Sprint	female	20.1	164.9	56.7	19.3	Malina
	male	20.1	178.2	72.8	5.4	Wilmore
	male	46.5	177.0	74.1	16.5	Barnard
Cross-country	female	15.6	164.2	51.1	15.3	Butts
	female	15.6	163.3	50.9	15.4	Butts
Race walking	male	26.7	178.7	68.5	7.8	Franklin
Discus	male	26.4	190.8	110.5	16.3	Wilmore
	male	28.3	186.1	104.7	16.4	Fahey
	female	21.1	168.1	71.0	25.0	Malina

Body Composition Values in Male and Female Athletes

Athletic Group or Sport	Sex	Age (yr)	Height (cm)	Weight (kg)	Relative Fat %	Reference
Jumpers and hurdlers	female	20.3	165.9	59.0	20.7	Malina
Shot put	male	22.0	191.6	126.2	19.6	Behnke
	male	27.0	188.2	112.5	16.5	Fahey
	female	21.5	167.6	78.1	28.0	Malina
Triathlon	male	—	—	—	7.1	Holly
	female	—	—	—	12.6	Holly
Volleyball	male	26.1	192.7	85.5	12.0	Puhl
	female	19.4	166.0	59.8	25.3	Conger
	female	19.9	172.2	64.1	21.3	Kovaleski
	female	21.6	178.3	70.5	17.9	Puhl
Weight lifting	male	24.9	166.4	77.2	9.8	Sprynarova
Power	male	25.5	173.6	89.4	19.9	Hakkinen
	male	26.3	176.1	92.0	15.6	Fahey
Olympic	male	25.3	177.1	88.2	12.2	Fahey
Body builders	male	25.6	176.9	87.6	13.4	Hakkinen
	male	27.6	178.8	88.1	8.3	Pipes
	male	29.0	172.4	83.1	8.4	Fahey
	female	27.0	160.8	53.8	13.2	Freedson
Wrestling	male	11.3	141.2	34.2	12.7	Sady
	male	15–18	172.3	66.3	6.9	Katch
	male	19.6	174.6	74.8	8.8	Sinning
	male	20.6	174.8	67.3	4.0	Stine
	male	22.0	—	—	5.0	Parizkova
	male	23.0	—	79.3	14.3	Taylor
	male	24.0	173.3	77.5	12.7	Hakkinen
	male	26.0	177.8	81.8	9.8	Fahey
	male	27.0	176.0	75.7	10.7	Gale

Maximal Oxygen Uptake (ml · kg^{-1} · min^{-1}) of Male and Female Athletes

Athletic Group or Sport	Sex	Age (yr)	Height (cm)	Weight (kg)	VO_{2max}	Reference
Baseball/softball	M	21	182.7	83.3	52.3	Novak
	M	26	185.4	87.5	41.6	Gurry
	M	28	183.6	88.1	52.0	Wilmore
Basketball	F	19	167.0	63.9	42.3	Conger
	F	19	169.1	62.6	42.9	Sinning
	F	19	173.0	68.3	49.6	Vaccaro
Centers	M	28	214.0	109.2	41.9	Parr
Forwards	M	25	200.6	96.9	45.9	Parr
Guards	M	25	188.0	83.6	50.0	Parr

Maximal Oxygen Uptake (ml · kg⁻¹ · min⁻¹) of Male and Female Athletes

Athletic Group or Sport	Sex	Age (yr)	Height (cm)	Weight (kg)	VO$_{2max}$	Reference
Bicycling	M	24	182.0	74.5	68.2	Gollnick
(competitive)	M	24	180.4	79.2	70.3	Hermansen
	M	25	180.0	72.8	67.1	Burke
	M	—	180.3	67.1	74.0	Burke
	M	—	—	—	74.0	Saltin
	M	—	—	—	69.1	Strømme
	F	20	165.0	55.0	50.2	Burke
	F	—	167.7	61.3	57.4	Burke
Canoeing/paddlers	M	18	—	66.5	71.2	Tesch
	M	19	173.0	64.0	60.0	Sidney
	M	20	179.9	76.3	60.1	Vaccaro
	M	22	190.5	80.7	67.7	Hermansen
	M	24	182.0	79.6	66.1	Rusko
	M	25	—	78.0	69.2	Tesch
	M	26	181.0	74.0	56.8	Gollnick
	F	18	166.0	57.3	49.2	Sidney
Dancing, ballet	M	28	175.0	64.0	59.3	Mostardi
	M	29	177.0	69.0	56.0	Schantz
	F	15	161.1	48.4	48.9	Clarkson
	F	25	165.0	50.0	48.6	Mostardi
	F	28	164.0	51.0	51.0	Schantz
General	F	21	162.7	51.2	41.5	Novak
Fencing	M	20	174.9	68.0	50.2	Vander
Football	M	19	186.8	93.1	56.5	Smith
	M	20	184.9	96.4	51.3	Novak
Defensive backs	M	25	182.5	84.8	53.1	Wilmore
Offensive backs	M	25	183.8	90.7	52.2	Wilmore
Linebackers	M	24	188.6	102.2	52.1	Wilmore
Offensive line	M	25	193.0	112.6	49.9	Wilmore
Defensive line	M	26	192.4	117.1	44.9	Wilmore
Quarterbacks/kickers	M	24	185.0	90.1	49.0	Wilmore
Golf	F	33	168.9	61.8	34.2	Crews
Gymnastics	M	20	178.5	69.2	55.5	Novak
	F	15	161.1	50.4	45.2	Moffatt
	F	15	159.7	48.8	49.8	Hermansen
	F	19	163.0	57.9	36.3	Conger
Ice hockey	M	11	140.5	35.5	56.6	Cunningham
	M	22	179.0	77.3	61.5	Rusko
	M	24	179.3	81.8	54.6	Seliger
	M	26	180.1	86.4	53.6	Wilmore
Jockey	M	31	158.2	50.3	53.8	Wilmore
Orienteering	M	25	179.7	70.3	71.1	Hermansen
	M	31	—	72.2	61.6	Knowlton
	M	52	176.0	72.7	50.7	Gollnick
	F	23	165.8	60.0	60.7	Hermansen
	F	29	—	58.1	46.1	Knowlton

Maximal Oxygen Uptake (ml · kg⁻¹ · min⁻¹) of Male and Female Athletes

Athletic Group or Sport	Sex	Age (yr)	Height (cm)	Weight (kg)	VO_{2max}	Reference
Pentathlon	F	21	175.4	65.4	45.9	Krahenbuhl
Racquetball/handball	M	24	183.7	81.3	60.0	Hermansen
	M	25	181.7	80.3	58.3	Pipes
Rowing	M	—	—	—	65.7	Strømme
	M	23	192.7	89.9	62.7	Mickelson
	M	24	180.0	71.8	72.0	Secher
	M	25	189.9	86.9	66.9	Hermansen
	M	26	192.0	93.0	63.0	Secher
Heavyweight	M	23	192.0	88.0	68.9	Hagerman
Lightweight	M	21	186.0	71.0	71.1	Hagerman
	F	23	173.0	68.0	60.3	Hagerman
Rugby	M	28	181.6	86.3	45.9	Maud
Skating, speed	M	—	181.0	73.6	64.4	van Ingen
	M	20	175.5	73.9	56.1	Maksud
	M	21	181.0	76.5	72.9	Rusko
	M	25	183.1	82.4	64.6	Hermansen
	F	20	168.1	65.4	52.0	Hermansen
	F	21	164.5	60.8	46.1	Maksud
Figure	M	21	166.9	59.6	58.5	Niinimaa
	F	17	158.8	48.6	48.9	Niinimaa
Skiing, alpine	M	16	173.1	65.5	65.6	Song
	M	21	176.0	70.1	63.8	Rusko
	M	21	178.0	78.0	52.4	Veicsteinas
	M	22	178.5	77.6	63.1	Brown
	M	22	177.8	75.5	66.6	Haymes
	M	26	176.6	74.8	62.3	Sprynarova
	F	19	165.1	58.8	52.7	Haymes
Cross-country	M	21	176.0	66.6	63.9	Niinimaa
	M	23	176.2	73.2	73.0	Haymes
	M	25	180.4	73.2	73.9	Hermansen
	M	26	174.0	69.3	78.3	Rusko
	M	—	—	—	72.8	Strømme
	F	20	163.4	55.9	61.5	Haymes
	F	24	163.0	59.1	68.2	Rusko
	F	25	165.7	60.5	56.9	Hermansen
	F	—	—	—	58.1	Strømme
Nordic	M	23	176.0	70.4	72.8	Rusko
	M	22	181.7	70.4	67.4	Haymes
Ski jumping	M	22	174.0	69.9	61.3	Rusko
Soccer	M	26	176.0	75.5	58.4	Raven
U.S. Junior	M	18	178.3	72.3	61.8	Kirkendall
Swimming	M	12	150.4	41.2	52.5	Cunningham
	M	13	164.8	52.1	52.9	Cunningham
	M	15	169.6	59.8	56.6	Cunningham
	M	15	166.8	59.1	56.8	Vaccaro
	M	20	181.4	76.7	55.7	Magel

Maximal Oxygen Uptake (ml · kg^{-1} · min^{-1}) of Male and Female Athletes

Athletic Group or Sport	Sex	Age (yr)	Height (cm)	Weight (kg)	VO$_{2max}$	Reference
	M	20	181.0	73.0	50.4	Charbonnier
	M	21	182.9	78.9	62.1	Novak
	M	21	181.0	78.3	69.9	Gollnick
	M	22	182.3	79.1	56.9	Sprynarova
	M	22	182.3	79.7	55.9	Cunningham
	F	12	154.8	43.3	46.2	Cunningham
	F	13	160.0	52.1	43.4	Cunningham
	F	15	164.8	53.7	40.5	Cunningham
Sprint	M	19	181.1	75.0	58.3	Shephard
Mid-distance	M	22	178.0	74.6	55.4	Shephard
Long-distance	M	21	179.0	74.9	65.4	Shephard
	F	19	168.0	63.8	37.6	Conger
Synchronized	F	20	166.2	55.8	43.2	Roby
Tennis	M	12	147.9	38.5	56.3	Buti
	M	42	179.6	77.1	50.2	Vodak
	F	12	150.9	42.9	52.6	Buti
	F	39	163.3	55.7	44.2	Vodak
Track and field runners	M	21	180.6	71.6	66.1	Novak
	M	22	177.4	64.5	64.0	Sprynarova
	M	23	177.0	69.5	72.4	Gollnick
Sprint	M	17–22	—	—	51.0	Thomas
	M	46	177.0	74.1	47.2	Barnard
Mid-distance	M	20	178.1	71.9	55.8	Wilmore
	M	25	180.1	67.8	70.1	Costill
	M	25	179.0	72.3	69.8	Rusko
Distance	M	10	144.3	31.9	56.6	Mayers
	M	26	177.1	63.1'	76.9	Pollock
	M	26	176.1	64.5	72.2	Hermansen
	M	26	178.9	63.9	77.4	Costill
	M	26	177.0	66.2	78.1	Rusko
	M	27	178.7	64.9	73.2	Costill
	M	32	177.3	64.3	70.3	Costill
	M	35	174.0	63.1	66.6	Costill
	M	36	177.3	69.6	65.1	Hagan
	M	40–49	180.7	71.6	57.5	Pollock
	M	55	174.5	63.4	54.4	Barnard
	M	50–59	174.7	67.2	54.4	Pollock
	M	60–69	175.7	67.1	51.4	Pollock
	M	70–75	175.6	66.8	40.0	Pollock
	M	—	—	—	72.5	Davies
	F	16	162.2	48.6	63.2	Burke
	F	16	163.3	50.9	50.8	Butts
	F	21	170.2	58.6	57.5	Hermansen
	F	25	165.7	52.3	59.8	Upton
	F	32	169.4	57.2	59.1	Wilmore
	F	38	165.1	54.1	55.5	Upton

Maximal Oxygen Uptake (ml · kg^{-1} · min^{-1}) of Male and Female Athletes

Athletic Group or Sport	Sex	Age (yr)	Height (cm)	Weight (kg)	VO$_{2max}$	Reference
	F	38	165.5	54.7	55.5	Upton
	F	44	161.5	53.8	43.4	Vaccaro
	F	—	—	—	58.2	Davies
Cross-country	F	16	163.3	50.9	50.8	Butts
Race walking	M	27	178.7	68.5	62.9	Franklin
Shot/discus	M	26	190.8	110.5	42.8	Wilmore
	M	27	188.2	112.5	42.6	Fahey
	M	28	186.1	104.7	47.5	Fahey
Triathlon	M	—	—	—	72.0	Holly
	F	—	—	—	58.7	Holly
Volleyball	M	25	187.0	84.5	56.4	Conlee
	M	26	192.7	85.5	56.1	Puhl
	F	19	166.0	59.8	43.5	Conger
	F	20	172.2	64.1	56.0	Kovaleski
	F	22	183.7	73.4	41.7	Spence
	F	22	178.3	70.5	50.6	Puhl
Weight lifting	M	25	171.0	81.3	40.1	Gollnick
	M	25	166.4	77.2	42.6	Sprynarova
Power	M	26	173.6	89.4	41.9	Hakkinen
	M	26	176.1	92.0	49.5	Fahey
Olympic	M	25	177.1	88.2	50.7	Fahey
Body builder	M	26	176.9	87.6	50.8	Hakkinen
	M	27	178.8	88.1	46.3	Pipes
	M	29	172.4	83.1	41.5	Fahey
Wrestling	M	11	141.2	34.2	54.0	Sady
	M	21	174.8	67.3	58.3	Stine
	M	23	—	79.2	50.4	Taylor
	M	24	173.3	77.5	57.8	Hakkinen
	M	24	175.6	77.7	60.9	Nagel
	M	26	177.0	81.8	64.0	Fahey
	M	27	176.0	75.7	54.3	Gale

REFERENCES

Adams, J., Mottola, M., Bagnall, K.M., & McFadden, K.D. (1982). Total body fat content in a group of professional football players. *Canadian Journal of Applied Sports and Science, 7,* 36–40.

Astrand, P.O., & Rodahl, K. (1986). *Textbook of work physiology* (3rd ed.). New York: McGraw-Hill Publishing Co.

Barnard, R.J., Grimditch, G.K., & Wilmore, J.H. (1979). Physiological characteristics of sprint and endurance Masters runners. *Medicine and Science in Sports, 11,* 167–171.

Bar-Or, O. (1975). Predicting athletic performance. *Physician and Sportsmedicine, 3* (#2), 80–85.

Behnke, A.R., & Wilmore, J.H. (1974). *Evaluation and regulation of body build and composition.* Englewood Cliffs, NJ: Prentice-Hall.

Bergh, U., Thorstensson, A., Sjodin, B., Hulten, B., Piehl, K., & Karlsson, J. (1978). Maximal oxygen uptake and muscle fiber types in trained and untrained humans. *Medicine and Science in Sports, 10,* 151–154.

Brown, C.H., & Wilmore, J.H. (1974). The effects of maximal resistance training on the strength and body composition of women athletes. *Medicine and Science in Sports, 6,* 174–177.

Brown, S.L., & Wilkinson, J.G. (1983). Characteristics of national, divisional, and club male alpine ski racers. *Medicine and Science in Sports and Exercise, 15,* 491–495.

Burke, E.J., & Brush, F.C. (1979). Physiological and anthropometric assessment of successful teenage female distance runners. *Research Quarterly, 50,* 180–187.

Burke, E.R. (1980). Physiological characteristics of competitive cyclists. *Physician and Sportsmedicine, 8* (#7), 78–84.

Burke, E.R., Cerny, F., Costill, D., & Fink, W. (1977). Characteristics of skeletal muscle in competitive cyclists. *Medicine and Science in Sports, 9,* 109–112.

Buti, T., Elliott, B., & Morton, A. (1984). Physiological and anthropometric profiles of elite prepubescent tennis players. *Physician and Sportsmedicine, 12* (#1), 111–116.

Butts, N.K. (1982). Physiological profile of high school female cross-country runners. *Physician and Sportsmedicine, 10,* 103–111.

Butts, N.K. (1982). Physiological profiles of high school female cross country runners. *Research Quarterly for Exercise and Sport, 53,* 8–14.

Charbonnier, J.P., Lacour, J.R., Riffat, J., & Flandrois, R. (1975). Experimental study of the performance of competition swimmers. *European Journal of Applied Physiology, 34,* 157–167.

Clarkson, P.M., Freedson, P.S., Keller, B., Carney, D., & Skrinar, M. (1985). Maximal oxygen uptake, nutritional patterns and body composition of adolescent female ballet dancers. *Research Quarterly for Exercise and Sport, 56,* 180–184.

Clement, D.B., Asmundson, C., Taunton, C., Taunton, J.E., Ridley, D., & Banister, E.W. (1979). The sport scientist's role in identification of performance criteria for distance runners. *Canadian Journal of Applied Sports Science, 4,* 143–148.

Coleman, A.E. (1981). Skinfold estimates of body fat in major league baseball players. *Physician and Sportsmedicine, 9* (#10), 77–82.

Conger, P.R., & Macnab, R.B.J. (1967). Strength, body composition, and work capacity of participants and nonparticipants in women's intercollegiate sports. *Research Quarterly, 38,* 184–192.

Conlee, R.K., McGown, C.M., Fisher, A.G., Dalsky, G.P., & Robinson, K.C. (1982). Physiological effects of power volleyball. *Physician and Sportsmedicine, 10* (#2), 93–97.

Costill, D.L. (1967). The relationship between selected physiological variables and distance running performance. *Journal of Applied Physiology, 28,* 251–255.

Costill, D.L., Bowers, R., & Kammer, W.F. (1970). Skinfold estimates of body fat among marathon runners. *Medicine and Science in Sports, 2,* 93–95.

Costill, D.L., Daniels, J., Evans, W., Fink, W., Krahenbuhl, G., & Saltin, B. (1976). Skeletal muscle enzymes and fiber composition in male and female track athletes. *Journal of Applied Physiology, 40,* 149–154.

Costill, D.L., Fink, W.J., & Pollock, M.L. (1976). Muscle fiber composition and enzyme activities of elite distance runners. *Medicine and Science in Sports, 8,* 96–100.

Costill, D.L., Thomason, H., & Roberts, E. (1973). Fractional utilization of the aerobic capacity during distance running. *Medicine and Science in Sports, 5,* 248–252.

Costill, D.L., & Winrow, E. (1970). Maximal oxygen intake among marathon runners. *Archives of Physical and Medical Rehabilitation, 51,* 317–320.

Crews, D., Thomas, G., Shirreffs, J.H., & Helfrich, H.M. (1984). A physiological profile of ladies' professional golf association tour players. *Physician and Sportsmedicine, 12* (#5), 69–76.

Cunningham, D.A., & Eynon, R.B. (1973). The working capacity of young competitive swimmers, 10–16 years of age. *Medicine and Science in Sports, 5,* 227–231.

Cunningham, D.A., Telford, P., & Swart, G.T. (1976). The cardiopulmonary capacities of young hockey players: Age 10. *Medicine and Science in Sports, 8,* 23–25.

Cureton, T.K. (1951). *Physical fitness of champion athletes.* Urbana, IL: University of Illinois Press.

Davies, C.T.M. (1971). Body composition in children: A reference standard for maximum aerobic power output on a stationary bicycle ergometer. In, Proceedings of the III International Symposium on Pediatric Work Physiology. *Acta Paediatrica Scandinavica* (Suppl) *217*, 136–137.

Davies, C.T.M., & Thompson, M.W. (1979). Aerobic performance of female marathon and male ultramarathon athletes. *European Journal of Applied Physiology, 41*, 233–245.

deGaray, A.L., Levine, L., & Carter, J.E.L. (Eds). (1974). *Genetic and anthropological studies of Olympic athletes.* New York: Academic Press.

Drinkwater, B.L. (1973). Physiological responses of women to exercise. *Exercise and Sport Sciences Reviews, 1*, 125–153.

Drinkwater, B.L. (1984). Women and exercise: Physiological aspects. *Exercise and Sport Sciences Reviews, 12*, 21–51.

Edstrom, L., & Ekblom, B. (1972). Differences in sizes of red and white muscle fibers in vastus lateralis of musculus quadriceps femoris of normal individuals and athletes: Relation to physical performance. *Scandinavian Journal of Clinical Laboratory Investigation, 30*, 175–181.

Ekblom, B. (1986). Applied physiology of soccer. *Sports Medicine, 3*, 50–60.

Fahey, T.D., Akka, L., & Rolph, R. (1975). Body composition and VO₂ max of exceptional weight-trained athletes. *Journal of Applied Physiology, 39*, 559–561.

Forsyth, H.L., & Sinning, W.E. (1973). The anthropometric estimation of body density and lean body weight of male athletes. *Medicine and Science in Sports, 5*, 174–180.

Franklin, B.A., Kaimal, K.P., Moir, T.W., & Hellerstein, H.K. (1981). Characteristics of national-class race walkers. *Physician and Sportsmedicine, 9* (#9), 101–108.

Freedson, P.S. Mihevic, P.M., Loucks, A.B., & Girandola, R.N. (1983). Physique, body composition, and psychological characteristics of competitive female body builders. *Physician and Sportsmedicine, 11* (#5), 85–93.

Gale, J.B., & Flynn, K.W. (1974). Maximal oxygen consumption and relative body fat of high-ability wrestlers. *Medicine and Science in Sports, 6*, 232–234.

Gollnick, P.D., Armstrong, R.B., Saubert IV, C.W., Piehl, K., & Saltin, B. (1972). Enzyme activity and fiber composition in skeletal muscle of untrained and trained men. *Journal of Applied Physiology, 33*, 312–319.

Gurry, M., Pappas, A., Michaels, J., Maher, P., Shakman, A., Goldberg, R., & Rippe, J. (1985). A comprehensive preseason fitness evaluation for professional baseball players. *Physician and Sportsmedicine, 13* (#6), 63–74.

Hagan, R.D., Smith, M.G., & Gettman, L.R. (1981). Marathon performance in relation to maximal aerobic power and training indices. *Medicine and Science in Sports and Exercise, 13*, 185–189.

Hagberg, J.M., & Coyle, E.F. (1983). Physiological determinants of endurance performance as studied in competitive racewalkers. *Medicine and Science in Sports and Exercise, 15*, 287–289.

Hagerman, F.C., Hagerman, G.R., & Mickelson, T.C. (1979). Physiological profiles of elite rowers. *Physician and Sportsmedicine, 7* (#7), 74–83.

Hakkinen, K., Alen, M., & Komi, P.V. (1984). Neuromuscular, anaerobic, and aerobic performance characteristics of elite power athletes. *European Journal of Applied Physiology, 53*, 97–105.

Haymes, E.M., & Dickinson, A.L. (1980). Characteristics of elite male and female ski racers. *Medicine and Science in Sports and Exercise, 12*, 153–158.

Hermansen, L. (1973). Oxygen transport during exercise in human subjects. *Acta Physiologica Scandinavica*, (Suppl) *399*, 1–104.

Hermansen, L., & Andersen, K.L. (1965). Aerobic work capacity in young Norwegian men and women. *Journal of Applied Physiology, 20*, 425–431.

Holly, R.G., Barnard, R.J., Rosenthal, M., Applegate, E., & Pritikin, N. (1986). Triathlete characterization and response to prolonged strenuous competition. *Medicine and Science in Sports and Exercise, 18*, 123–127.

Katch, F.I., & Michael, E.D. (1971). Body composition of high school wrestlers according to age and wrestling weight category. *Medicine and Science in Sports, 3*, 190–194.

Kirkendall, D.T. (1985). The applied sport science of soccer. *Physician and Sportsmedicine, 13* (#4), 53–59.

Knowlton, R.G., Ackerman, K.J., Fitzgerald, P.I., Wilde, S.W., & Tahamont, M.V. (1980). Physiological and performance characteristics of United States championship class orienteers. *Medicine and Science in Sports and Exercise, 12*, 164–169.

Kovaleski, J.E., Parr, R.B., Hornak, J.E., & Roitman, J.L. (1980). Athletic profile of women college volleyball players. *Physician and Sportsmedicine, 8* (#2), 112–118.

Krahenbuhl, G.S., Wells, C.L., Brown, C.H., & Ward, P.E. (1979). Characteristics of national and world class female pentathletes. *Medicine and Science in Sports, 11*, 20–23.

Lewis, S., Haskell, W.L., Klein, H., Halpern, J., & Wood, P.D. (1975). Prediction of body composition in habitually active middle-aged men. *Journal of Applied Physiology, 39*, 221–225.

Magel, J.R., & Faulkner, J.A. (1967). Maximum oxygen uptakes of college swimmers. *Journal of Applied Physiology, 22*, 929–933.

Maksud, M.G., Wiley, R.L., Hamilton, L.H., & Lockhart, B. (1970). Maximal VO₂, ventilation, and heart rate of

Olympic speed skating candidates. *Journal of Applied Physiology, 29,* 186–190.

Malina, R.M., Harper, A.B., Avent, H.H., & Campbell, D.E. (1971). Physique of female track and field athletes. *Medicine and Science in Sports, 3,* 32–38.

Malina, R.M., & Rarick, G.L. (1973). Growth, physique and motor performance. In G.L. Rarick (Ed). *Physical activity, human growth and development* (pp. 125–153). New York: Academic Press.

Maud, P.J., & Shultz, B.B. (1984). The U.S. national rugby team: A physiological and anthropometric assessment. *Physician and Sportsmedicine, 12* (#9), 86–99.

Mayers, N., & Gutin, B. (1979). Physiological characteristics of elite prepubertal cross-country runners. *Medicine and Science in Sports, 11,* 172–176.

Mickelson, T.C., & Hagerman, F.C. (1982). Anaerobic threshold measurements of elite oarsmen. *Medicine and Science in Sports and Exercise, 14,* 440–444.

Moffatt, R.J., Surina, B., Golden, B., & Ayres, N. (1984). Body composition and physiological characteristics of female high school gymnasts. *Research Quarterly for Exercise and Sport, 55,* 80–84.

Mostardi, R.A., Porterfield, J.A., Greenberg, B., Goldberg, D., & Lea, M. (1983). Musculoskeletal and cardiopulmonary characteristics of the professional ballet dancer. *Physician and Sportsmedicine, 11* (#12), 53–61.

Nagel, F.J., Morgan, W.P., Hellickson, R.O., Serfass, R.C., & Alexander, J.F. (1975). Spotting success traits in Olympic contenders. *Physician and Sportsmedicine, 3,* 31–36.

Nicholas, J.A., & Hershman, E.B. (Eds). (1984). *Profiling.* (Clinics in Sports Medicine, Volume 3, #1) Philadelphia: W.B. Saunders Company.

Niinimaa, V. (1982). Figure skating: What do we know about it? *Physician and Sportsmedicine, 10* (#1), 51–56.

Niinimaa, V., Dyon, M., & Shephard, R.J. (1978). Performance and efficiency of intercollegiate cross-country skiers. *Medicine and Science in Sports, 10,* 91–93.

Novak, L.P., Hyatt, R.E., & Alexander, J.F. (1968). Body composition and physiologic function of athletes. *Journal of the American Medical Association, 205,* 764–770.

Novak, L.P., Magill, L.A., & Schutte, J.E. (1978). Maximal oxygen intake and body composition of female dancers. *European Journal of Applied Physiology, 39,* 277–282.

Parizkova, J. (1973). Body composition and exercise during growth and development. In G.L. Rarick (Ed.) *Physical activity, human growth and development.* New York: Academic Press. (pp. 97–124).

Parizkova, J., & Poupa, D. (1963). Some metabolic consequences of adaptation to muscular work. *British Journal of Nutrition, 17,* 341–345.

Parr, R.B., Wilmore, J.H. Hoover, R., Bachman, D., & Kerlan, R.K. (1978). Professional basketball players:

Athletic profiles. *Physician and Sportsmedicine, 6* (#4), 77–84.

Pipes, T.V. (1979). Physiological characteristics of elite body builders. *Physician and Sportsmedicine, 7* (#3), 116–122.

Pipes, T.V. (1979). The racquetball pro: A physiological profile. *Physician and Sportsmedicine, 7* (#10), 91–94.

Pollock, M.L. (1973). The quantification of endurance training programs. *Exercise and Sport Sciences Reviews, 1,* 155–188.

Pollock, M.L. (1977). Submaximal and maximal working capacity of elite distance runners. Part I. Cardiorespiratory aspects. *New York Academy of Science, 301,* 310–322.

Pollock, M.L., Miller, H.S., & Wilmore, J. (1974). Physiological characteristics of champion American track athletes 40 to 75 years of age. *Journal of Gerontology, 29,* 645–649.

Prince, F.P., Hikida, R.S., & Hagerman, F.C. (1977). Muscle fiber types in women athletes and non-athletes. *Pflugers Archives, 371,* 161–165.

Puhl, J., Case, S., Fleck, S., & Van Handel, P. (1982). Physical and physiological characteristics of elite volleyball players. *Research Quarterly for Exercise and Sports, 53,* 257–262.

Raven, P.B., Gettman, L.R., Pollock, M.L., & Cooper, K.H. (1976). A physiological evaluation of professional soccer players. *British Journal of Sports Medicine, 10,* 209–216.

Roby, F.B., Buono, M.J., Constable, S.H., Lowdon, B.J., & Tsao, W.Y. (1983). Physiological characteristics of champion synchronized swimmers. *Physician and Sportsmedicine, 11* (#4), 136–147.

Rusko, H., Havu, M., & Karvinen, E. (1978). Aerobic performance capacity in athletes. *European Journal of Applied Physiology, 38,* 151–159.

Sady, S.P., Thomson, W.H., Berg, K., & Savage, M. (1984). Physiological characteristics of high-ability prepubescent wrestlers. *Medicine and Science in Sports and Exercise, 16,* 72–76.

Saltin, B., & Astrand, P.O. (1967). Maximal oxygen uptake in athletes. *Journal of Applied Physiology, 28,* 353–358.

Schantz, P.G., & Astrand, P.O. (1984). Physiological characteristics of classical ballet. *Medicine and Science in Sports and Exercise, 16,* 472–476.

Secher, N.H. (1983). The physiology of rowing. *Journal of Sports Science, 1,* 23–53.

Secher, N.H., Vaage, O., Jensen, K., & Jackson, R.C. (1983). Maximal aerobic power in oarsmen. *European Journal of Applied Physiology, 51,* 155–162.

Seliger, V., Kostka, V., Grusova, D., Kovac, J., Machovcova, J., Pauer, M., Pribylova, A., & Urbankova, R. (1972). Energy expenditure and physical fitness of ice-hockey players. *International Zeitschrift Angewandte Physiology, 30*, 283–291.

Shephard, R.J., Godin, G., & Campbell, R. (1974). Characteristics of sprint, medium, and long-distance swimmers. *European Journal of Applied Physiology, 32*, 99–103.

Sidney, K., & Shephard, R.J. (1973). Physiological characteristics and performance of the white-water paddler. *European Journal of Applied Physiology, 32*, 55–70.

Sinning, W.E. (1973). Body composition, cardiorespiratory function, and rule changes in women's basketball. *Research Quarterly, 44*, 313–321.

Sinning, W.E. (1974). Body composition assessment of college wrestlers. *Medicine and Science in Sports, 6*, 139–145.

Sinning, W.E., & Lindberg, G.D. (1972). Physical characteristics of college-age women gymnasts. *Research Quarterly, 43*, 226–234.

Smith, D.P., & Byrd, R.J. (1976). Body composition, pulmonary function and maximal oxygen consumption of college football players. *Journal of Sports Medicine, 16*, 301–308.

Song, T.M.K. (1982). Relationship of physiological characteristics to skiing performance. *Physician and Sportsmedicine, 10* (#12), 96–102.

Spence, D.W., Disch, J.G., Fred, H.L., & Coleman, A.E. (1980). Descriptive profiles of highly skilled women volleyball players. *Medicine and Science in Sports and Exercise, 12*, 299–302.

Sprynarova, S., & Parizkova, J. (1971). Functional capacity and body composition in top weight-lifters, swimmers, runners and skiers. *International Zeitschrift Angewandte Physiology, 29*, 184–194.

Stine, G., Ratliff, R., Shierman, G., & Grana, W.A. (1979). Physical profile of the wrestlers at the 1977 NCAA championships. *Physician and Sportsmedicine, 7* (#11), 98–105.

Stromme, S.B., Ingjer, F., & Meen, H.D. (1977). Assessment of maximal aerobic power in specifically trained athletes. *Journal of Applied Physiology, 42*, 833–837.

Tanner, J.M. (1964). *The physique of the Olympic athlete.* London: George Allen and Unwin Ltd.

Taylor, A.W., Brassard, L., Proteau, L., & Robin, D. (1979). A physiological profile of Canadian Greco-Roman wrestlers. *Canadian Journal of Applied Sport Sciences, 4*, 131–134.

Tesch, P., Piehl, K., Wilson, G., & Karlsson, J. (1976). Physiological investigations of Swedish elite canoe competitors. *Medicine and Science in Sports, 8*, 214–218.

Thorstensson, A., Larsson, L., Tesch, P., & Karlsson, J. (1977). Muscle strength and fiber composition in athletes and sedentary men. *Medicine and Science in Sports, 9*, 26–30.

Upton, S.J., Hagan, R.D., Lease, B., Rosentswieg, J.,

Gettman, L.R., & Duncan, J.J. (1984). Comparative physiological profiles among young and middle-aged female distance runners. *Medicine and Science in Sports and Exercise, 16*, 67–71.

Upton, S.J., Hagan, R.D., Rosentswieg, J., & Gettman, L.R. (1983). Comparison of the physiological profiles of middle-aged women distance runners and sedentary women. *Research Quarterly for Exercise and Sport, 54*, 83–87.

Vaccaro, P., Clarke, D.H., & Morris, A.F. (1980). Physiological characteristics of young well-trained swimmers. *European Journal of Applied Physiology, 44*, 61–66.

Vaccaro, P., Clarke, D.H., & Wrenn, J.P. (1979). Physiological profiles of elite women basketball players. *Journal of Sports Medicine, 19*, 45–54.

Vaccaro, P., Dummer, G.M., & Clarke, D.H. (1981). Physiological characteristics of female masters swimmers. *Physician and Sportsmedicine, 9* (#12), 75–78.

Vaccaro, P., Gray, P.R., Clarke, D.H., & Morris, A.F. (1984). Physiological characteristics of world class white-water slalom paddlers. *Research Quarterly for Exercise and Sport, 55*, 206–210.

Vaccaro, P., Morris, A.F., & Clarke, D.H. (1981). Physiological characteristics of masters female distance runners. *Physician and Sportsmedicine, 9* (#7), 105–108.

Vander, L.B., Franklin, B.A., Wrisley, D., Scherf, J., Kogler, A.A., & Rubenfire, M. (1984). Physiological profile of national-class National Collegiate Athletic Association fencers. *Journal of the American Medical Association, 252*, 500–503.

van Ingen Schenau, G.J., de Groot, G., & Hollander, A.P. (1983). Some technical, physiological and anthropometrical aspects of speed skating. *European Journal of Applied Physiology, 50*, 343–354.

Veicsteinas, A., Ferretti, G., Margonato, V., Rosa, G., & Tagliabue, D. (1984). Energy cost of and energy sources for alpine skiing in top athletes. *Journal of Applied Physiology, 56*, 1187–1190.

Vodak, P.A., Savin, W.M., Haskell, W.L., & Wood, P.D. (1980). Physiological profile of middle-aged male and female tennis players. *Medicine and Science in Sports and Exercise, 12*, 159–163.

Wickkiser, J.D., & Kelly, J.M. (1975). The body composition of a college football team. *Medicine and Science in Sports, 7*, 199–202.

Wilmore, J.H. (1974). Alterations in strength, body composition and anthropometric measurements consequent to a 10-week weight training program. *Medicine and Science in Sports, 6*, 133–138.

Wilmore, J.H. (1983). Body composition in sport and exercise: Directions for future research. *Medicine and Science in Sports and Exercise, 15*, 21–31.

Wilmore, J.H. (1984). The assessment of and variation in aerobic power in world class athletes as related to specific sports. *American Journal of Sports Medicine, 12,* 120–127.

Wilmore, J.H., & Bergfeld, J.A. (1979). A comparison of sports: Physiological and medical aspects. In R.H. Strauss (Ed.) *Sports medicine and physiology.* Philadelphia: W.B. Saunders.

Wilmore, J.H., & Brown, C.H. (1974). Physiological profiles of women distance runners. *Medicine and Science in Sports, 6,* 178–181.

Wilmore, J.H., Brown, C.H., & Davis, J.A. (1977). Body physique and composition of the female distance runner. *Annals of the New York Academy of Science, 301,* 764–776.

Wilmore, J.H., Parr, R.B., Haskell, W.L., Costill, D.L., Milburn, L.J., & Kerlan, R.K. (1976). Football pros' strengths—and CV weakness—charted. *Physician and Sportsmedicine, 4* (#10), 45–54.

Clinical Signs Associated with Nutrition Deficiencies

Body Area	Normal Appearance	Clinical Sign(s)	Nutritional Deficiency Indicated
Hair	Shiny, firm, not easily plucked	Hair dull and dry, lack of shine, thinness and sparseness, depigmentation (flag sign), straightness of previously curly hair, easy pluckability	Kwashiorkor; less commonly, marasmus (protein-calorie)
Face	Uniform skin color, smooth, healthy appearance, not swollen	Depigmentation: skin dark over cheeks and eyes, moon face	Protein-calorie, protein
		Scaling of skin around nostrils, nasolabial seborrhea	Riboflavin or niacin, pyridoxine
Eyes	Bright, clear, shiny, healthy pink moist membranes, no prominent blood vessels	Pale conjunctiva	Anemia: iron, folate, or B_{12}
		Bitot's spots, night blindness, conjunctiva and corneal xeroxis (drying), keratomalacia	Vitamin A
		Redness and fissuring of eyelid corners (angular palpebritis)	Riboflavin, pyridoxine, niacin

Source: Data from McLaren and Burman, *Textbook of Pediatric Nutrition*, 2nd ed., p. 95, © 1982, Churchill Livingstone; Walker and Hendricks, *Manual of Pediatric Nutrition*, p. 30, © 1985, W.B. Saunders Company; R.M. Ruskind and R.J. Varma, Assessment of Nutritional Status of Children, *Pediatrics in Review* 5, pp. 199–200, © 1984, American Academy of Pediatrics; and H.M. Sandstead and W.N. Pearson, Clinical Evaluation of Nutritional Status, in *Modern Nutrition in Health and Disease*, R.S. Goodhart and M.E. Shils, eds., © 1973, Lea & Febiger.

Body Area	Normal Appearance	Clinical Sign(s)	Nutritional Deficiency Indicated
Lips	Smooth, not chapped	Redness and swelling of mouth or lips, especially at corners of mouth (cheilosis) and angular stomatitis, angular scars	Riboflavin, niacin, iron, pyridoxine
Mouth		Ageusia, dysgeusia	Zinc
Tongue	Deep red in appearance, not smooth or swollen	Glossitis	Niacin, folate, riboflavin, iron, vitamin B_{12}
		Scarlet and raw	Nicotinic acid
		Magenta tongue	Riboflavin
Teeth	Bright, no cavities, no pain	Pitted, grooved teeth	Vitamin D
		Missing or erupting abnormally, gray or black spots (fluorosis), mottled	Fluoride
		Cavities	Poor hygiene and fluoride
		Mottled enamel	Excess fluoride
Gums	Healthy red, do not bleed, not swollen	Spongy, bleeding gums, swollen	Ascorbic acid (vitamin C)
Glands	Face not swollen	Thyroid enlargement	Iodine
		Parotid enlargement	Starvation (protein-calorie)
Skin	No signs of rashes, swelling, dark or light spots	Dryness of the skin (xerosis), sandpaper feel of skin (follicular hyperkeratosis)	Vitamin A or essential fatty acid
		Petechiae ecchymoses	Ascorbic acid and vitamin D
		Red, swollen pigmentation of exposed areas (pellagrous dermatosis)	Nicotinic acid and tryptophan
		Flakiness of the skin, lack of fat under skin	Kwashiorkor, essential fatty acid
		Scrotal and vulvar dermatosis	Riboflavin
Nails	Firm, pink	Nails spoon shaped (koilonychia)	Iron

Body Area	Normal Appearance	Clinical Sign(s)	Nutritional Deficiency Indicated
Muscles and skeletal system	Good muscle tone, some fat under skin, can walk or run without pain	Muscle wasting	Starvation, kwashiorkor, marasmus
		Knock knees or bow legs	Vitamin D
		Thoracic rosary	Vitamin D, ascorbic acid
		Musculoskeletal hemorrhage	Ascorbic acid
Organ Systems:			
Gastrointestinal	No palpable organs or masses	Hematomegaly (fatty infiltration)	Protein
Cardiovascular	Normal heart rhythm, no murmur, normal blood pressure for age	Cardiac enlargement, tachycardia	Thiamine
Nervous system	Psychological stability, normal reflexes	Psychomotor changes, mental confusion	Kwashiorkor (protein), thiamine, nicotinic acid
		Sensory loss, motor weakness, loss of vibration, loss of ankle movement, knee jerks, calf tenderness	Thiamine, vitamin B_{12} deficiency

Laboratory Tests and Normal Ranges for Adults and Children Affected by Exercise or Related Conditions

Test	Normal Value	Response to Exercise	Rationale
Hemoglobin (inner core of the RBC[†] in a given volume)	Male 13.5–18 g/dL (140–180 g/L)	Decrease	Anemias, iron deficiency, excessive fluid intake
	Female 12–16 g/dL (115–155 g/L)	Increase	High altitude, burns, dehydration
	Athlete 16–18 g/dL		
	Child 11–16 g/dL		
Hematocrit (proportion of packed cells in a given volume)	Male 40%–54% (0.40–0.54)	Decrease	Anemias
	Female 36%–46% (0.36–0.46)	Increase	Dehydration; diarrhea; drug influence: antibiotics
	Child 36%–38% (0.36–0.38)		
RBCs	Male 4.6–6.0 m/cu mm by 10–12/L	Decrease	Excessive fluid intake, intravascular hemolysis
	Female 4.0–5.0		
	Child 3.8–5.5	Increase	High altitude, dehydration
Blood volume	70–100 mL/kg of body weight	Increase	Response to regular strenuous exercise, altitudes
Plasma volume	30–50 mL/kg of body weight	Increase	Response to strenuous exercise
MCV[‡]	Male 80–98 cu μ	Decrease	Excessive fluid intake > 80, iron deficiency anemia
	Female 80–98 cu μ		
	Child 82–92 cu μ	Increase	Dehydration > 98, pernicious anemias

Source: Data from *Eat to Compete: A Guide to Sports Nutrition* (pp 266–269) by MS Peterson and K Peterson with permission of Year Book Medical Publishers, Inc., © 1988. Adapted from Kee JL, *Laboratory and Diagnostic Tests with Nursing Implications.* New York, Appleton-Century-Crofts, 1983; Monsen ER: The journal adopts SI units for clinical laboratory values. *J Am Diet Assoc* 1987;87:356; Tilkian SM, Conover MB, Tilkian AG: *Clinical Implications of Laboratory Tests.* St. Louis, C.V. Mosby Co, 1979; Krebs PS, Scully BC, Zinkgraf SA: The acute and prolonged effects of marathon running on 20 blood parameters. *Phys Sports Med* 1983;11:66; Martin DE, Vroom DH, May DF, et al: Physiological changes in elite male distance runners training. *Phys Sports Med* 1986;14:152.

Test	Normal Value	Response to Exercise	Rationale
Serum iron	Male 80–180 µg/dL (14–32 µmol/L)	Increase	Excessive hemolysis (red blood cell destruction); drug influence: excessive iron supplements
	Female 60–160 µg/dL(11–29 µmol/L)	Decrease	Blood loss, dietary deficiency
TIBC§ (measures serum iron bound with transferrin)	Adult 250–450 µg/dL (45–82 µmoles/L) or 16% saturation	Increase	Iron deficiency anemia, acute and chronic blood loss
		Decrease	Pernicious anemia; drug influence: ACTH‖, steroids
SGOT¶	Adult 5–40 µ/mL	Increase	Infections; strenuous exercise; vitamin dosage; drug influence: antibiotics, narcotics, antihypertensives, cortisone, indomethecin
		Decrease	Aspirin use, salicylates
Haptoglobin	Adult 30–160 mg/dL	Decrease	Hemolysis, pernicious anemias
Ferritin	Male 18–300 µg/dL Female 10–270 µg/dL or 60 µg/L < 12 depletion > 200 overload	Decrease	Bone marrow and liver storage of iron
Serum cholesterol	Adult 150–220 mg/dL (5.20–5.85 mmol/L)	Decrease	Increased fat oxidation, also in malnutrition, anemia
VLDL#	60 mg/dL	Decrease	
LDL**	Adult 50–190 mg/dL (1.3–4.9 mmol/L)	Decrease	
Triglycerides	Adult > 150 mg/dL (< 1.80 mmol/L)	Decrease	Increased fat oxidation, protein malnutrition
	Child 10–140 mg/dL	Increase	Hypertension; uncontrolled diabetes; high-carbohydrate diet; drug influence: estrogens, alcohol
HDL††	Male 30–70 mg/dL (0.80–1.80 mmol/L)	Decrease	Steroid use
	Female 30–90 mg/dL (0.80–2.35 mmol/L)	Increase	Increase in hepatic enzyme activity, increased production due to exercise, or both
Bilirubin	Adult 0.1–1.2 mg/dL (2–18 µmoles/L) Child 0.2–0.8 mg/dL)	Increase	RBC destruction; drug influence: steroids, increased vitamin A, C, and K, antibiotics
		Decrease	Iron deficiency, anemia, large amounts of caffeine, aspirin

Test	Normal Value	Response to Exercise	Rationale
Serum potassium	Adult 3.5–5.0 mEq/L Child 3.5–5.5 mEq/L	Decrease	Vomiting and diarrhea; dehydration; crash dieting; starvation; stress and trauma; injuries; burns; increased glucose ingestion; laxative abuse; drug influence: diuretics, thiazides, steroids, antibiotics, insulin, laxatives
		Increase	Acute renal failure, crushing injuries, and burns (with kidney shutdown)
Serum sodium	Adult 135–145 mEq/L (or 135–145 mmol/L)	Increase	Dehydration; severe vomiting and diarrhea; congestive heart failure; drug influence: cough medicines, cortisones, antibiotics, laxatives
		Decrease	Vomiting, increased perspiration, reduced Na in diet, burns, tissue injury, large amounts of water
Serum magnesium	Adult 1.6–2.4 mEq/L	Decrease	Loss of gastrointestinal fluids, use of diuretics
Uric acid	Male 3.5–7.8 mg/dL Female 2.8–6.8 mg/dL Child 2.5–5.5 mg/dL	Decrease	Folic acid deficiency; burns; drug influence: ACTH
		Increase	Dehydration; nitrogen catabolism; stress, increased protein; weight reduction diets; gout; drug influence: megadose of vitamin C, diuretics, thiazides, aspirin, ACTH
Fasting glucose	Adult 65–110 mg/dL (3.9–6.1 mmol/L) Child 60–100 mg/dL	Decrease	Hypoglycemic response to excessive glucose/sucrose solutions, extended strenuous exercise
		Increase	Stress, crushing injury, burns, infections, hypothermia, mild exercise, dumping syndrome, diabetes

[†] RBC = red blood cell
[‡] MCV = mean corpuscular volume
[§] TIBC = total iron-binding capacity
[‖] ACTH = adrenocorticotropic hormone
[¶] SGOT = serum glutamic oxaloacetic transaminase
[#] VLDL = very low-density lipoprotein
[**] LDL = low-density lipoprotein
[††] HDL = high-density lipoprotein

Index

Notes

Notes

Notes

Notes

Notes

Notes

Notes

Notes